MODERN MANAGEMENT OF PREMENSTRUAL SYNDROME

MODERN MANAGEMENT OF PREMENSTRUAL SYNDROME

Edited by

SAMUEL SMITH, M.D., F.A.C.O.G.

Director, Division of Reproductive Endocrinology-Infertility
Department of Obstetrics and Gynecology, Sinai Hospital of Baltimore

Assistant Professor, Department of Obstetrics and Gynecology
The Johns Hopkins Medical School

Assistant Professor, Department of Obstetrics and Gynecology
University of Maryland Medical School

ISAAC SCHIFF, M.D.

Chief of Vincent Memorial Gynecology Service
The Women's Care Division of the Massachusetts General Hospital

Joe Vincent Meigs Professor and Chairman, Department of Gynecology
Harvard Medical School

Norton Medical Books

W · W · Norton & Company
New York · London

The text of this book is composed in Sabon. Composition by ComCom. Manufacturing by Arcata Graphics. Book design by Jacques Chazaud.

DRUG DOSAGE

The authors and publishers have exerted every effort to insure that drug selection and dosage set forth in this text are in accord with current recommendations and practice at the time of publication. However, in the view of ongoing research, changes in government regulations, and the constant flow of information relating to drug therapy and drug reactions, the reader is urged to check the package insert for each drug for any change in indications and dosage and for added warnings and precautions. This is particularly important when the recommended agent is a new and/or infrequently used drug.

First Edition

Library of Congress Cataloging-in-Publication Data

Modern management of premenstrual syndrome / Samuel Smith, Isaac
Schiff, editor[s].
    p. cm.
  ISBN 0-393-71018-1
  1. Premenstrual syndrome. I. Smith, Samuel, 1955– .
  [DNLM: 1. Premenstrual Syndrome—diagnosis. 2. Premenstrual
Syndrome—therapy. WP 560 M689]
  RG165.M63   1993
  618.1'72—dc20
  DNLM/DLC
  for Library of Congress   92-48663
                                   CIP

W. W. Norton & Company, Inc., 500 Fifth Avenue, New York, N.Y. 10110
W. W. Norton & Company, Ltd., 10 Coptic Street, London WC1A 1PU

1 2 3 4 5 6 7 8 9 0

*We dedicate this text to
our patients from whom
we have learned so much.*

CONTENTS

INTRODUCTION

DIAGNOSIS AND PHYSIOLOGY

MANAGEMENT

SUMMARY

EDITORS

Samuel Smith, MD

Director, Division of Reproductive Endocrinology-Infertility,
Department of Obstetrics and Gynecology, Sinai Hospital of
Baltimore, Baltimore, Maryland

Academic Appointments for Dr. Smith:

  Assistant Professor
  Department of Gynecology and Obstetrics
  The Johns Hopkins Medical School
  Baltimore, Maryland

  Assistant Professor
  Department of Obstetrics and Gynecology
  University of Maryland Medical School
  Baltimore, Maryland

Isaac Schiff, MD

Chief of Vincent Memorial Gynecology Service, The Women's
Care Division of the Massachusetts General Hospital, Boston,
Massachusetts

Academic Appointment for Dr. Schiff:

  Joe Vincent Meigs Professor and Chairman
  Department of Gynecology
  Harvard Medical School
  Boston, Massachusetts

CONTRIBUTORS

Yogesh Bakhai, MD

Clinical Assistant Professor, Department of Psychiatry, State
University of New York at Buffalo, Erie County Medical Center,
Buffalo, New York

Ashok Balasubramanyam, MD

Clinical and Research Fellow in Medicine, Endocrine Division,
Massachusetts General Hospital, Harvard Medical School,
Boston, Massachusetts

Robert L. Barbieri, MD

Professor and Chairman, State University of New York at Stony
Brook, School of Medicine, Department of Obstetrics and
Gynecology, Health Sciences Center, Stony Brook, New York

Robert F. Casper, MD

Professor, Director, Division of Reproductive Sciences, Department
of Obstetrics and Gynecology, Toronto General Hospital,
Toronto, Ontario, Canada

Ellen W. Freeman, PhD

Research Associate Professor, Department of Obstetrics and
Gynecology, Hospital of the University of Pennsylvania, Human
Behavior Unit, Philadelphia, Pennsylvania

Susanna Goldstein, MD

Assistant Professor, Department of Psychiatry, College of
Physicians and Surgeons of Columbia University, New York,
New York

Uriel Halbreich, MD

Professor of Psychiatry, Research Professor of OB/GYN, Director
of Biobehavioral Research, University of Buffalo, State University
of New York, Department of Psychiatry, School of Medicine and
Biomedical Sciences, Faculty of Health Sciences, Erie County
Medical Center, Buffalo, New York

Keith Isaacson, MD

Assistant Professor of Obstetrics, Gynecology and Reproductive
Biology, Massachusetts General Hospital, Harvard Medical School,
Boston, Massachusetts

David L. Keefe, MD

Division of Reproductive Endocrinology, Department of Obstetrics
and Gynecology, Yale University School of Medicine, New Haven,
Connecticut

Ken Muse, MD

Associate Professor, Division of Reproductive Endocrinology,
University of Kentucky, Chandler Medical Center, Kentucky
Center for Reproductive Medicine, Department of Obstetrics and
Gynecology, Lexington, Kentucky

Frederick Naftolin, MD, PhD

Chairman, Department of Obstetrics and Gynecology, Yale
University School of Medicine, New Haven, Connecticut

David R. Rubinow, MD

Chief, Section on Behavioral Endocrinology, Biological Psychiatry Branch, National Institute of Mental Health, Bethesda, Maryland

Peter J. Schmidt, MD

Chief, Unit on Reproductive Endocrine Studies, Section on Behavioral Endocrinology, Biological Psychiatry Branch, National Institute of Mental Health, Bethesda, Maryland

Heather Shapiro, MD

Assistant Professor, Division of Reproductive Sciences, Department of Obstetrics and Gynecology, The University of Toronto, Toronto, Ontario, Canada

Steven J. Sondheimer, MD

Associate Professor—OB/GYN, Department of Obstetrics and Gynecology, University of Pennsylvania Medical Center, Division of Human Reproduction, Philadelphia, Pennsylvania

John W.W. Studd, MD

Consultant, Premenstrual Tension Clinic, Dulwich Hospital, East Dulwich Grove, London, England

Kathleen Ulman, PhD

Instructor in Psychology, Department of Psychiatry, Harvard Medical School, Women's Health Associates, Massachusetts General Hospital, Boston, Massachusetts

Neale R. Watson, MB, BS

Research Registrar, Premenstrual Tension Clinic, Dulwich Hospital, East Dulwich Grove, London, England

Judith J. Wurtman, PhD

Research Scientist, Department of Brain and Cognitive Science, Clinical Research Center, Massachusetts Institute of Technology, Cambridge, Massachusetts

PREFACE

Sixty years after Frank's pioneering description of agitated, irritable patients, premenstrual syndrome (PMS) remains an enigma. Literally dozens of papers include statements such as "the etiology of premenstrual syndrome is unknown" and "agreement on definition and criteria are needed." Clinicians, researchers, and patients are confused and frustrated by the lack of consensus as to definition, diagnosis, etiology, and treatment.

In this text, we provide a practical guide for managing patients with premenstrual syndrome. We have enlisted the help of a renowned group of collaborators who have formulated clear, concise, and scholarly presentations that should be of great practical significance to any physician who treats women with PMS. The first eight chapters review the diagnosis and differential diagnosis of PMS, the physiology of the normal menstrual cycle, the neurobiologic basis of mood, the etiology of PMS, parallels between PMS and psychiatric illness, and the relationship of medical illness to the menstrual cycle. The next eight chapters review PMS therapy. Nutritional modification, measures to improve physical symptoms, psychotropic medications, ovulation suppression, estrogen, progesterone, psychotherapy, and surgical management are discussed. The last chapter describes the editors' approach to the evaluation and therapy of PMS.

We are certain that this text will improve your level of understanding of PMS and will better enable you to improve the quality of life of women with PMS.

ACKNOWLEDGMENT

Preparation of this text would not have been possible without the administrative and secretarial support of Elaine Urquhart. We are indebted to her for her patience and diligence.

INTRODUCTION

CHAPTER 1

Premenstrual Syndrome: Controversy and Consensus

Samuel Smith and Isaac Schiff

Premenstrual syndrome (PMS) has been a recognized clinical entity for many years, but there is still tremendous controversy regarding its epidemiology, definition, diagnosis, pathophysiology, and treatment. In the last decade, scientific inquiry has brought us closer to understanding PMS and answering these basic questions.

EPIDEMIOLOGY

PMS is thought to be extremely prevalent. However, most studies examine groups of women who are not representative of the general female reproductive-age population, including college students, gynecology clinic patients, and general medical patients. A recent door-to-door survey of 179 women residing in five different neighborhoods identified classic PMS symptoms in 30% to 40% of the study population, with 5% to 10% of the women reporting severe symptoms.[1] Larger population-based surveys also suggest that about 30% of women have PMS and 2% to 10% are severely affected.[2,3]

Contrary to popular belief, PMS is not just a disease of older women. Teenagers and young women report severe PMS as frequently as older women do.[4] However, most women who seek treatment for PMS are in their thirties or forties. It is unknown why PMS is first experienced by some women in their teens and other women in their middle reproductive years.

Little is known about the natural history of PMS. Retrospective data suggest that PMS temporarily resolves during pregnancy and may permanently remit during menopause. There are currently no prospective longitudinal studies that follow PMS patients over many years, including their menopause. The list of functional impairments associated with PMS is impressive—poor performance in school, reduced work efficiency, work absences, marital discord, divorce, child abuse, loss of friendships, loss of employment, increased rates of criminal activity, suicide attempts, and alcohol abuse. However, data are lacking to accurately describe the prevalence of these functional impairments in women with PMS and unaffected controls. The limited data available, however, do not support the concept that work absence is more common in PMS patients.[3] Therefore, more research is needed to clarify these issues.

CLASSIFICATION AND DIAGNOSIS OF DISEASE

Any mood, physical, or behavioral symptom is considered to be a menstrually related change if it appears in the luteal phase of the menstrual cycle and disappears shortly after the onset of the next menstruation. This definition implies that the symptom does not exist during the second week of the menstrual cycle. Menstrually related changes vary in severity from nonexistent to disabling. Cross-sectional population surveys suggest that at least 50% of menstruating women report some mild menstrually related change(s) that they perceive as nondistressing. These changes are commonly termed *molimina,* and are considered to be a normal experience.[5]

Diagnostic Criteria

Menstrually related changes severe enough to cause physical or emotional distress and/or functional impairment are abnormal. A cross-discipline review of the medical literature leads to the conclusion that premenstrual syndrome is a menstrually related disorder. Although there is no uniformly accepted definition of PMS, various diagnostic criteria are widely accepted:

1. Cyclic, recurrent physical, emotional, and/or behavioral symptoms are present in the luteal phase of the menstrual cycle that remit shortly after the onset of menstruation.
2. The luteal phase symptoms are present in the majority of menstrual cycles.
3. The luteal phase symptoms do not simply represent a worsening of a chronic physical or emotional disorder.
4. Luteal phase symptoms are severe enough to cause physical or emotional distress, or deterioration in psychosocial functioning.
5. The recurrent, cyclic nature of the disorder can be confirmed by prospective daily monitoring by the woman and/or her "significant other" for at least two menstrual cycles.

Whether PMS can occur in the anovulatory female is controversial. Anecdotal reports of cyclic, recurrent emotional disturbances in menopausal women exist. However, the cyclicity of symptoms is usually briefer than that observed in menstruating women and may merely represent a rapidly cycling affective disorder. The same is true concerning anecdotal reports of PMS in oligoovulatory women with polycystic ovarian syndrome.

It is also unclear whether PMS can be diagnosed in women who present for medical evaluation while on oral contraceptives. Virtually all PMS research to date excludes women who are using oral contraceptives. Yet, some women who use oral contraceptives demonstrate cyclic, recurrent symptoms that are similar to PMS. These women are usually advised to discontinue oral contraception to see if they have PMS when they resume ovulatory menstrual cycles. It is unclear whether those women who refuse to discontinue oral contraceptives should be diagnosed with PMS.

Classification of Disease

The *International Classification of Disease—9th Revision* (ICD-9) categorizes medical conditions according to a variety of factors—known etiology, presumed etiology, organs or body systems involved in the principal manifestations of the disorder, historical precedent, and others. Even when etiology is understood, a disease is usually classified by its principal manifestations, instead of by etiological features it may share with disorders classified elsewhere in the ICD-9.

There are many medical disorders that may occur regularly during the luteal phase of the menstrual cycle or during menstruation. These diseases include, but are not limited to, menstrual migraine, catamenial seizures, flare-ups of dermatologic conditions, irritable bowel syndrome, and asthma. The hypothesis that some underlying mechanism triggers these diverse phenomena is not widely accepted. The idea to classify people with very different menstrually related medical disorders, for example, irritable bowel syndrome and epilepsy, with the same diagnosis based on presumed etiology is also not widely accepted. It is unlikely that the same pathophysiologic mechanism causes all of these conditions to become linked to phases of the menstrual cycle. Moreover, inappropriately grouping these disorders together may be counterproductive to research aimed at evaluating risk factors, longitudinal course, etiology, and therapy. We also intuitively realize that women affected with menstrually related migraine or cyclic luteal phase irritable bowel syndrome are more likely to obtain optimum evaluation and treatment by a headache or gastrointestinal specialist, respectively, than in a PMS clinic.

The classification of PMS as a menstrually related condition versus a mental/psychiatric disorder is still subject to ongoing controversy. The ICD-9 currently includes premenstrual tension syndrome as a genitourinary system disorder. The *Diagnostic and Statistical Manual-III-Revised* (DSM-III R) lists the late luteal phase dysphoric disorder (LLPDD) in the appendix as a condition deserving further study. Although there is evidence to suggest that reproductive endocrine factors play a role in the expression of PMS symptoms, there is still no evidence for a specific reproductive endocrine trigger evoking these symptoms. There is also no evidence that the menstrual cycle is aberrant. Consequently, many psychiatrists argue that PMS should be classified as a mental disorder, particularly in light of clues suggesting a possible shared pathophysiology between PMS and major mood disorders. That notwithstanding, reproductive endocrine events associated with ovulation appear to be important for the expression of PMS, and approximately 60% of patients present with disturbing physical and emotional symptoms.[6] Consequently, many are reluctant to classify PMS as a mental disorder. LLPDD is regarded as a subset of PMS characterized by severe functional impairment and is easier to accept as a psychiatric diagnosis.

PATHOPHYSIOLOGY

Ovarian Hormones

Ovarian hormones are considered very important to the pathophysiology of PMS. Multiple, separate lines of investigation support this and point to the dynamic variation in steroid hormone levels in ovulatory cycles as critical for the expression of PMS. Consequently, current research criteria and definitions infer that PMS is diagnosed only in ovulatory females, and it may be diagnosed after hysterectomy in the absence of menstruation.

Epidemiologic data show that the onset of PMS is frequently in the postpubertal years and that it resolves after spontaneous or surgical menopause. PMS is also not seen in patients with hypoestrogenic amenorrhea or hyperandrogenic oligoovulation (polycystic ovarian syndrome). Similarly, pregnancy is not associated with PMS despite very high levels of gonadal hormones, and neither is postpartum lactational amenorrhea. Thus, cyclic recurrent symptoms mimicking PMS are not seen in states of amenorrhea, regardless of the circulating levels of gonadal hormones.

Neurons throughout the human, primate, and subprimate brain have the ability to concentrate estradiol and progesterone. Specific receptors for estradiol and progesterone are found throughout the central nervous system (CNS), and these hormones also bind nonspecifically to synaptic plasma membranes. The topography of estrogen- and progesterone-binding neurons has been documented in the rat and rhesus monkey. Estradiol and progesterone concentrate in a variety of CNS areas, most notably the hypothalamus, striatum, preoptic area, amygdala, hippocampus, and cerebral cortex. Moreover, estrogen- and progesterone-binding neurons are in close relationship to the monoaminergic neuronal systems innervating these same regions (see Chapter 6).

Estradiol, progesterone, and/or their metabolites interact with and modulate activity of some dopaminergic, serotonergic, GABAergic, acetylcholinergic, noradrenergic, and endogenous opioid peptide pathways that are involved in mood and behavior. A growing body of literature indicates that estrogen and progesterone influence synthesis, metabolism, uptake, turnover, and reception of these neurotransmitters and neuromodulators. Direct evidence that estradiol and progesterone influence cerebral cortex function also exists. For example, estradiol decreases electroshock seizure threshold and progesterone acts as an anticonvulsant and sedative-hypnotic (see Chapter 6).

Controlled pharmacologic trials suggest that eliminating ovulation and cyclic ovarian activity effectively treats PMS. Danazol is an extremely effective therapy when administered at dosages high enough to induce anovulation.[7] Gonadotropin-releasing hormone agonists (GnRHa) also eliminate PMS symptoms when administered at dosages sufficient to induce hypoestrogenic amenorrhea.[8–10] Interestingly, in one clinical trial, three women who were receiving placebo became spontaneously anovulatory, and also asymptomatic.[10] Subcutaneous estradiol implants and 0.2 mg/day transdermal estradiol patches also suppress ovulation, and despite high circulating estradiol levels, PMS symptoms improve.[11]

Another line of investigation evaluates the role of gonadal hormones in exacerbating PMS symptoms. Women have dropped out of GnRHa studies because their PMS symptoms worsened during the first two weeks of the active drug, presumably due to the high sex steroid milieu created during the initial "flare" phase of GnRHa administration.[10] Studies utilizing transdermal estradiol to inhibit ovulation also report an initial worsening of symptoms in some subjects as the serum levels dramatically rise before achievement of a steady state.[11] Low dosage estrogen-progestin replacement therapy is often combined with GnRHa therapy to prevent osteoporosis from developing. These patients seldom have an exacerbation of PMS complaints.[9] However, high dosages of estrogen-progestin replacement will elicit PMS symptoms in GnRHa-treated patients. Studies also document that menopausal women receiving cyclic estrogen-progestin therapy may develop significant cyclicity in both mood and physical symptoms, primarily limited to the progestin phase; this too is a dosage-dependent phenomenon.[12–14]

Recent data indicate that women experience more severe PMS in cycles with high luteal phase plasma estradiol and progesterone production.[15] Elimination of late luteal phase progesterone secretion with RU-486 does not significantly reduce PMS symptoms. That two RU-486-treated patients did show lower late luteal phase symptoms is interesting, but this may be a placebo response.[16]

These lines of data support the concept that cyclic ovarian activity and ovulation are critical to the pathophysiology of PMS. However, a variety of data also suggest that PMS cannot be explained solely by gonadal steroid effects.

Factors Other than Ovarian Hormones

Basal levels of steroid hormones, gonadotropins, and sex hormone-binding globulin in PMS subjects are similar to those of control subjects.[17] In addition, the concentrations of 5-alpha reduced metabolites of progesterone, which have GABA-agonist effects, are not significantly different in PMS patients. Therefore, PMS does not seem to be related to abnormal circulating hormonal levels. PMS subjects also do not demonstrate abnormalities in the response of gonadotropins to GnRH.[18]

Several biologic factors are different in PMS patients compared to controls. These include:

1. Increased prevalence of abnormal thyroid-stimulating hormone (TSH) responses to thyrotropin-releasing hormone (TRH).[19]
2. Decreased whole blood serotonin and platelet serotonin uptake.[20,21]
3. Decreased intracellular magnesium concentration.[22]
4. Phase-advanced basal body temperature minimal.[23]
5. Phase-advanced offset of melatonin secretion.[24]
6. Decreased slow wave sleep.[25]

All of these differences may be observed in both the follicular and luteal phases. In fact, reduced levels of late luteal phase beta-endorphin is the only consistently observed cycle phase-specific difference between PMS and control subjects.[26–28] It is therefore unlikely that any of these biologic factors explain the cyclic nature of PMS. A more popular explanation is that these biologic differences are related to the vulnerability to experience PMS, and that PMS occurs as a result of the interaction of vulnerability factors with specific triggering or cuing factors. Thus, reproductive endocrine signals may be

occurring in the context of a special sensitivity that is required for the expression of PMS.

Psychophysiologic responses are clearly influenced by the context within which they occur. Expectations of subjects and environmental variables have been shown to modify neurobehavioral responses to stimuli. Thus, a woman's environment and emotional or experiential states may significantly modify affective, physical, and behavioral responses to physiologic stimuli. Factors such as lifestyle stresses, history of physical, sexual, or emotional abuse, and a sense of "learned helplessness" contribute significantly to vulnerability, as do the previously mentioned biologic factors.

Studies with RU-486 demonstrate that PMS symptoms are not dependent on the late luteal phase.[16] When administered to PMS patients in the late luteal phase, RU-486 induces menstruation and a follicular phase hormonal milieu characterized by typical PMS symptoms. These data suggest that PMS symptoms are triggered by events occurring prior to the mid-late luteal phase of the cycle. However, another explanation suggests that PMS may represent an autonomous mood state disorder that has become linked to, or entrained by, the menstrual cycle. This is an important point of controversy. Research studies in which RU-486 is administered in the late follicular phase or early luteal phase may help to identify where in the menstrual cycle the cue for PMS symptom expression occurs, and whether PMS is actually an autonomous disorder that has become entrained by the menstrual cycle. Quite likely, a small percentage of PMS patients will be found to have an autonomously cycling mood disorder; these women would not be expected to improve with GnRH-agonist therapy.

ETIOLOGY

Sixty years after Frank's report on premenstrual tension, the etiology of PMS is still obscure. However, the focus of research has changed in the last decade. Previously, etiologic theories proposed that discrete abnormalities caused PMS. For example, progesterone deficiency, estrogen excess, pyridoxine deficiency, serotonin deficiency, endogenous opioid deficiency, hyperprolactinemia, genetic factors, hypoglycemia, fluid retention, endogenous hormone allergy, and psychogenic factors have all been advanced to explain the etiology of PMS.[5] However, the multifactorial-multiorgan nature of PMS has made it all but impossible to prove a single inciting etiologic cause for the disorder. Current research into the pathophysiology and etiology of PMS is focusing on the interaction of cuing factors and context or vulnerability factors. The precise role of reproductive endocrine hormones in this interactive process remains to be clarified.

THERAPEUTIC OPTIMISM

The primary treatment for PMS consists of some combination of nutritional modification, lifestyle modification, stress reduction, education, counseling, and support.[29] If these measures do not reduce the severity of symptoms sufficiently, then medical management is indicated.

In the past, progesterone suppositories, pyridoxine, and diuretics were the medications most commonly used by gynecologists to treat PMS. Lithium was frequently used by psychiatrists but was never scientifically proven effective. These drug therapies helped some women, but only a minority. Physicians have been slow to abandon these therapies because of a lack of effective alternatives.

Since 1984, a variety of medications have been proven to be superior to placebo for the treatment of PMS. GnRH-agonists are especially effective in eliminating both physical and emotional symptoms.[8–10] GnRH-agonist therapy may be supplemented with low dosage hormone replacement therapy.[9] Several psychotropic agents now have documented superiority compared to placebo. Alprazolam,[30,31] buspirone,[32] and fluoxetine,[33,34] used in the treatment of anxiety and depressive disorders, are all significantly more effective than placebo for the marked irritability, anger, depressed mood, and anxiety of PMS. In fact, PMS has often been likened to an angry, anxious, atypical depression.

Current research is attempting to identify clinical predictors of differential response to the various psychotropic medications. Because serotonin deficiency is associated with cravings for carbohydrates and sweets, food cravings may be a clinical predictor for response to serotonin agents such as fluoxetine.

SUMMARY

There is great reason to have therapeutic optimism when we think about PMS. In the last 10 years, truly effective medical therapy for PMS has been established. An increasing emphasis on the interaction of vulnerability factors and cuing factors has made clinicians and researchers intelligently focus on psychologic, environmental, and biologic phenomena simultaneously. PMS is truly becoming a multidiscipline disorder, and communication between psychiatrists and reproductive endocrinologists is changing the way both groups of physicians view PMS. Now, more than ever before, women can receive comprehensive management that will truly enhance the quality of their lives.

ACKNOWLEDGMENT

The authors express their gratitude to Uriel Halbreich, MD, for inviting us to participate in a Study Group on Menstrually Related Disorders at the 1991 annual meeting of the American College of Neuropsychopharmacology. Participants included Dr. Halbreich, John Bancroft, MD, Jean Endicott, PhD, Barbara L. Parry, MD, Robert L. Reid, MD, David R. Rubinow, MD, and Peter J. Schmidt, MD. Much of this chapter's content is derived from our Study Group Session.

REFERENCES

1. Woods N, Most A, Dery GK. Prevalence of perimenstrual symptoms. *Am J Pub Health.* 1982;72:1257.
2. Van Keep PA, Lehert P. The premenstrual syndrome—an epidemiologic and statistical exercise. In: Van Keep PA, Utian WH, eds. *The Premenstrual Syndrome.* Lancaster, England: MTP Press Limited; 1981.
3. Andersch B, Wenderstram G, Hahn L, et al. Premenstrual complaints: prevalence of premenstrual symptoms in a Swedish urban population. *J Psychosom Obstet Gynaecol.* 1986;5:39.
4. Rivera-Tovar AD, Frank E. Late luteal phase dysphoric disorder in young women. *Am J Psychiatry.* 1990;147:1634.
5. Reid RL. Premenstrual syndrome. *Curr Prog Obstet Gynecol Fertil.* 1985;8(2):1.
6. Freeman EW, Sondheimer S, Weinbaum PH, et al. Evaluating premenstrual symptoms in medical practice. *Obstet Gynecol.* 1985;65:500.
7. Halbreich U, Rojansky N, Palter S. Elimination of ovulation and menstrual cyclicity (with danazol) improves dysphoric premenstrual syndrome. *Fertil Steril.* 1991;56:1066.
8. Muse KN, Cetel NS, Futterman LA, et al. The premenstrual syndrome: effects of "medical ovariectomy." *N Engl J Med.* 1984;311:1345.
9. Mortola JF, Girton L, Fischer U. Successful treatment of severe premenstrual syndrome by combined use of gonadotropin-releasing hormone agonist and estrogen/progestin. *J Clin Endocrinol Metab.* 1991;72:252A.
10. Hammarback S, Backstrom T. Induced anovulation as treatment

of premenstrual tension syndrome: a double-blind cross-over study with GnRH-agonist versus placebo. *Acta Obstet Gynecol Scand.* 1988;67:159.

11. Watson NR, Studd JWW. Use of oestrogen in treatment of the premenstrual syndrome: a comparison of the routes of administration. *Contemp Rev Obstet Gynaecol.* 1990;2:117.

12. Hammarback S, Backstrom T, Holst J, et al. Cyclical mood changes as in the premenstrual tension syndrome during sequential estrogen-progestagen postmenopausal replacement therapy. *Acta Obstet Gynecol Scand.* 1985;64:393.

13. Magos AL, Brewster E, Singh R, et al. The effects of norethisterone in postmenopausal women on oestrogen replacement therapy: a model for the premenstrual syndrome. *Br J Obstet Gynecol.* 1986;93:1290.

14. Kirkham C, Hahn PM, Vugt AV, et al. A randomized, double-blind, placebo-controlled, cross-over trial to assess side effects of medroxyprogesterone acetate in hormone replacement therapy. *Obstet Gynecol.* 1991;78:93.

15. Hammarback S, Damber JE, Backstrom T. Relationship between symptom severity and hormone changes in women with premenstrual syndrome. *J Clin Endocrinol Metab.* 1989;68:125.

16. Schmidt PJ, Nieman LK, Grover GN, et al. Lack of effect of induced menses on symptoms in women with premenstrual syndrome. *N Engl J Med.* 1991;324:1174.

17. Rubinow DR, Hoban C, Grover GN, et al. Changes in plasma hormones across the menstrual cycle in patients with menstrually related mood disorder and in control subjects. *Am J Obstet Gynecol.* 1988;158:5.

18. Facchinetti F, Martignoni E, Sola D, et al. Transient failure of central opioid tonus and premenstrual symptoms. *J Reprod Med.* 1988;33:633.

19. Roy-Byrne PP, Rubinow DR, Hoban MC, et al. TSH and prolactin responses to TRH in patients with premenstrual syndrome. *Am J Psychiatry.* 1987;144:480.

20. Rapkin AJ, Edelmuth E, Chang LC, et al. Whole blood serotonin in premenstrual syndrome. *Obstet Gynecol.* 1987;70:533.

21. Ashby CR, Carr LA, Cook CL, et al. Alteration of 5-HT uptake by plasma fractions in the premenstrual syndrome. *J Neural Transm.* 1990;79:41.

22. Facchinetti F, Borella P, Fioroni L, et al. Reduction of monocyte's magnesium in patients affected by premenstrual syndrome. *J Psychosom Obstet Gynecol.* 1990;11:221.

23. Severino SK, Wagner DR, Moline ML, et al. High nocturnal body temperature in premenstrual syndrome and late luteal phase dysphoric disorder. *Am J Psychiatry.* 1991;148:1329.

24. Parry BL, Berga SL, Kripke DF, et al. Altered waveform of plasma nocturnal melatonin secretion in premenstrual depression. *Arch Gen Psychiatry.* 1990;47:1139.

25. Parry BL, Mendelson WB, Duncan WC, et al. Longitudinal sleep EEG, temperature, and activity measurements across the menstrual cycle in patients with premenstrual depression and in age-matched controls. *Psychiatry Res.* 1989;30:285.

26. Chuong CJ, Coulam CB, Kao PC, et al. Neuropeptide levels in premenstrual syndrome. *Fertil Steril.* 1985;44:760.

27. Giannini AJ, Martin DM, Turner CE. Beta-endorphin decline in late luteal phase dysphoric disorder. *Int J Psychiatry Med.* 1990; 20:279.

28. Facchinetti F, Genazzani A, Martignoni E, et al. Neuroendocrine correlates of premenstrual syndrome: changes in the pulsatile pattern of plasma LH. *Psychoneuroendocrinology.* 1990;15:269.

29. Smith S, Schiff I. The premenstrual syndrome—diagnosis and management. *Fertil Steril.* 1989;52:527.

30. Smith S, Rinehart JS, Ruddock VE, et al. Treatment of premenstrual syndrome with alprazolam: results of a double-blind, placebo-controlled, randomized crossover trial. *Obstet Gynecol.* 1987;70:37.

31. Harrison WM, Endicott J, Nee J. Treatment of premenstrual dysphoria with alprazolam: a controlled study. *Arch Gen Psychiatry.* 1990;47:270.

32. Rickels K, Freeman E, Sondheimer S. Buspirone in treatment of premenstrual syndrome. *Lancet.* 1989;1:777.

33. Rickels K, Freeman E, Sondheimer S, et al. Fluoxetine in the treatment of premenstrual syndrome. *Curr Ther Res.* 1990;48: 161.

34. Stone A, Pearlstein T, Brown W. Fluoxetine in the treatment of late luteal phase dysphoric disorder. *J Clin Psychiatry.* 1991;52: 290.

DIAGNOSIS
AND
PHYSIOLOGY

CHAPTER 2

Diagnosis of Premenstrual Syndrome

Samuel Smith

Premenstrual syndrome (PMS) has been well defined as "the cyclic recurrence, in the luteal phase of the menstrual cycle, of a combination of distressing physical, psychological, and/or behavioral changes of sufficient severity to result in deterioration of interpersonal relationships, and/or interference with normal activities."[1] There are three important components to this definition. First, there is a specific temporal relationship of symptoms to menstruation; symptoms present during the luteal phase of the menstrual cycle are absent during the follicular phase of the cycle. Second, symptoms must be severe enough to interfere with some aspect of lifestyle. Third, PMS is a repetitive phenomenon; symptoms are present month after month, to some degree. The diagnosis of PMS is in doubt unless all three components of the definition are present.[2]

DIAGNOSTIC CRITERIA

PMS is currently considered a gynecologic disorder in the *International Classification of Diseases*—9th Revision (ICD-9), a reference text that standardizes the classification of disease throughout the United States.[3] Unfortunately, there are no uniformly accepted diagnostic criteria for PMS, nor is there even a uniformly accepted working definition.[4,5] This often leads to poor communication between researchers and clinicians, and reduces the generalizability of conclusions obtained in research studies, because each research group utilizes slightly different diagnostic criteria for inclusion of subjects into protocols.[6] Thus, confusion and lack of consensus in the medical literature complicate the clinical diagnosis of PMS.

In 1983 the National Institute of Mental Health (NIMH) convened a workshop in which guidelines for the diagnosis of PMS were offered.[7-10] The NIMH group recommended that PMS be diagnosed when the intensity of symptoms changes at least 30% in the 6 days prior to menstruation (premenstrual period) compared to days 5 to 10 of the menstrual cycle (postmenstrual period) for 2 consecutive months. The workshop did not designate that any particular core symptoms be present; this acknowledged that the clinical presentation of PMS is quite diverse. The temporal relationship of symptoms to menstruation was specified, as was the magnitude of change in symptom severity. However, the NIMH guidelines were vague in defining the level of postmenstrual symptoms that would exclude PMS because they were more typical of chronic affective disorder, and many patients with mild premenstrual symptoms that did not interfere with their ability to function could be diagnosed with PMS. In addition, the 1983 guidelines did not designate which symptoms or how many symptoms needed to change.[7-10]

Recognizing these limitations, an NIMH advisory committee was established in 1985 to develop a diagnostic category for PMS to be included in the *Diagnostic and Statistical Manual of Mental Disorders,* Third Edition—Revised (DSM-III-R).[6,10] Late luteal phase dysphoric disorder (LLPDD), a subset of PMS in which mood disturbance is the primary complaint, was added as an Appendix to the DSM-III-R.[11] Clearly defined diagnostic criteria were developed for LLPDD (Table 1) to facilitate communication between researchers and clinicians and to enhance the generalizability of results from research protocols. Although LLPDD is a severe subset of PMS, the diagnostic criteria for LLPDD can be extrapolated and utilized to diagnose PMS.

SYMPTOMS OF PMS

The symptoms of PMS are diverse and potentially disabling. There are more than 150 psychologic, physical, and behavioral symptoms associated with PMS.[12] Some of the more common PMS symptoms are listed in Table 2. Emotional symptoms are the most common complaints that lead patients to treatment.[13] Depression, irritability, anxiety, and mood swings are the most common emotional symptoms. The most common physical, or somatic, complaints are headache, bloating or swelling, and cramps. Food cravings are the most common behavioral symptom.[13] Approximately 58% of

patients present with disturbing emotional and physical symptoms; 37% present with distressing emotional symptoms with absent or mild physical symptoms; and about 5% present with distressing physical symptoms with absent or mild emotional symptoms.[13]

Symptom Subgroups

PMS symptoms sometimes appear to cluster together. Consequently, various investigators have used statistical techniques to identify PMS symptom subgroups. Moos developed the 47-item retrospective Menstrual Distress Questionnaire (MDQ) which encompassed eight symptom subgroups: pain, concentration, behavioral change, autonomic reactions, water retention, negative affect, arousal, and control.[14,15] The majority of Moos' symptom subgroups focus on somatic changes. Emotional and behavioral symptoms were included under two of the eight categories. Approximately 50% of Moos' normative population was taking oral contraceptives, and almost 10% were pregnant, thus reducing the Moos MDQ applicability to PMS diagnosis.[14,15] Despite these shortcomings, the MDQ has remained a commonly utilized symptom rating scale for assessing menstrual cycle symptoms.

Abraham divided 19 menstrual cycle symptoms into four premenstrual tension (PMT) subgroups: those characterized by anxiety and irritability (PMT-A); by

Table 1
Diagnostic Criteria for Late Luteal Phase Dysphoric Disorder[11]

A. In most menstrual cycles during the past year, symptoms in section B (below) occurred during the last week of the luteal phase and remitted within a few days after onset of the follicular phase. In menstruating females, these phases correspond to the week before, and a few days after, the onset of menses. (In nonmenstruating females who have had a hysterectomy, the timing of luteal and follicular phases may require measurement of circulating reproductive hormones.)

B. At least five of the following symptoms have been present for most of the time during each symptomatic late luteal phase, at least one of the symptoms being either 1, 2, 3, or 4:
    1. Marked affective lability (eg, feeling suddenly sad, tearful, irritable, or angry).
    2. Persistent and marked anger or irritability.
    3. Marked anxiety, tension, feelings of being "keyed up," or "on edge."
    4. Markedly depressed mood, feelings of hopelessness, or self-deprecating thoughts.
    5. Decreased interest in usual activities (eg, work, friends, hobbies).
    6. Easy fatigability or marked lack of energy.
    7. Subjective sense of difficulty in concentrating.
    8. Marked change in appetite, overeating, or specific food cravings.
    9. Hypersomnia or insomnia.
    10. Other physical symptoms, such as breast tenderness or swelling, headaches, joint or muscle pain, a sensation of "bloating," or weight gain.

C. The disturbance seriously interferes with work or with usual social activities or relationships with others.

D. The disturbance is not merely an exacerbation of the symptoms of another disorder, such as major depression, panic disorder, dysthymia, or a personality disorder (although it may be superimposed on any of these disorders).

E. Criteria A, B, C, and D are confirmed by prospective daily self-ratings during at least two symptomatic cycles. (The diagnosis may be made provisionally prior to this confirmation.)

Table 2
Common PMS Symptoms[a]

Emotional	Physical	Behavioral
Anxiety*	Headache*	Food cravings*
Irritability*	Migraines	Increased appetite*
Labile moods*	Breast tenderness*	Increased alcohol intake
Depression	Swelling of extremities	Decreased motivation
Anger*	Bloatedness*	Decreased efficiency
Sadness	Fatigue*	Avoid activities
Crying easily*	Abdominal cramps	Staying at home
Nervous tension	Aches and pains	Sleep changes
Overly sensitive*	Weight gain	Changes in libido
	Skin problems	Reduced cognitive function
	Hot flashes*	Social isolation*
	Gastrointestinal*	Poor concentration*
	Dizziness*	Forgetfulness*
	Palpitation*	

[a]Items labeled with an asterisk (*) are included in the *Calendar of Premenstrual Experiences.*[23]

symptoms of water retention (PMT-H); by depressed affect and cognitive impairment (PMT-D); and by increased appetite and food cravings (PMT-C)[16] (Table 3). PMS patients most commonly demonstrate PMT-A and PMT-H symptoms, with PMT-D and PMT-C symptoms somewhat less frequently described.[13] In addition, PMS patients seldom present with only PMT-D or PMT-C symptoms; they are usually seen in combination with anxiety-related and water retention symptoms.[13]

Rubinow and Roy-Byrne identified nine PMS symptom subgroups: affective, cognitive, pain, neurovegetative, autonomic, central nervous system, fluid/electrolyte, dermatological, and behavioral.[5] It is clear that statistical techniques, and perhaps clinical experience, have been employed by various researchers to create symptom categories. Each investigator's results depend on the control group and PMS population from which data were obtained and the statistical methods used for analysis. Symptom subgroups are largely artificial con-structs, attempts to devise standard methods for assessing menstrually related symptoms. As such, they are primarily tools for assessing research data.

DIAGNOSIS

PMS encompasses many symptoms; however, there are no symptoms that are unique to and diagnostic of PMS. The diagnosis of PMS depends on the temporal relationship between symptoms and menstruation, and the severity of symptoms.[2]

Affective symptoms such as irritability, anxiety, and depression, behavioral symptoms such as appetite changes, sleep changes, and lowered performance, and physical symptoms such as fatigue are not specific to PMS and characterize many psychiatric disorders. In fact, 40% to 60% of women who are referred or who seek treatment for PMS may be found to have general-

Table 3
Premenstrual Tension (PMT) Symptom Subgroups[16]

PMT-A	PMT-H	PMT-D	PMT-C
Nervous tension	Weight gain	Depression	Craving sweets
Mood swings	Swelling of extremities	Forgetfulness	Increased appetite
Irritability	Breast tenderness	Crying easily	Heart pounding
Anxiety	Abdominal bloating	Confusion	Headache
		Insomnia	Fatigue
			Dizziness

ized psychiatric disorders,[9,17–19] and in some series only 20% to 25% of women were found to have PMS.[18,19] The most common Axis I psychiatric diagnoses made are minor and major depressive syndromes, especially atypical and hostile subtypes, and adjustment disorders.[18,19] In addition, approximately 10% of women seeking PMS care have DSM-III-R Axis II personality disorders.[19] Many of the Axis I psychiatric disorders demonstrated worsened symptoms in the premenstrual period.[17–19] It is essential, therefore, to distinguish PMS from chronic psychiatric or adjustment disorders that demonstrate premenstrual worsening of symptoms. This is the major differential diagnosis for PMS. It is also important to look for psychiatric disorders coexisting with severe PMS because one series documented that more than one-third of women with LLPDD had a concurrent Axis I or II psychiatric diagnosis.[20]

There is frequently a large discrepancy between recalled, retrospective data and information obtained prospectively throughout the menstrual cycle.[4,9,21,22] Thus it is imperative that the physician prospectively confirm the temporal aspects of symptoms with some form of daily reporting.

Daily Symptom Reporting

The main feature distinguishing PMS from chronic psychiatric disorders is the presence of at least one asymptomatic week in the follicular phase of every menstrual cycle. A variety of techniques are available to assess symptoms on a daily basis—symptom calendars or rating scales, visual analog scales, self-report inventories, and psychiatric rating scales.[2] Daily symptom calendars (DSC) or daily rating forms (DRF) are the most useful in clinical practice (Fig. 1). The DSC allows a patient to record her symptoms and their severity each day of the month. Basal body temperature (BBT) and weight may also be recorded to document the onset of the luteal phase and cyclic fluctuation in weight. Symptoms are generally graded on a 4-point scale—0 (absent), 1 (mild), 2 (moderate), and 3 (severe)—daily throughout two consecutive menstrual cycles. A variety of DSCs and DRFs are available to facilitate prospective documentation of symptoms. For example, Reid[1] developed the Prospective Record of the Impact and Severity of Menstrual Symptoms, which incorporates symptoms, lifestyle impact, and information regarding life events and medication. Mortola et al[23] developed the Calendar of Premenstrual Experiences (CPE) and demonstrated that their calendar successfully distinguished PMS subjects from controls; the CPE had a 2.8% false-negative rate and 0% false-positive rate

when used for two consecutive cycles. Many physicians choose to create their own calendars.

Temporal Patterns of Symptoms

The temporal relationship of symptoms to menstruation is easily determined by prospective recording. Several patterns are commonly observed.[24] First, many patients demonstrate affective symptoms throughout the month, frequently with increased symptoms during the late luteal phase (Fig. 2). These patients demonstrate total symptom scores greater than 40 on cycle days 3 to 9 using the CPE.[23] They usually suffer from a chronic affective disorder, often with premenstrual worsening of symptoms. Appropriate management consists of informing the patient that her symptoms do not fulfill the temporal criteria for PMS, followed by referral for complete psychiatric evaluation.

A second pattern commonly seen is illustrated in Fig. 3. Many women demonstrate symptoms during the luteal phase of the cycle that are mild and do not interfere with their level of psychosocial functioning. Their CPE scores are consistently less than 42 during the last 7 days of the menstrual cycle.[23] Although there is a premenstrual pattern to symptoms, these women do not fulfill the severity criteria for PMS; rather, they have mild moliminal symptoms. These women often respond well to education, support, and over-the-counter products. Many state that their symptoms are improved and less disturbing after a 2-month period of evaluation and education.[19]

Third, there are some women who have symptoms that "come and go" but bear no consistent temporal relationship to the menstrual cycle. These women may have a rapidly cycling affective disorder and require psychiatric evaluation.[24]

Finally, there are women who are essentially symptom free during the follicular phase and sufficiently symptomatic during the luteal phase to experience interference with interpersonal relationships and work efficiency, fulfilling the diagnostic criteria for PMS (Fig. 4). CPE luteal phase scores are greater than 42.[23] Two months of prospective symptom recording are satisfactory to confirm the diagnosis of PMS, although the diagnosis may be provisionally made after one menstrual cycle.

Uncommonly, PMS may be superimposed on a chronic affective disorder (Fig. 5). These women are differentiated from those with chronic affective disorders because of the emergence in the luteal phase of a variety of physical symptoms, usually related to water retention or pain, that are not present during the follicular phase. These women require a coordinated treat-

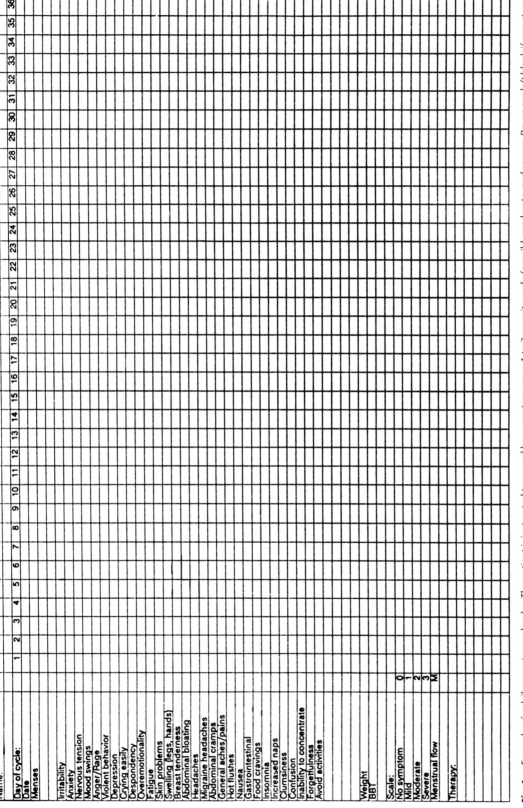

Fig. 1 Example of a daily symptom calendar. The patient is instructed to record her symptoms on a 1 to 3 severity scale for mild, moderate, and severe. Boxes are left blank if symptom severity is zero. The author is grateful to Ms. Bernadette Budniakiewicz for developing this symptom calendar.

Name: _____

Day of cycle:	1	2	3	4	5	6	7	8	9	10	11	12	13	14	15	16	17	18	19	20	21	22	23	24	25	26	27	28	29	30	31	32	33	34	35	36
Date																																				
Menses	M	M	M	M	M																								M							
Irritability	2	2	2	2	2	2	2	2	1	1	2	2	2	2	1	2	1	1	2	3	3	2	2	3	3	3	3	3	2							
Anxiety	2	2	2	2	2	2	2	2	1	1	2	3	3	3	1	2	1	1	2	3	3	2	2	3	3	3	3	3	2							
Nervous tension	2	2	2	2	2	2	2	2	1	1	2	3	3	3	1	3	1	1	2	3	3	3	3	3	3	3	3	3	2							
Mood swings	2	2	2	2	2	2	2	2	1	1	2	2	2	2	1	2	1	1	3	1	2	2	2	3	2	3	3	2	2							
Anger/Rage	2	2	2	2	2	2	2	2	1	1	2	2	2	2	1	2	1	1	3	2	2	2	2	3	3	3	2	2	2							
Violent behavior																																				
Depression	2	2	2	2	2	2	2	2	1	1	2	2	2	2	1	2	1	1	2	2	2	2	2	3	3	3	3	3	2							
Crying easily	2	2	2	2	2	2	2	2	1	1	2	2	2	2	1	2	1	1	2	2	2	2	2	3	3	3	3	3	3							
Despondency	2	2	2	2	2	2	2	2	1	1	2	2	2	2	1	2	1	1	2	2	2	2	2	3	3	3	3	3	2							
Overemotionality	2	2	2	2	2	2	2	2	1	1	2	2	2	2	1	2	1	1	2	2	2	2	2	3	3	3	3	3	2							
Fatigue																																				
Skin problems																																				
Swelling (legs, hands)																																				
Breast tenderness																																				
Abdominal bloating																																				
Headaches																																				
Migraine headaches																																				
Abdominal cramps																																				
General aches/pains																																				
Hot flushes																																				
Nausea																																				
Gastrointestinal																																				
Food cravings																																				
Insomnia																																				
Increased naps																																				
Clumsiness																																				
Confusion																																				
Inability to concentrate																																				
Forgetfulness																																				
Avoid activities																																				
Weight																																				
BBT																																				

Scale:
No symptom 0
Mild 1
Moderate 2
Severe 3
Menstrual flow M

Therapy: _____

Fig. 2   Example of a symptom calendar that demonstrates emotional symptoms throughout the month and increased late luteal phase symptom severity.

Fig. 3 Example of a symptom calendar that demonstrates mild luteal phase symptoms.

Fig. 4 Example of a symptom calendar consistent with the diagnosis of PMS.

Name:

Day of cycle:		1	2	3	4	5	6	7	8	9	10	11	12	13	14	15	16	17	18	19	20	21	22	23	24	25	26	27	28	29	30	31	32	33	34	35	36
Date																																					
Menses		M	M	M	M																									M							
Irritability		2	2	2	2	2	2	2	2	2	2	2	2	2	2	2	2	2	2	2	2	2	2	2	2	2	2	3	3	3							
Anxiety																			1	2	2	2	2	2	2	2	2	2	2	2							
Nervous tension		2	1	1															1	2	2	2	2	2	2	2	2	2	2	2							
Mood swings		2	1	1															1	2	2	2	2	2	2	2	2	2	2	2							
Anger/Rage		2	2	2	2	2	2	2	2	2	2	2	2	2	2	2	2	2	2	2	2	2	2	2	2	2	2	2	2	2							
Violent behavior																																					
Depression		2	2	2	2	2	2	2	2	2	2	2	2	2	2	2	2	2	2	2	3	2	2	2	2	3	2	2	2	2							
Crying easily																																					
Despondency																																					
Overemotionality																																					
Fatigue																			1	2	1	1	1	3	2	2	2	2	2	2							
Skin problems		2	2	1																																	
Swelling (legs, hands)																																					
Breast tenderness		1																	1	2	2	2	2	3	3	3	3	3	3	3							
Abdominal bloating		2	1																1	2	2	2	3	2	3	2	2	3	2	2							
Headaches																																					
Migraine headaches																																					
Abdominal cramps																																					
General aches/pains																			2	2	2	2	2	2	2	2	2	2	2	2							
Hot flushes																																					
Nausea																																					
Gastrointestinal																																					
Food cravings		2	3	3	2	1	1	1	1	1	2	2	2	2	2	2	2	2	3	3	3	3	3	3	3	3	3	3	3	3							
Insomnia																			3	1	1	3	2	2	1	3	1	1	1	1							
Increased naps																																					
Clumsiness		1																		1	1	2	2	2	2	2	2	2	2	2							
Confusion		2	1																	1	1	1	1	2	2	2	2	2	2	3							
Inability to concentrate																																					
Forgetfulness		2	2	1																	1.	1	1	2	2	2	1	3	3	3							
Avoid activities		2	1	1																1	1	2	2	2	2	2	2	2	2	2							
Weight		167	166		164		164		164		164		165		168		168		172		172		177		179		181		182								
BBT																																					
Scale:																																					
No symptom	0																																				
Mild	1																																				
Moderate	2																																				
Severe	3																																				
Menstrual flow	M																																				
Therapy:																																					

Fig. 5 Example of a symptom calendar in which PMS appears to be superimposed on a chronic affective disorder.

ment effort between psychiatrist and gynecologist (or other primary physician).

Psychologic Questionnaires

Many physicians and clinics use psychologic questionnaires to distinguish PMS from chronic affective disorders. Follicular and luteal phase symptoms are compared to identify whether there is a clear-cut difference between the luteal phase and follicular phase. These assessments are often completed retrospectively by patients as a means of screening out women who describe follicular phase symptoms.

A variety of questionnaires are available for office use. Moos' MDQ is commonly used. It requires a woman to grade 47 symptoms on a 1 to 6 severity scale. Scores below 70 in the follicular phase and greater than 90 during the luteal phase are suggestive of PMS; the minimum score for this questionnaire is 47. [14,15]

Halbreich et al[25,26] developed the Premenstrual Assessment Form (PAF), which uses 95 symptoms assessed on a 1 to 6 scale. It was developed for initial screening and evaluation of premenstrual symptoms, and was designed to reflect Halbreich and coworkers' concept of premenstrual changes as diversified clusters of phenomena. The PAF is usually applied as a retrospective report for the last three menstrual cycles, although it may be used prospectively. The PAF can categorize dysphoric premenstrual symptoms into entities such as the full depressive syndrome (with atypical, hostile, anxious-agitated, and withdrawn subtypes), organic mental syndrome, and impulsive syndrome. It categorizes physical premenstrual changes into water retention syndrome, general discomfort syndrome, and the increased well-being syndrome. The PAF also designates criteria for impairment in social functioning. [25,26] The authors recognize that the PAF is primarily a screening tool that requires confirmation by prospective daily rating of symptoms.

Steiner et al[27] developed a simple self-rating scale for PMS screening consisting of 36 "yes or no" questions. Patients with PMS generally have fewer than 6 "yes" answers in the follicular phase and more than 14 "yes" responses in the luteal phase. Patients can complete this questionnaire in a matter of minutes.

A variety of psychiatric self-report inventories are available to assess emotional symptoms during the follicular and luteal phases of the cycle. Some commonly utilized inventories are the Beck Depression Inventory, Hamilton Depression Rating Scale, Spielberger State Anxiety Scale, Profile of Mood States, Hopkins Symp-

tom Checklist, and Schedule for Affective Disorders and Schizophrenia (SADS). These questionnaires are most useful when a patient demonstrates follicular phase symptoms and appears to have a chronic affective disorder. They may be utilized in combination with a psychiatric interview to diagnose mental disorders. However, these inventories are primarily used in research protocols to help delineate study and control populations.

Data obtained from daily symptom records correlate highly with scores on various psychiatric rating scales during the same cycle phase. [23] Moreover, it is much more practical to have patients prospectively record symptoms on a DSC than to prospectively record data from inventories. The latter method is more cumbersome for the patient, more limited in the scope of symptoms that can be assessed, and results in the collection and interpretation of many data sheets over a month as opposed to a single menstrual calendar sheet. Visual analog self-ratings for individual symptoms are used in some research settings, but they have limited application for clinical practice at present. [28–30]

Lastly, the Minnesota Multiphasic Personality Inventory (MMPI) may be employed to assess patients presenting with premenstrual complaints. [24,31] The MMPI is a 550-item, self-report questionnaire that can be used to profile a patient's personality functioning and general mental health. PMS subjects demonstrate significant menstrual cycle phase-related changes in MMPI response patterns; luteal phase responses tend to demonstrate increased stress, tension, depression, oversensitivity, and social discomfort than follicular phase responses. [31] Because the MMPI takes so long to complete, it is mainly used to screen patients in the follicular phase for psychologic stress and dysfunction, profiles indicating a need for complete psychiatric evaluation.

Diagnosis of PMS after Hysterectomy

A small number of cases of PMS are diagnosed after hysterectomy. Backstrom et al[32] recorded daily symptom ratings prior to and following hysterectomy in six women with prospectively confirmed PMS. Ovarian activity was monitored with urinary estrogen and pregnanediol levels. Cyclic changes in mood and physical symptoms persisted after hysterectomy and were maximal in the late luteal phase of the cycle. However, in the absence of menstruation, most patients did not recognize the cyclical nature of the symptoms. [32]

Clearly, PMS can occur in nonmenstruating women

who have undergone hysterectomy but retain ovarian function. In these cases the follicular and luteal phase of the cycle may be determined by basal body temperature charting or measurement of ovarian steroid concentrations in serum, urine, or saliva. The temporal relationship of symptoms to the ovarian cycle phase can then be followed prospectively.

SUMMARY

Many women report a variety of emotional, physical, and behavioral changes associated with the luteal phase of the menstrual cycle. For the majority of women, these cyclic changes are not severe enough to cause interference with psychosocial functioning. Those women who report cyclic luteal phase symptoms that remit during menstruation and that are severe enough to affect their level of psychosocial or occupational functioning may have PMS. However, quite often information obtained through patient history is not confirmed when symptoms are monitored prospectively. Consequently, daily self-ratings for at least two consecutive cycles are required to confirm the diagnosis of PMS; during this time the temporal relationship of symptoms to menstruation and their severity are monitored prospectively. Symptoms that do not disappear within a few days after onset of menstruation suggest that the premenstrual changes represent an exacerbation of a chronic psychiatric disorder.

LLPDD represents a subset of PMS that is characterized by severe impairment in social, family, or work function predominantly due to severe emotional symptoms. It is currently included in the appendix of the DSM-III-R to facilitate systematic clinical assessment and research.[11]

REFERENCES

1. Reid RL. Premenstrual syndrome. *Curr Probl Obstet Gynecol Fertil.* 1985;8:1.
2. Smith S, Schiff I. The premenstrual syndrome—diagnosis and management. *Fertil Steril.* 1989;52:527.
3. United States Department of Health and Human Resources. *International Classification of Diseases—Nineth Revision, Clinical Modification, Volume I.* Washington, DC: Public Health Services—Health Care Financing Administration; 1980:523.
4. Halbreich U, Endicott J. Methodological issues in studies on premenstrual changes. *Psychoneuroendocrinology.* 1985;10:15.
5. Rubinow DR, Roy-Byrne P. Premenstrual syndromes: overview from a methodologic perspective. *Am J Psychiatry.* 1984;141:163.
6. Spitzer RL, Severino SK, Williams JBW, et al. Late luteal phase dysphoric disorder and DSM-III-R. *Am J Psychiatry.* 1989;146:892.
7. Anderson M, Severino SK, Hurt SW, et al. Premenstrual syndrome research: using the NIMH guidelines. *J Clin Psychiatry.* 1988;49:484.
8. Osofsky HJ, Keppel W, Kuczmierczyk AR. Evaluation and clinical management of premenstrual syndrome in clinical psychiatric practice. *J Clin Psychiatry.* 1988;49:494.
9. Rubinow DR, Hoban C, Roy-Byrne P, et al. Premenstrual syndromes: past and future research strategies. *Can J Psychiatry.* 1985;30:469.
10. Blumenthal SJ, Nadelson CC. Late luteal phase dysphoric disorder (premenstrual syndromes): clinical implications. *J Clin Psychiatry.* 1988;49:469.
11. American Psychiatric Association. *Diagnostic and Statistical Manual of Mental Disorders,* Third Edition Revised. Washington, DC: APA;1987:367–369.
12. Hamilton JA, Parry B, Alagna S, et al. Premenstrual mood changes: a guide to evaluation and treatment. *Psychiatric Annals.* 1984;14:426.
13. Freeman EW, Sondheimer S, Weinbaum PH, et al. Evaluating premenstrual symptoms in medical practice. *Obstet Gynecol.* 1985;65:500.
14. Moos RH. The development of a menstrual distress questionnaire. *Psychosom Med.* 1968;30:853.
15. Moos RH. Typology of menstrual cycle symptoms. *Am J Obstet Gynecol.* 1968;103:390.
16. Abraham GE. Nutritional factors in the etiology of the premenstrual tension syndromes. *J Reprod Med.* 1983;28:446.
17. Harrison WM, Rabkin JG, Endicott J. Psychiatric evaluation of premenstrual changes. *Psychosomatics.* 1985;26:789.
18. Yuk VJ, Jugdutt AV, Cumming CE, et al. Towards a definition of PMS: a factor analytic evaluation of premenstrual change in noncomplaining women. *J Psychosom Res.* 1990;34:439.
19. Gise LH, Lebovits AH, Paddison PL, et al. Issues in the identification of premenstrual syndromes. *J Nerv Mental Dis.* 1990;178:228.
20. Harrison WH, Endicott J, Nee J, et al. Characteristics of women seeking treatment of premenstrual syndrome. *Psychosomatics.* 1989;30:405.
21. Sampson GA, Prescott P. The assessment of the symptoms of premenstrual syndrome and their response to therapy. *Br J Obstet Gynaecol.* 1981;38:399.
22. Endicott J, Halbreich U. Retrospective report of premenstrual depressive changes: factors affecting confirmation by daily ratings. *Psychopharm Bull.* 1983;18:109.
23. Mortola JF, Girton L, Beck L, et al. Diagnosis of premenstrual syndrome by a simple, prospective, and reliable instrument: the calendar of premenstrual experiences. *Obstet Gynecol.* 1990;76:302.
24. Keye WR. General evaluation of premenstrual symptoms. *Clin Obstet Gynecol.* 1987;30:396.
25. Halbreich U, Endicott J, Schacht S, et al. The diversity of premenstrual changes as reflected in the Premenstrual Assessment Form. *Acta Psychiatr Scand.* 1982;65:46.
26. Halbreich U, Endicott J, Lesser J. The clinical diagnosis and classification of premenstrual changes. *Can J Psychiatry.* 1985;30:489.
27. Steiner M, Haskett RF, Carroll BJ. Premenstrual tension syndrome: the development of research criteria and new rating scales. *Acta Psychiatr Scand.* 1980;62:177.
28. Casper RF, Powell AM. Premenstrual syndrome: documentation by a linear analog scale compared to two descriptive scales. *Am J Obstet Gynecol.* 1986;155:862.

29. Rubinow DR, Roy-Byrne P, Hoban MC, et al. Premenstrual mood changes, characteristic patterns in women with and without premenstrual syndrome. *J Affective Disord*. 1986;10:85.

30. Rabin DS, Schmidt PJ, Campbell G, et al. Hypothalamic-pituitary-adrenal function in patients with the premenstrual syndrome. *J Clin Endocrinol Metab*. 1990;71:1158.

31. Chuong CJ, Colligan RC, Coulam CB, et al. The MMPI as an aid in evaluating patients with premenstrual syndrome. *Psychosomatics*. 1988;29:197.

32. Backstrom CT, Boyle H, Baird DT. Persistence of symptoms of premenstrual tension in hysterectomized women. *Br J Obstet Gynaecol*. 1981;88:530.

Principles of Psychiatric Assessment for Differential Diagnosis of Premenstrual Syndrome

Yogesh Bakhai and Uriel Halbreich

Recent publicity on premenstrual syndrome (PMS) in the mass media has been followed by an increased awareness of its existence and by a tendency of women with a variety of symptoms to relate them to PMS.[1] Premenstrual symptoms are diverse and of variable intensity. There are more than 200 physical and psychological symptoms reported by women.[2,3] Psychological symptoms are generally related to anxiety and depression. They include sadness and various shades of depression, tension, anxiety, impulsivity, aggression, mood swings, irritability, crying, loneliness, and low self-esteem. Changes in sleep, energy, activity, and appetite are very common, as are reduced concentration and changes in cognitive function. Conversely, it was shown that some premenstrual changes can actually be positive, such as increased energy and efficiency as well as increased affection and sexual desire.[4]

Because many of these symptoms, when grouped together, resemble psychiatric syndromes or disorders, it is important to differentiate them from other mental disorders. Therefore a detailed psychiatric evaluation should be included in any evaluation of premenstrual syndrome.

OVERVIEW OF THE PROBLEM OF DIFFERENTIAL DIAGNOSIS

Some of the mental disorders that should be ruled out before diagnosis of dysphoric PMS include major depressive disorder, atypical depression, dysthymic disorder, organic mood disorder, impulse control disorder, bipolar disorder, various personality disorders, anxiety disorders, panic disorder, and others.

Not only are premenstrual symptoms similar to those of psychiatric disorders, but some psychiatric disorders (eg, depressive disorders, panic disorder, obsessive compulsive disorder, bulimia, alcoholism, and borderline personality disorder) can be exacerbated premenstrually.[5]

There is an established epidemiological and statistical association between dysphoric premenstrual changes and lifetime history of affective disorders[6–8]; there is little association between physical premenstrual changes and lifetime history of depression. Other studies of women who seek treatment for PMS reported a higher prevalence of lifetime history of anxiety disorders and substance abuse compared to women with no premenstrual dysphoric changes.[9,10] There is also a reported increased risk of suicide[11] and child abuse during the premenstrual period. These findings suggest that women seeking treatment for dysphoric premenstrual changes might be at a higher risk of suicide and aggression, particularly if they have been suffering from current psychiatric illness, which is an additional reason for a careful psychiatric evaluation.

The interpretation of studies reporting a high prevalence of mental disorders in women seeking treatment for PMS might be questioned if complete psychiatric evaluations were not performed or reported, since symptoms of many mental disorders may be exacerbated premenstrually. Furthermore, women with persistent mental disorders may find it more acceptable to attribute their distress to premenstrual syndrome than to acknowledge that they have chronic mental problems.

Therefore, the diagnosis of dysphoric premenstrual syndrome is one of exclusion; the patient should be diagnosed as "not currently mentally ill."[12] That is, the patient should not meet criteria for any major mental disorder, as defined by some of the widely acceptable diagnostic manuals, usually the *Diagnostic and Statistical Manual-III-Revised* (DSM-III-R) of the American Psychiatric Association (APA),[13] or the *International Code of Diagnosis,* 9th and 10th editions (ICD 9 and 10).[14] For research protocols, any diagnosable entity in the *Research Diagnostic Criteria* (RDC)[15] should be excluded.

Indeed, in order to effectively rule out mental disorders as they are defined in these manuals, some knowledge of their structure and philosophy is required. In the United States the DSM system is used almost exclusively and is gaining popularity in other countries as well; we will focus here on that manual.

CLASSIFICATION OF MENTAL DISORDERS

Classification of mental disorders serves the purpose of communication, control, and comprehension. With the DSM-III, the APA emphasized phenomenology and data-derived criteria with the explicit wish to avoid controversial theories and interpretations.

The current diagnostic classification of the APA is descriptive and is primarily based on phenomenology. Symptoms and signs are grouped into diagnostic entities and then into classes on the basis of shared clinical features, and not based on etiology or pathophysiology that is usually unknown.

This diagnostic system, introduced in 1980 with the DSM-III, is a departure from the previous APA DSMs that were based mostly on psychodynamic concepts. It was felt that the state of knowledge (or lack of knowledge) is such that an atheoretical framework is preferable.

Specific diagnostic criteria and guidelines for making each diagnosis were developed to enhance inter-interviewer diagnostic reliability. Therefore, DSM-III and its revision, DSM-III-R, serve as useful tools for clinical decisions and research. The DSM-III-R (approved in 1986) is comparable to the *International Diagnostic Manual* ICD-9 CM. The DSM-III-R is aimed to make the classification clinically useful, reliable, and acceptable among various groups of different theoretical orientation. It was designed to be suitable in research, and is consistent with data from research studies.

Meanwhile, an ICD-10 has been developed and the APA is developing a compatible DSM-IV that follows the same atheoretical, descriptive concept of DSM-III. We believe that the rapid succession of diagnostic manuals is an indication of the rapid progress in the field. The accumulation of knowledge will certainly lead to further updates and then to major changes in the diagnostic system. Therefore, an understanding of diagnostic principles is important. They might be more significant than current semischematic criteria.

A multiaxial diagnostic system that provides a biopsychosocial approach to psychiatric assessment was first introduced in the DSM-III. A complete diagnosis is ideally based on five axes.

Axis I contains most of the major mental disorders except personality disorders and developmental disorders, which are included in Axis II. Axis III includes physical disorders and conditions that might contribute to mental dysfunction (eg, hypertension). Axis IV describes severity of psychosocial stressors (eg, death of a spouse); and Axis V is a global assessment of functioning. It includes the Global Assessment Scale (GAS),[16] which provides criteria to assess functioning and scores patients from 0 to 100 (100 is highest level of functioning).

DIFFERENTIAL DIAGNOSIS OF DYSPHORIC PMS FROM CURRENT MENTAL OR OTHER MEDICAL DISORDERS

Axis I and Axis II Mental Disorders

Several mental disorders and symptoms of physical disorders can resemble dysphoric PMS, as follow:

1. Major mood disorders, including major depressive disorder, atypical depression, depressive disorder not otherwise specified (NOS), dysthymic disorder, bipolar disorder, cyclothymic disorder, and recurrent depressive disorder.
2. Anxiety disorders, including generalized anxiety disorder, panic disorder, and others.
3. Personality disorders, such as borderline and histrionic disorders.
4. Substance abuse disorders (mainly abuse of psychoactive drugs).
5. Somatoform disorders, such as conversion disorder and hypochondriasis.
6. Eating disorders, especially bulimia.
7. Several physical disorders, including endocrine disorders such as hypothyroidism or hyperthyroidism, nonspecific infections, some malignancies, autoimmune disorders, and seizure disorder.

Many of these disorders are exacerbated only during the luteal phase of the menstrual cycle, and episodes are long enough that women might meet diagnostic criteria for mental disorders even if symptoms are limited to the luteal and perimenstrual periods. We will not attempt to determine whether these episodes are truly PMS. For the purpose of this chapter, it is important to realize that psychiatric disorders and PMS may co-exist.

Late Luteal Phase Dysphoric Disorder

The DSM-III-R is the first APA diagnostic manual that includes the diagnostic entity of premenstrual syndrome. Following a lengthy debate,[17] PMS was named late luteal phase dysphoric disorder (LLPDD). It is included in the DSM-III-R as an appendix, as a provisional proposed diagnostic category that requires further studies. The DSM-III-R criteria for LLPDD are as follows:

A. In most menstrual cycles during the past year, symptoms in section B (below) occurred during the last week of the luteal phase and remitted within a few days after onset of the follicular phase. In menstruating females, these phases correspond to the week before, and a few days after, the onset of menses. (In nonmenstruating females who have had a hysterectomy, the timing of luteal and follicular phases may require measurement of circulating reproductive hormones.)

B. At least five of the following symptoms have been present for most of the time during each symptomatic late luteal phase, at least one of the symptoms being either 1, 2, 3, or 4:
   1. Marked affective lability (eg, feeling suddenly sad, tearful, irritable, or angry).
   2. Persistent and marked anger or irritability.
   3. Marked anxiety, tension, feelings of hopelessness, or self-deprecating thoughts.
   4. Markedly depressed mood, feelings of hopelessness, or self-deprecating thoughts.
   5. Decreased interest in usual activities (eg, work, friends, hobbies).
   6. Easy fatigability or marked lack of energy.
   7. Subjective sense of difficulty in concentrating.
   8. Marked change in appetite, overeating, or specific food cravings.
   9. Hypersomnia or insomnia.
   10. Other physical symptoms, such as breast tenderness or swelling, headaches, joint or muscle pain, a sensation of "bloating," or weight gain.

C. The disturbance seriously interferes with work or with usual social activities or relationships with others.

D. The disturbance is not merely an exacerbation of the symptoms of another disorder, such as major depression, panic disorder, dysthymia, or a personality disorder (although it may be superimposed on any of these disorders).

E. Criteria A, B, C, and D are confirmed by prospective daily self-ratings during at least two symptomatic cycles. (The diagnosis may be made provisionally prior to this confirmation.)

These criteria are still debatable and are not fully accepted. It is uncertain at present what the DSM-IV criteria will be. However, the DSM system is internationally influential, and whatever criteria are developed will have an impact on the field.

Authors' Criteria for Premenstrual Syndrome

Our diagnostic criteria are somewhat different. As previously published,[18,19] we believe that although the attempt to define a diagnostic entity on the basis of phenomenology is consistent with current common sense thinking, the application of the approach to premenstrual changes is not successful; hence a different approach is needed. The definition of premenstrual changes should be based on temporal occurrence, not on phenomena. Any symptom may occur premenstrually, and as long as it occurs cyclically and is essentially limited to the premenstrual period, it is a premenstrual change. In some women, premenstrual changes consist of many diverse symptoms; in others, only a single change may appear. Also, though many women have negative changes premenstrually, some women have positive changes (mostly increased energy, productivity, and libido).[4] Hence, to avoid giving a negative connotation to a diversified set of phenomena, the term "premenstrual changes" is preferred.

The criteria for such changes are as follows.[19]

Any physical, mood, or behavioral phenomenon or phenomena are considered to be premenstrual changes if:

1. There is a consistent, cyclic appearance or change in intensity of function(s), symptom(s), or sign(s) during the late luteal phase of the menstrual cycle (1 to 7 days prior to onset of the menses).
2. Function(s), symptom(s), or sign(s) disappear or return to the usual level of intensity shortly after the beginning of the next menstrual cycle.
3. The changes do not exist in the same form or intensity during the second week of the menstrual cycle (midfollicular phase).
4. The consistent, recurrent appearance and the exclusivity to the luteal phase are confirmed by prospective daily monitoring by the woman or significant other.

It should be reemphasized that the definition of premenstrual changes and their distinction are based on the timing of the appearance and disappearance of changes and not on their description or character. In other words, the main diagnostic issue is "when" rather than "what."

Sometimes, premenstrual changes cluster into syndromes. Even though we have demonstrated consistent typologic clusters that characterize these changes in individual women,[4] this clustering is not yet confirmed. However, the use of the term "a premenstrual syndrome" is unjustified because of the demonstrated diversity of the changes.

The first criterion for premenstrual syndrome is a consistent, cyclic recurrence of a cluster of symptoms or signs during the late luteal phase of the menstrual cycle.

The second, third, and fourth criteria are the same as for premenstrual changes.

Some degree of premenstrual change is normal. Between 20% and 80% of women report some changes, the wide range mainly due to varied definitions of premenstrual change and different methods of data gathering. In the reports showing greater prevalence of changes, it is clear that most women had only mild changes that did not interfere with their daily functioning. In approximately 5% to 8% of women, however, the negative changes are severe enough to cause functional and social impairment. In such cases, the term "premenstrual disorder" would be appropriate. The criteria for premenstrual disorder are the same as for premenstrual change with the addition of a fifth criterion:

The changes cause a significant impairment in work or social functioning that seriously interferes with usual activities or social interactions.

In such cases, in which premenstrual changes reach the magnitude of a disorder, treatment is warranted.

PSYCHIATRIC ASSESSMENT— INTERVIEW

Initial Interview

The evaluation of patients seeking treatment for PMS might differ in various clinical and nonclinical settings. Although the focus here is on a clinical setting, we will also describe some current diagnostic tools that are applied mostly in research.

The psychiatric interview should be based on a clear knowledge of phenomenology with understanding of current theories on psychopathology and psychodynamics. In the psychiatric interview, like all medical interviews, one person is suffering and desires relief; the other person is expected to provide that relief. It is the patient's hope of obtaining relief from her suffering that motivates her to seek treatment[20] and fully cooperate with the examiner. Therefore even when the interview and initial examination are performed for research purposes, treatment options should be considered.

Optimally, the initial interview should be scheduled for two sessions, including one during the premenstrual period in order to obtain a direct observation of any possible symptoms, and another session during the midfollicular phase, when no symptoms are expected. Preferably the complete interview is performed during the nonsymptomatic phase, with a short supplemental interview during the symptomatic phase. This is because during the premenstrual period some women tend to over report severity of past and lifetime events. If only a single session is possible, a premenstrual visit is preferred for direct observation.

A complete psychiatric interview should contain information and knowledge so as to form a psychiatric report and diagnosis. A full psychiatric report consists of (a) identifying information, (b) chief complaint, (c) history of present illness, (d) past psychiatric history, (e) medical history, (f) personal history (includes a childhood history, current social, employment, personal issues), (g) family history, and (h) a complete mental status examination, including appearance, mood, affect, thought process, thought content, perception, orientation, memory, insight, and judgment.

This information is best collected with a structured or semistructured interview. This is not limited to research assessments. In clinical assessments there is also a distinct trend toward a more standardized way of ascertaining or obtaining data rather than just utilizing a uniform post hoc recording format.[20] The antecedents of this trend were probably in the development of the Research Diagnostic Criteria (RDC) and the operationally defined DSM-III Criteria for diagnosing psychiatric disorders. Rating devices are needed to capture clinical information to determine if the criteria are met to justify a diagnosis.

Structured Interviews

One of the most widely used structured interviews has been the schedule for affective disorders and schizophrenia (SADS).[21] It is an assessment tool that provides a set of predetermined questions on specific symptoms and signs, but also encourages the interviewer to use his or her judgment for evaluation of answers and the need for additional questions. It follows the DSM-III, with the primary purpose of providing sufficient information to classify patients into relatively homogeneous subgroups for the purpose of research. These classifications were explicated by the research diagnostic criteria (RDC),[15] which specified symptomatic criteria for 23 psychiatric disorders.

The SADS provides extensive but incomplete coverage of Axis I disorders, pays little attention to Axis II and IV, and uses a separate scale, the Global Assessment Scale (GAS),[16] to provide information relevant to Axis V. Its main advantage is its extensiveness and flexibility. The detailed evaluation of many symptoms allows for programming decision trees that can accommodate different diagnostic systems. This is quite an advantage in an era when the psychiatric diagnostic system is in flux and is frequently changing. However, the lack of direct relationship between the SADS and the DSM-III is more severe in the revised version. The difficulties in establishing a uniform relationship between SADS and DSM-III-R have led Spitzer and associates to replace the SADS. Utilizing the same semistructured interview format and item rating procedures, Spitzer et al[22] developed the structured clinical interview for diagnosis (SCID), which directly orients the diagnostic process to Axes I[22] and II[23] categories of the DSM-III-R.

The main advantage of the SCID, being tailored to the DSM-III-R entities, is also its main weakness. Most of the DSM-III-R categories are based on decision trees with inclusion and exclusion criteria, as well as a specific number of symptoms that are needed for a diagnosis of a particular entity. Once it is apparent that these criteria are not going to be met, the interviewer is then instructed to skip to another set of questions. This seemingly efficient method may result in a lack of information that might be needed for another set of diagnostic criteria. Information gathered with the SCID might not be sufficient for conversion of DSM-III-R diagnoses to DSM-IV.

SADS and SCID interviews usually take a few hours (2 to 4) to complete. They also require specific training in their formal application and assessment and a good knowledge of psychopathology. There is a training program for interviewers using structured interview assessment manuals to improve reliability. The prior knowledge and experience needed for a proper performance of SADS and SCID make them inadequate for large-scale applications, as is needed in screening of large population groups and other epidemiological studies. A practical tool for that purpose is the Diagnostic Interview Schedule (DIS).[24]

The DIS is a structured interview that was developed for use by trained lay interviewers. It requires minimal prior psychiatric knowledge and judgment, and its information can provide DSM-III as well as RDC diagnoses. As is the case with the SADS, it can provide data for a given day, episode, and lifetime diagnoses.

The assessment instruments described so far provide information on the entire episode of a disorder or on parts and lifetime history. They do not include questions on the clinical situation on a given day, nor do they provide tools for assessment of changes within an episode or during treatment. For this purpose, the SADS-C (change) was developed.[25] It is structured according to the same conceptual framework as the SADS and contains 45 items pertinent to the past week. The same questions can be asked for the past 24 or 48 hours. Therefore SADS-C interviews performed in various time periods can be compared to each other to monitor change over time. The SADS-C allows for extracted scores of Hamilton Depression Rating Scale. This will be described later.

In a clinical setting, the assessment (may it be structured or just a methodological interview and examination) results in a diagnosis as well as an evaluation of severity of specific symptoms. Sometimes the severity of a specific symptom or syndrome requires referral to a specialist. For instance, psychiatric referral is needed if a severe major depressive disorder (MDD) is diagnosed, even if its severity fluctuates along the menstrual cycle.

Targeted Rating Scales

Specific diagnostic aspects can be elucidated with targeted rating scales. Rating scales may be discussed based on "who is doing the rating" (eg, self-report by the patient, informant-rated scale, professional-rated observation, professional-rated interview) and the source of rated material (observation of the patient in the clinical setting, information from the interview). Each of these types has advantages and disadvantages. It is usually advantageous to gather information from several sources to cover a range of relevant areas; therefore several different types of rating scales may be employed in an individual situation. Most of these scales can now be completed and analyzed using a computer program. Some are interactional with the user and can further improve the data entry and analysis.

Self-Report Scales

Self-report scales are appealing because they report the opinion of the patient. They might be useful in assessing subjective internal states that are not apparent to an observer and sensitive in detecting more subtle pathology such as mild depression. Other advantages of self-rating scales include the limited investment of professional time and expense and the chance for patients to complete and return them to the physician in between visits.

There are also several disadvantages. Some people are unable or unwilling to complete the scales. The scales are also subject to variability based on the educational, social, and cultural background of the patient.

The PMS evaluation is even more complicated because patients tend to attribute unrelated symptoms to PMS,[26] and about half of retrospectively self-reported complaints are not confirmed. An observation by a person close to the patient is helpful in such cases. Indeed another form of self-report, a prospective daily monitoring, is needed here. *Informant-rated scales* might consist of the same items as self-rating scales and might complement them. *Observant-rating scales* are completed by professionals based on observation of the patient in the clinical setting. Advantages of such scales are increased objectivity and reliability, but they require professional time and expense and the patient is not observed in her natural environment.[27]

Professional-rated scales can be based on unstructured, semistructured, or structured interview formats based on information from either patients or other informants. During the face-to-face interview, professionals can encourage cooperation, clarify questions, and otherwise use individual clinical judgment to aid in completing the scale. However, the use of clinical judgment and an excessive amount of inference can decrease the reliability and validity of a scale. The use of completely structured interviews in which the specific order and wording of questions is standardized can reduce variability. Structured interviews can be more awkward for the patient than standard clinical interviews.

PSYCHIATRIC ASSESSMENT—
GENERAL SCREENING SCALES

SCL-90 (Symptom Checklist)

The SCL-90 (symptom checklist)[28] is designed to provide preliminary information about a broad range of complaints related to mental disorders and syndromes. It can be completed in a quarter of an hour and scored by computer. The items can be combined into nine symptom scales according to syndromal clusters, and three global indices may be compiled. The SCL-90 is deficient in items representing symptoms of atypical depression, which are quite prevalent among women with dysphoric PMS. Therefore we modified it by an addition of an atypical depression scale consisting of 10 relevant items. This modified SCL-90 can be used for initial screening to distinguish normal from abnormal subjects. We also use it as a measure of mental state pertinent to the "last 24 hours" to evaluate changes over time.

Rating Scales for Anxiety

For some time the measurement of anxiety was almost exclusively based on the Minnesota Multiphasic Personality Inventory (MMPI)[29] and a number of different anxiety measures derived from this scale.

Because of the notion that normal and pathological anxiety are different and do not constitute a continuum, the MMPI and its derivatives are gradually being replaced by other instruments designed primarily to qualify levels of pathology in patients with diagnostically different anxiety disorders.

Two frequently used observer-rated instruments (mostly in psychopharmacological research) are the Hamilton Anxiety Scale[30] and brief outpatient psychopathology scale. Hamilton's Anxiety Scale is based on his scale for depression. Frequently used self-reports include the Hopkins symptom checklist or HSCL-90[31] and global health questionnaire. Self-Rating Anxiety Scale[32] is a companion self-report instrument that assesses a wide range of anxiety-related behaviors: fear, panic, physical symptoms of fear, panic nightmares, and cognitive effects.

One of the most widely used self-rating scales for anxiety is the State-Trait Anxiety Inventory (STAI) developed by Spielberger.[33] It consists of two self-reported lists of items. One of these is pertinent to general or lifetime anxiety and is designed to evaluate trait; the other one is focused on current symptoms and is an evaluation of state anxiety. Despite the distinction between the state and trait questionnaires, the answers to the trait questions might be influenced by the state of anxiety. This was demonstrated by us[34] with another trait instrument for anxiety, the Taylor's Manifest Anxiety Scale (MAS).[35] Women reported higher levels of trait anxiety during the symptomatic late luteal phase compared to their reports during the nonsymptomatic midfollicular phase.

The semistructured anxiety disorders interview schedule is used to differentiate subcategories of anxiety disorders as well as to rule out affective disorders and other DSM III major disorders.[36] This differentiation is important for treatment choices. For example, it is important to distinguish agoraphobia with panic, generalized anxiety disorder, and panic disorder because each disorder is optimally treated with different therapeutic approaches.

Rating Scales for Affective Symptoms and Mood Disorders

There are many more scales for assessing depression than for assessing mania. Different scales for depression emphasize the cognitive, physiological, behavioral, or affective components of these syndromes. Among the most frequently employed rating scales for the assessment of depression are the Hamilton Depression Rating Scale (HDRS),[37] the Newcastle Scale,[38] the Beck Depression Inventory,[39] and the Zung Self-Rating Scale for Depression.[40] The first two are completed on the basis of clinical interview, and the last two are self-assessment scales. Other frequently used scales include Brief Depression Rating Scale,[41] Carroll's Rating Scale of Depression,[42] and many others.

Beck Depression Inventory (BDI)

The BDI is a self-administered depression rating scale that primarily emphasizes cognitive aspects of depression. The 21 items of the inventory were selected to represent symptoms commonly associated with a depressive disorder. Ratings of each item are based on a forced choice of one of four statements listed in the order of symptom severity. Item categories include mood, pessimism, crying spells, guilt, self-hate, irritability, social withdrawal, inhibition, sleep and appetite disturbances, and loss of libido.

Hamilton Depression Rating Scale (HDRS)

The HDRS emphasizes physiological aspects of depression and is a clinician-rated scale. The clinician rates the patient in a semistructured interview and adds any other information available to him. It was designed to use mostly with patients who are already diagnosed as having a depressive disorder. The total score is the sum of all the scores on all the items (eg, a score of zero indicates the absence of the symptoms measured in the scale, and a score of 74 indicates the maximum presence of symptoms).

There are several versions of the HDRS that differ from each other on the number of items. Therefore, the number of items should be indicated when results are reported. Usually a score of 10 or more is considered to be abnormal and a score of more than 20 indicates quite severe depression.

The HDRS does not include items indicative of atypical depression, which occurs frequently among women with dysphoric PMS. Therefore, for evaluation of menstrually related disorders another score should be added. As has been already mentioned, the HDRS can be extracted from the SADS and SADS-C.

The suicidal potential of patients is greatest in those suffering from depression. In addition to the clinical interview, self-report instruments that focus on evaluation of risk factors, including previously reported predictions of suicidal behavior, may be clinically useful. Evaluation of suicidal tendency is especially important in outpatients seeking PMS evaluation. The Suicide Intent Scale[43] and the Index of Potential Suicide[44] are two instruments that evaluate suicide potential.

As mentioned previously, there are a limited number of rating scales that focus on mania. Many of the symptoms of mania can be measured by the Brief Psychiatric Rating Scale (BPRS)[45] or SADS. The Manic State Rating Scale (MSRS)[46] is a 26-item observer-rated scale that is useful with bipolar patients. Eleven items reflecting elation-grandiosity and paranoid destructive features of manic patients have produced the most consistent results. The scale has demonstrated adequate reliability and concurrent validity and reflects clinical change. Nonetheless, a SADS or SAD-C provides similar information.

PSYCHIATRIC ASSESSMENT OF PSYCHOSIS

Major aspects of psychosis can be measured by comprehensive scales like the BPRS or the Nurses' Observation Scale for inpatient evaluation (NOSIE).[47] The BPRS is a clinician-rated scale that is completed based on an unstructured interview and observation of the patient's present condition. The NOSIE was developed to be based on behavior of hospitalized psychiatric patients observed over a 3-day period. The total score is a sum of the scores for each item. Either BPRS or NOSIE may be utilized to evaluate cases of premenstrual psychotic episodes. They are seldom used in routine clinical outpatient evaluations of suspected PMS patients.

Personality Tests

Several widely used and psychometrically dependable instruments are available for the assessment of personality. Popular tests of this sort include the 16-Personality Factor Inventory,[48] Eysenek Personality Inventory,[49] Millon Clinical Multiaxial Inventory (MCMI),[50] and semistructured interviews that are constructed to assess (by the patient's report and clinical judgment of the interviewer) the presence of DSM-III-R Axis II disorders; for example, Personality-disorder Examination,[51] Structured Clinical Interview, and the Structural Analysis of Social Behavior.[52]

A very promising tool for assessment of personality characteristics and disorders is the Tridimensional Personality Questionnaire (TPQ) developed by Cloninger.[53] It is based on assessment of three proposed continuous dimensions of personality—novelty seeking, harm avoidance, and reward dependence—which may interact with each other. The combinations of extremes on each continuous dimension provide for a categorical description of most current personality disorder entities. Theoretically, specific personality dimensions derived from the TPQ might be associated with changes in monoamine neurotransmitters that are putatively involved in modulation of mood and behavior. This makes the TPQ an intriguing instrument for future research.

INSTRUMENTS FOR ASSESSMENT OF PMS

Premenstrual Assessment Form (PAF)

The PAF is a self-rating retrospective questionnaire that was developed for initial screening and evaluation of PMS.[34] Following initial developmental work, 95 items were selected for the current version of the PAF. They are descriptive of premenstrual changes in physical condition, mood, and behavior. The items are rated in a six-point scale from "no change" to "extreme change."

The emphasis in the PAF is on change from usual state. It allows for evaluation of categorical subtypes of PMS as well as dimensions of behaviors. As with any retrospective questionnaire, about half of the women who report premenstrual symptoms do not prospectively confirm the proper temporal relationship of symptoms to menstruation. Therefore, the PAF is properly used only for screening purposes. Versions of the PAF were developed as state questionnaires pertinent to the middle follicular and late luteal phases. Their reliability as compared to daily ratings is quite high, and they can be used in lengthy follow-ups when compliance with daily monitoring of symptoms might be low.

There are many other retrospective questionnaires for assessment of PMS; some of them also have "current state" variants. Most widely used is the Moos' Menstrual Distress Questionnaire,[54] which underwent extensive developmental work and is convenient to use. However, it does not allow for detailed evaluation of subtypes of dysphoric PMS, which might be pertinent

Table 1
Assessment of Dysphoric Premenstrual Syndromes

A. For Research Studies
  1. Initial phone screening
  2. First clinical interview during a nonsymptomatic period
    I. a. Schedule for Affective Disorders and Schizophrenia (SADS)
        b. Research Diagnostic Criteria (RDC)
        c. Family History—RDC (FH-RDC)
        d. Demographic form
    II. Self-reported retrospective questionnaires
        a. Premenstrual Assessment Form (PAF)
        b. Medical and treatment history
        c. Reproductive and menstrual history
        d. Screening for mental disorders (eg, modified SCL-90)
  3. Prospective confirmation of complaints—Daily Rating Forms filled out for two menstrual cycles (at least 6 weeks)
  4. Optional—collateral observation report by a "significant other"
  5. Second clinical interview during a reported premenstrual period
B. Assessments for Clinical Purposes Only
  1. Self-reported retrospective questionnaires
  2. Daily Rating Forms filled out for at least two menstrual cycles
  3. A clinical interview during the reported premenstrual period

for treatment choice and evaluation of pathophysiology and treatment response.

Daily Rating Form (DRF)

The DRF was developed for the purpose of confirming retrospective findings.[55] It includes 18 items that emphasize dysphoric changes and major physical changes. It can also be modified to monitor other selected individual changes. DRFs help to differentiate dysphoric PMS from chronic disorders that might exacerbate premenstrually, dysmenorrhea (during the menstruation), and other menstrually related symptoms and syndromes. Daily Ratings Forms are required for the

Table 2
Relevant Psychiatric Assessment Instruments Used by Our Group

Procedures	Derived Measures
A. SADS, RDC	Lifetime and current diagnoses of mental disorder. Summary scale scores and individual items of relevance for evaluation of severity of lifetime and current mental disorders
B. SADS-C	Measurement of change in condition in last 24 hours. Severity of disorders and specific symptoms. Extracted HDRS
C. SCID	Diagnostic entities in Axes I and II of DSM-III-R
D. FH-RDC	Presence or absence of evidence of mental disorders in relatives, and cause of death of relatives
E. Modified SCL-90	Initial screening for presence or absence of mental disorders
F. BDI	Total score: intensity of depression. Subscales, for subtypes, especially cognitive aspects
G. HDRS	Severity of depression. Observer ratings. Is extracted from the SADS-C
H. Hamilton Anxiety Scale	Severity of anxiety
I. BPRS	Summary of clinical interview. Total score and 5 factors scores
J. Global Assessment Scale (GAS)	Interviewer-rated scale Level of functioning on Axis V of DSM-III-R (rated from 0 to 99, with 99 being the highest)
K. NOSIE	Observation over a 3-day period. Total score
L. PAF	Initial screening for PMS. Subtypes of PMS, dimensional evaluations, and severity of specific items
M. DRF	Prospective confirmation of retrospective reports, temporal pattern of complaints. Syndromal clusters

final diagnoses of PMS. There are numerous forms for prospective monitoring of symptoms but most of them are variations on the same principles.

The Process of Assessment of PMS

Although the assessment of PMS is discussed in detail in another chapter, we will briefly describe our procedures for evaluating PMS patients.

For initial screening and evaluation, the PAF is used. Following the completion of PAF, a prospective DRF for PMS is filled out for at least 6 weeks, including at least 2 late luteal symptomatic periods and two midfollicular nonsymptomatic periods. DRFs confirm or refute the reports on PAF. All patients undergo thorough psychiatric and physical evaluations.

We summarize our assessment of patients reporting dysphoric premenstrual syndrome in Table 1 and the psychiatric assessment instruments that we use in Table 2.

SUMMARY

Many women with psychiatric symptoms prefer to be diagnosed with PMS than a major psychiatric disorder, because PMS is a more "socially acceptable" disease. However, approximately half of women who believe they have PMS actually have Axis I or II psychiatric disorders. It is critical to differentiate PMS from major mental disorders so that women can receive proper treatment. Careful psychiatric assessment, as described in this chapter, is often required to accomplish this task.

ACKNOWLEDGMENT

The preparation of this chapter was supported in part by NIMH Grant RO1MH45242.

REFERENCES

1. Halbreich U, Endicott JP, Lesser J. The clinical diagnosis and classification of premenstrual changes. *Can J Psych.* 1985;30:489–497.
2. Smith S, Schiff I. The premenstrual syndrome—diagnosis and management. *Fertil Steril.* 1989;4:527–543.
3. Halbreich U, Endicott J, Nee J. The diversity of premenstrual changes as reflected in the Premenstrual Assessment Form. *Acta Psych Scand.* 1982;65:46–65.
4. Halbreich U, Endicott J, Nee J. Premenstrual depressive changes: value of differentiation. *Arch Gen Psychiatry.* 1982;40:535–542.
5. Harrison W, Endicott J, Nee J, et al. Characteristics of women seeking treatment of premenstrual syndrome. *Psychosomatics.* 1989;4:405–411.
6. DeJong R, Rubinow DR, Roy-Byrne P, et al. Premenstrual mood disorder and psychiatric illness. *Am J Psychiatry.* 1985;142:1359–1361.
7. Halbreich U, Endicott J. Relationship of dysphoric premenstrual changes to depressive disorders. *Acta Psychiatr Scand.* 1985;71:331–338.
8. MacKenzie TB, Wilcox K, Barron H. Lifetime prevalence of psychiatric disorders in women with premenstrual difficulties. *J Affective Disorders.* 1986;10:15–19.
9. Stout AL, Steege JF, Blazer DC, et al. A comparison of lifetime psychiatric diagnosis in premenstrual syndrome clinic and community sample. *J Nerv Ment Dis.* 1986;174:517–521.
10. Keye WR, Hammond DC, Strong J. Medical and psychological characteristics of women presenting with premenstrual symptoms. *Obstet Gynecol.* 1986;68:634–637.
11. Tonks CM, Rack PH, Rose MJ. Attempted suicide and menstrual cycle. *J Psychosom Res.* 1969;11:319–323.
12. Halbreich U, Bakhai Y, Bacon KB, et al. The normalcy of self-proclaimed "Normal Volunteers." *Am J Psychiatr.* 1989;146:1052–1055.
13. American Psychiatric Association. *Diagnostic and Statistical Manual—DSM III-Revised.* Washington DC: 1987.
14. World Health Organization. *International Classification of diseases.* 9th and 10th Editions. U.S. Government Printing Office, Washington, DC: 1986, 1990.
15. Spitzer RL, Endicott J, Robins E. Research diagnostic criteria: rationale and reliability. *Arch Gen Psychiatry.* 1978;35:773–782.
16. Endicott J, Spitzer RI, Fleiss J, et al. The Global Assessment Scale. *Arch Gen Psychiatry.* 1976;33:766–771.
17. Spitzer RL, Severino SK, Williams JBW, et al. Late luteal phase dysphoric disorder and DSM III-R. *Am J Psychiatry.* 1989;146:892–896.
18. Halbreich U, Endicott J. Methodological issues in studies of premenstrual changes. *Psychoneuro Endocrinol.* 1985;10:15–32.
19. Halbreich U, Alt I, Paul L. Premenstrual changes: impaired hormonal homeostasis. *Endocrine Metab Clin N Am.* 1988;17:173–194.
20. Mackinnon RA, Michels R. In: *Textbook of the Psychiatric Interview in Clinical Practice.* Philadelphia: W. B. Saunders; 1971.
21. Endicott J, Spitzer RC. A diagnostic interview: the schedule of affective disorders and schizophrenia. *Arch Gen Psychiatry.* 1978;35:837–844.
22. Spitzer R, Williams J, Gibben M. *Structured clinical interview for DSM III-R* (SCID). New York State Psychiatric Institute, Biometrics Research Department; 1987.
23. Spitzer R, Williams J. *Structured clinical interview for DSM III-R. Personality disorders.* (SCID-II). New York State Psychiatric Institute, Biometrics Research Department; 1985.
24. Robins LN, Helzer JE, Croughan J, et al. National Institute of Mental Health Diagnostic Interview Schedule: its history, characteristics, and validity. *Arch Gen Psychiatry.* 1981;38:381–389.
25. Endicott J, Spitzer R. Schedule for affective disorders and schizophrenia: regular and change versions. In: Sartorius N, Ban TA, eds. *Assessment of Depression.* New York, NY: Springer-Verlag; 1978:316–333.
26. Endicott J, Halbreich U. Retrospective report of premenstrual depressive changes: factors affecting confirmation by daily ratings. *Psychopharmacological Bull.* 1982;18:109–112.
27. Grebb JA. Psychiatric rating scales. In: *Textbook of Comprehensive Psychiatry.* Baltimore, Md: Williams & Wilkins; 1989:534–552.

28. Derogatis LR. *The SCL-90L Clinical Psychometric Research.* Baltimore, Md: The Johns Hopkins University School of Medicine; 1977.

29. Dahlstrom WA, Welsh GS, Dahlstrom LE. *An MMPI Handbook* (Volumes 1 and 2). Minneapolis, Minn: University of Minnesota Press; 1972.

30. Hamilton M. The assessment of anxiety states by rating. *Br J Med Psych.* 1959;32:50–55.

31. Lippman RS, Covi L, Shapiro AK. HSCL-90. *J Affec Dis.* 1979;1:9–24.

32. Zung WWK. Self-Rating Anxiety Scale. *Psychosomatics.* 1971;12:371–379.

33. Spielberger CD, Grorsuch RL, Lushene RE. *Manual for the State-Trait Anxiety Inventory.* Palo Alto, Ca: Consulting Psychological Press; 1970.

34. Halbreich U, Kas D. Variations in the Taylor MAS of women with premenstrual syndrome. *J Psychosomatic Res.* 1977;21:391–393.

35. Taylor JA. Taylor's Manifest Anxiety Scale. *J Exp Psychology.* 1951;42:183–188.

36. DiNardo PA, O'Brien GT, Barlow DM, et al. Reliability of DSM-III anxiety disorder categories using a new structured interview. *Arch Gen Psychiatry.* 1983;40:1070–1075.

37. Hamilton M. A rating scale for depression. *J Neurol Neurosurgery Psychiatry.* 1960;23:51–56.

38. Carney MWP, Roth M, Garside RF. *Br J Psychiatry.* 1965;111:659–674.

39. Beck AT, Ward CH, Mendelson J, et al. *Arch Gen Psychiatry.* 1968;4:561–571.

40. Zung WWK. Depression Rating Scale. *Arch Gen Psychiatry.* 1965;12:63–70.

41. Kellener R. Brief depression rating scale. In: Sartorius N, et al., eds. *The Textbook of Assessment of Depression.* Berlin, Heidelberg, New York; 1986.

42. Carroll BJ, Feinberg M, Smouse PE, et al. Carroll's rating scale for depression. *Br J Psychiatry.* 1981;138:194–200.

43. Beck AT, Schuyler D, Herman I. Development of suicidal intent scales. In: Beck AT et al., eds. *Prediction of Suicide.* Charles Press; 1974.

44. Zung WWK. Index of Potential Suicide: a rating scale for suicide prevention. In: Beck et al., eds. *Prediction of Suicide.* Charles Press; 1974.

45. Overall JE, Gorham DR. The Brief Psychiatric Rating Scale. *Psychiatry Res.* 1962;10:799–812.

46. Beigel A, Murphy D, Bunney W. The Manic State Rating Scale: Scale construct, reliability and validity. *Arch Gen Psychiatry.* 1971;25:256–262.

47. Horigfeld Gr, Klett CT. The Nurses' Observation Scale for Inpatient Evaluation. *J Clin Psychiatry.* 1965;21:65–71.

48. Cattell RB, Eber HW, Tatsuoka MM. *Handbook for the Sixteen Personality Factor Inventory.* Champaign, Ill: Institute for Personality and Ability Testing; 1970.

49. Eysenck HJ, Eysenck SB. The structure and measure of personality. San Diego, Ca: RR Knapp; 1969.

50. Millon T. *Millon Clinical Multiaxial Inventory,* 3rd ed. Minneapolis, Minn: Interpretive Scoring Systems; 1983.

51. Loranger A, Susman V, Oldham J, et al: Personality disorder examination (PDE). (Unpublished manuscript.) New York Hospital, Cornell Medical Center, White Plains, NY; 1985.

52. Benjamin LS. Structured analysis of social behavior. *Psychol Rev.* 1974;81:392–425.

53. Cloninger CB. A systematic method for clinical description and classification of personality variants. *Arch Gen Psychiatry.* 1987;44:573–588.

54. Moos R. The development of a menstrual distress questionnaire. *Psychosom Med.* 1968;30:853–867.

55. Endicott J, Nee J, Cohen J, et al. Premenstrual changes: patterns and correlates of daily ratings. *J Affect Dis.* 1986;10:127–135.

CHAPTER 4

Physiology of the Normal Menstrual Cycle

Robert L. Barbieri

The centerpiece of research in reproductive biology is the delineation of the mechanisms that control the physiology of the normal menstrual cycle. The complex communication required to integrate the functions of the brain, hypothalamus, pituitary, ovary, and uterus to produce the normal menstrual cycle is still not completely understood. In this chapter the physiology of the menstrual cycle is discussed at three levels: Level I, the integrative interactions between the hypothalamus, pituitary, ovary, and the uterus; Level II, the effects of adrenal, thyroid, and pancreatic hormones on the menstrual cycle; and Level III, molecular mechanisms by which ovarian hormones modulate neural events. Prior to addressing these three levels of control, important definitions and descriptive statistics of the menstrual cycle are reviewed.

DEFINITIONS AND DESCRIPTIVE STATISTICS

The menstrual cycle can be divided into three main phases: the follicular, ovulatory, and luteal phases (Fig. 1). By definition, the first day of menstrual bleeding is the first day of the follicular phase, and marks the transition from the previous luteal phase to the new follicular phase. In an idealized 28-day menstrual cycle, days 1 to 14 represent the follicular phase, and days 14 to 28 represent the luteal phase. The ovulatory phase consists of a 36-hour period beginning with the onset of the luteinizing hormone (LH) surge and ending with ovulation. The ovulatory phase is the terminal portion of the follicular phase, but is an extremely dynamic interval, thereby deserving treatment as a separate entity.

"Follicular" is derived from the Latin term for small fluid-filled bag or sac. This is quite appropriate because more than 90% of the mass of a preovulatory follicle consists of follicular fluid secreted by the granulosa cells. During the follicular phase of the cycle, an ovarian follicle containing a healthy egg grows from 4 mm to 24 mm in diameter. At ovulation (day 14), the follicle ruptures and releases the egg and follicular fluid into the peritoneal cavity or directly onto the tubal epithelium. After ovulation, the follicle becomes a corpus luteum. In contrast to the follicle, the corpus luteum is a solid structure that does not contain fluid. The term "luteal" is derived from the Latin word for "yellow body" and, appropriately, the corpus luteum is orange-yellow in color because it is rich in lipids (cholesterol esters). The corpus luteum has a preprogrammed life span of approximately 12 to 14 days. If a pregnancy occurs, the life span of the corpus luteum will be extended by the action of chorionic gonadotropin (hCG) secreted by the placenta. If a pregnancy does not occur, the corpus luteum regresses, estrogen and progesterone production decreases, the epithelium of the endometrium is dis-

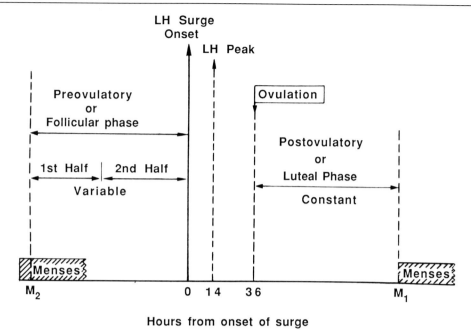

Fig. 1 Schematic outline of important events in menstrual cycle: follicular, ovulatory, and luteal phases. (Reprinted from Yen SSC, Jaffe RB. *Reproductive Endocrinology.* Philadelphia: WB Saunders; 1986, with permission.)

rupted, and menses begins. The regression of the corpus luteum and the onset of menses mark the beginning of a new menstrual cycle and the reinitiation of follicular growth.

The length of the menstrual cycle depends on a large number of variables including age, parity, nutritional intake, body composition, exercise status, and psychosocial stress. Treolar and colleagues[1] reported the results of one of the most extensive studies of menstrual interval and regularity of menstrual interval using alumnae of the University of Minnesota as the study subjects. The data were collected prospectively over 30 years and included more than 275,000 menstrual cycles. For most women, menses started for the first time at age 13 years (normal range, 10 to 16 years) and stopped by age 50 years (normal range, 45 to 55 years). Between 20 and 40 years of age, women had the greatest regularity of cycle length, with more variability in the immediate postmenarchal and premenopausal years. The median "normal" cycle length declined from a median of 28.9 (± 2.75) days at age 20 years to a median of 26.8 (± 2) days by age 40 years (Table 1). The cycle length usually

Table 1
Median and 5% Upper and Lower Bounds on Menstrual Interval in Days from 275,947 Menstrual Cycles[a]

Chronological Age (yr)	Menstrual Interval (days)		
	5% Lower Bound	Median	5% Upper Bound
17	22	28	40
25	23	28	37
33	22	27	34
41	22	26	32
49	15	27	>80

[a]Adapted from Treloar AE, Boynton RE, Behn BG, et al. Variation of human menstrual cycle through reproductive life. *Int J Fert.* 1967;12:77–126.

varied by 1 to 2 days each month, and only 50% of women had a cycle length within the 26- to 30-day range that encompassed the so-called typical 28-day interval. Cycle lengths less than 24 days are considered polymenorrhea, and those more than 35 days are considered oligomenorrhea. Cycles less than 24 days or greater than 35 days in length are often anovulatory.[2]

The average duration of menstruation is between 3 and 7 days, and a duration shorter (hypomenorrhea) or longer (hypermenorrhea) is considered abnormal. The amount of menstrual flow is usually 80 ml or less. Women vary widely from one another in the amount of blood lost at menstruation, but each woman is fairly consistent from month to month in her individual blood loss when checked by reliable measurements. This pattern has been established for women in several parts of the world in which the average loss and variation are strikingly similar. When menstrual blood loss exceeded 80 ml in an individual, there was a good correlation with anemia (hemoglobin value less than 12 g) and with low plasma iron values.[3]

CONTROL OF THE MENSTRUAL CYCLE: LEVEL 1

Complete characterization of the menstrual cycle is a nearly impossible task; like a series of ever-smaller boxes, one nested within another, as soon as a major discovery is made and one box opened, a new box appears to challenge the investigator. In this chapter, the menstrual cycle is discussed as a series of nested levels of organization. Level 1 focuses on the four primary components required to organize the menstrual cycle: the arcuate nucleus of the hypothalamus, the pituitary gonadotrope, the ovary, and the uterus. Level 2 focuses on secondary systems that modulate the function of these primary components. For example, the limbic system, adrenal, thyroid, and pancreas all play roles in the regulation of the menstrual cycle. Level 3

reviews data concerning the molecular interaction between products of the ovary and the brain. The four primary components contributing to the control of the menstrual cycle are discussed in Table 2.

The Hypothalamus

In the human, the arcuate nucleus of the hypothalamus is the site of the majority of neuronal cell bodies, which synthesize the decapeptide gonadotropin releasing hormone (GnRH).[4] GnRH is transported down the axons of these neurons from the arcuate nucleus to the median eminence. At the median eminence the axons terminate on the capillaries of the portal circulation. The portal circulation is a vascular system designed to transport substances secreted into the median eminence of the hypothalamus directly to the pituitary. The portal circulation consists of two capillary beds, one in the median eminence and one in the pituitary, which are connected by a venous system. The two-capillary-bed system limits the amount of GnRH that reaches the systemic circulation.

The GnRH neurons of the median eminence are *neuroendocrine transducers*. These neurons receive neurochemical signals (norepinephrine, dopamine, endorphin) and transduce them into an endocrine output (pulsatile GnRH). Current data suggest that endorphin and dopamine inhibit GnRH release and norepinephrine stimulates GnRH release.

The microcircuitry and the relative anatomic inaccessibility of the hypothalamus make it difficult to directly study the arcuate nucleus in living humans. Most invasive studies of the neuroendocrinology of the arcuate nucleus have utilized nonhuman primates or rodents. In monkeys, in an estrogen- and progestogen-deficient state, hypothalamic endorphin production is very low. Estrogen alone, or progesterone alone, does not dramatically stimulate hypothalamic endorphin production. However, estrogen plus progesterone act synergistically to produce a large increase in hypothalamic endorphin production which, in turn, suppresses

Table 2
Primary Components Controlling the Menstrual Cycle (Level 1)

Organ	Structure	Function
Hypothalamus	Arcuate nucleus	Pulsatile GnRH secretion
Pituitary	Gonadotrope	Pulsatile LH, FSH secretion
Ovary	Follicle (theca and granulosa cells)	Secretion of estradiol, progesterone, androgens, and inhibin
Uterus	Endometrium	Cyclic growth and shedding

GnRH production.[5] Therefore, in the luteal phase of the menstrual cycle, the production of progesterone plus estrogen by the corpus luteum increases hypothalamic endorphin, which decreases GnRH, LH, and follicle-stimulating hormone (FSH) production. This decrease in gonadotropins prevents the development of new follicles. At the end of the luteal phase of the cycle, the demise of the corpus luteum, and the associated decrease in estrogen and progesterone causes a decrease in hypothalamic endorphin production which results in an increase in GnRH, LH, and FSH production, and stimulates the development of follicles.

In the rodent, dopamine (inhibits GnRH) and norepinephrine (stimulates GnRH) clearly play important roles in the control of GnRH secretion. In humans, substantial evidence, much of it indirect, also suggests that dopamine and norepinephrine control GnRH secretion. For example, neuroepinephrine neurons with cell bodies in the locus ceruleus contain nuclear estradiol and androgen receptors and project into the arcuate nucleus.[6] In addition, the infusion of dopamine appears to decrease LH secretion in women.[7]

GnRH is secreted in a pulsatile manner, and the GnRH pulse frequency and amplitude are critical variables monitored by the pituitary gonadotrope. In a classic series of endocrine ablation-replacement experiments, Knobil and colleagues[8] demonstrated the importance of the pulsatile release of GnRH in the control of pituitary gonadotropin secretion. Radiofrequency lesions of the arcuate nucleus were made in Rhesus monkeys, thereby ablating most GnRH-secreting neurons. The ablation of the arcuate nucleus resulted in a decrease of circulating LH and FSH to undetectable concentrations. Replacement of GnRH by intravenous pulses of GnRH restored normal patterns of LH and FSH secretion. Replacement of GnRH by chronic continuous infusion resulted in abnormally low LH and FSH secretion. These experiments demonstrated the importance of the pulsatile nature of GnRH secretion in the regulation of LH and FSH release. In addition, these and other experiments have demonstrated that GnRH is absolutely necessary, but not sufficient, for the stimulation of normal, ovulatory menstrual cycles. In women with amenorrhea and low endogenous GnRH production, exogenous replacement of GnRH at normal pulse frequency and amplitude results in the restoration of normal ovulatory menstrual cycles.[9]

Since GnRH is released in pulses or secretory bursts, its secretion can be characterized by knowing its pulse frequency and amplitude. However, since hypothalamic GnRH does not enter the systemic circulation, most studies of GnRH pulse frequency in humans are based on an analysis of LH pulses in the peripheral circulation. In the follicular phase of the menstrual cycle, the arcuate nucleus releases a pulse of GnRH every 1 to 1.5 hours.[10] Each pulse of GnRH induces the pituitary to release a pulse of LH and FSH. In the midluteal phase of the menstrual cycle, the arcuate nucleus releases a pulse of GnRH every 3 to 4 hours.[10] The decrease in GnRH pulse frequency in the luteal phase of the cycle may be due, in part, to high hypothalamic endorphin tone. For example, in women, the administration of naloxone, at 1.6 mg/h, an opiate receptor antagonist, during the mid-luteal phase of the menstrual cycle produces an increase in LH pulse frequency implying an increase in GnRH pulse frequency.[11] Administration of naloxone in the mid-follicular phase of the cycle does not typically produce an increase in LH pulse frequency.[11] These studies imply that hypothalamic endorphin tone is high in the luteal phase but not in the follicular phase, and that endorphin suppresses GnRH pulse frequency.

GnRH pulse frequency is a critical factor in the regulation of the menstrual cycle. A low GnRH pulse amplitude or pulse frequency in the follicular phase does not usually stimulate enough pituitary LH and FSH secretion to produce normal follicular development. Therefore, a low GnRH pulse frequency (eg, one pulse every 4 hours) is often associated with anovulation and infrequent or absent menses. Many elite women athletes and many lean women have low GnRH pulse amplitude and/or frequency and are anovulatory. High GnRH pulse frequency is also associated with menstrual abnormalities. For example, in women with the polycystic ovary syndrome, GnRH pulse frequency is as high as one pulse every 0.5 hours. This high GnRH pulse frequency may cause partial pituitary desensitization resulting in high LH secretion, low or low-normal FSH secretion, and anovulation.[12] Normal ovulatory cycles require that GnRH pulse frequency be maintained within a relatively narrow range.

The Pituitary Gonadotropin

During embryogenesis the pituitary develops from both neural tissue (posterior pituitary) and from oral ectoderm (anterior pituitary). The pituitary gland resides within a bony cavity (sella turcica) at the base of the brain just below the hypothalamus. It is separated from the central nervous system by the diaphragm sella, a condensation of the dura mater overlying the sella turcica. The pituitary is connected to the hypothalamus by the pituitary stalk which transverses a small perforation in the diaphragm of sella.

The anterior pituitary secretes at least six major protein hormones: luteinizing hormone (LH), follicle-stimulating hormone (FSH), thyrotropin (TSH), growth hormone (GH), adrenocorticotropin (ACTH), and prolactin. The main contribution of the pituitary to the regulation of the menstrual cycle is the secretion of pulses of LH and FSH in response to pulses of hypothalamic GnRH. In turn, LH and FSH stimulate the growth and development of ovarian follicles. The pituitary response to GnRH is modulated in part by circulating steroids and inhibin. For example, just prior to ovulation, the dominant antral follicle produces large amounts of estradiol, but very little progesterone. The pituitary responds to this high-estrogen, low-progesterone environment by secreting relatively large amounts of LH in response to a fixed GnRH stimulus.[13] This preovulatory, estradiol-induced, sensitization of the pituitary to GnRH helps create the massive preovulatory LH surge.

A major question in reproductive endocrinology is how *one* hormone (GnRH) differentially regulates the secretion of two hormones, LH and FSH. A partial answer to this question is that hormones secreted by the ovary (steroids, inhibin) feed back on the pituitary to differentially modulate LH and FSH secretion. In addition, the pulse frequency of GnRH may contribute to the differential regulation of LH and FSH.

LH and FSH are glycoproteins and consist of noncovalently associated alpha and beta subunits. The alpha subunits of LH, FSH, TSH, and hCG are essentially identical. Therefore, it is the beta subunit of these hormones that confers biological specificity. The half-lives of LH, FSH, and hCG are determined in part by the degree of glycosylation of the proteins. Within the gonadotropin family, the greater the degree of glycosylation, the longer the half-life. Of the gonadotropins, hCG has 4 times more carbohydrate residues than FSH and 20 times more carbohydrate residues than LH.[14] Therefore, the rank order of the half-life of the gonadotropins is hCG (20 h) > FSH (4 h), > LH (<1 h). The gonadotropins stimulate the ovary by binding to specific cell-surface receptors and causing an increase in the production of cyclic AMP. Although the gonadotropins are secreted in a pulsatile form, the pulse signal is *not* a critical determinant of the gonadotropin signal. The ovary responds well to a "constant" infusion of gonadotropin. The critical component of the gonadotropin signal is the mean integrated concentration of hormone. Within the physiological range, the greater the mean concentration of gonadotropin, the greater the ovarian response.

The Ovarian Follicle

The functional unit of the lung is the alveolus. The functional unit of the kidney is the nephron. The functional unit of the ovary is the follicle. The structure–function relationships of the ovarian follicle are outlined in Fig. 2 and Table 3.

The number of ovarian primordial follicles becomes permanently fixed in the second trimester of fetal life.[15] From birth onward, no new follicular units can be generated. The primordial follicle consists of an oocyte surrounded by a single layer of flattened granulosa cells. The granulosa cells are separated from the systemic circulation and the remainder of the ovary by a basement membrane that consists of extracellular matrix (type IV collagen, laminin, and fibronectin). This unique structural separation of the ovarian follicle from the remainder of the ovary allows each follicle to create its own unique microenvironment. The follicle that develops the microenvironment most optimal to growth will be the follicle that ovulates.[16,17] Follicles that develop a microenvironment that does not support

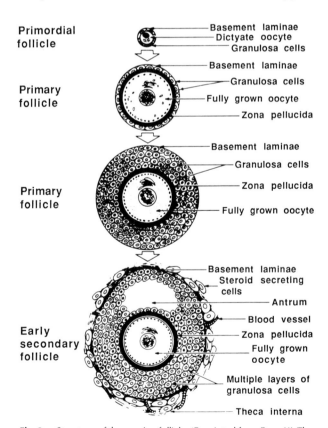

Fig. 2 Structure of the ovarian follicle. (Reprinted from Ryan KJ. The endocrine pattern and control of the ovulatory cycle. In: Insler V, Lunenfeld B, eds. *Infertility: Male and Female.* New York: Churchill Livingstone; 1986, with permission.)

Table 3
Structure–Function Relationships in the Ovarian Follicle

Structure	Function	
	Stimulus	Response
Stroma	LH	Androgen production
Theca	LH	Androgen production
Granulosa cells	FSH	Conversion of androgen to estrogen
Oocyte	Proteins, small regulatory nucleotides, phospholipids	Arrest of meiosis until LH surge

growth fail to achieve dominance and become atretic (follicular demise). For every 100 follicles that enter a growth trajectory, only 1 follicle achieves dominance and ovulates. The remaining 99 follicles undergo atresia and die.[15]

As noted above, the number of primordial follicles becomes permanently fixed in the second trimester of fetal life. From birth onward, follicles leave the resting pool of primordial follicles and start on a growth trajectory. The factors that stimulate primordial follicles to enter a growth phase are unclear. During the first stage of follicular growth, the primordial follicle grows into a preantral follicle (see Fig. 2). During this stage, the granulosa cells change their shape from flattened cells to cuboidal cells, and they begin to replicate at a rapid rate. In addition, the oocyte increases in size. An interesting feature of the human ovary is that the rate at which primordial follicles leave the resting pool and enter a growth trajectory can best be described by an exponential function. The key characteristic of an exponential function is that for any given time period "t", a fixed *percentage* of the primordial follicles remaining in the ovary are lost to a pool of growing follicles. Therefore, as the ovary "ages" fewer and fewer primordial follicles are allowed to enter the growth pool per time period "t".[15] In this manner the aging ovary conserves, or rations, its ever-dwindling follicular store. Since the loss of primordial follicles is an exponential function, the removal of one entire ovary (50% of all follicles) does not significantly change the age at which menopause (depletion of all follicles) occurs. Approximately 90% of all ovarian follicles must be destroyed to significantly change the timing of the menopause.[15]

Under the stimulation of LH and FSH, the preantral follicle grows into an antral follicle. The antral follicle consists of five key components: (1) theca, (2) basement membrane, (3) granulosa cells, (4) follicular (antral) fluid, and (5) oocyte. The thecal tissue is derived from the primitive mesenchyme of the ovary (stroma). The

theca forms the outer shell of the follicle. The theca contains LH receptors, but *no* FSH receptors. The main secretory product of the theca is the weak androgen, androstenedione.[16] The basement membrane consists of type IV collagen, laminin, and fibronectin. As noted above, no blood vessels cross the basement membrane. Therefore, the follicular components on the inner side of the basement membrane (granulosa cells, antral fluid, oocyte) are bathed in a microenvironment unique to that particular follicle. The granulosa cells contain FSH and LH receptors, and their main steroid products are progesterone and estradiol.[16] The granulosa cells participate in the generation of the follicular fluid. The follicular fluid concentration of progesterone, androgens, and estrogens is approximately 100 to 1000 times greater than the circulating concentration of these hormones. High intrafollicular concentrations of estrogen are required for optimal granulosa cell growth. The granulosa cells are directly connected to the oocyte by gap junctions. The granulosa cells thereby control the nutritional and hormonal environment of the oocyte.

For the antral follicle to grow, the theca and the granulosa cells must work in concert to produce an optimal microenvironment. This physiologic interdependency is often described as the *two-cell theory* of follicular function. One clear example of the two-cell theory is the biochemistry of follicular estrogen production. The theca cells contain the enzyme complex 17-alpha-hydroxylase, 17,20-lyase, and are able to convert progesterone to a weak androgen androstenedione (Fig. 3). However, the theca is very inefficient at converting androstenedione to estradiol. In contrast, the granulosa cells do not contain the 17-alpha-hydroxylase, 17,20-lyase complex and cannot synthesize androstenedione. The granulosa cells contain large amounts of the aromatase enzyme system which can convert androstenedione to estrone. Therefore, the theca and granulosa cells must interact to produce estrogen. The theca responds to LH stimulation by converting choles-

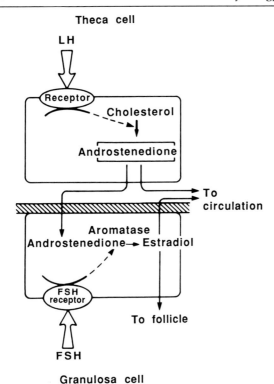

Theca cell

LH

Receptor

---Cholesterol

Androstenedione

→ To circulation

Aromatase
Androstenedione → Estradiol

FSH receptor

To follicle

FSH

Granulosa cell

Fig. 3 Diagrammatic representation of the relationship between theca and granulosa cells. Androstenedione production from the theca is controlled by LH. Androstenedione diffuses to the granulosa cell where aromatization to estrogen is controlled by FSH. (Reprinted from Ryan KJ. The endocrine pattern and control of the ovulatory cycle. In: Insler V, Lunenfeld B, eds. *Infertility: Male and Female.* New York: Churchill Livingstone; 1986, with permission.)

terol to androstenedione. In turn, the granulosa cells respond to FSH stimulation by converting the thecal androstenedione to estradiol. Evidence is accumulating that, in addition to interacting to produce estrogen, the theca and granulosa cells stimulate the growth of the follicle by sending protein (paracrine) signals back and forth across the basement membrane. Proteins that may be involved in this cross-talk between the theca and granulosa cells include: insulin-like growth factor I, renin, angiotensin II, epidermal growth factor, and fibroblast growth factor.

A second major principle of ovarian physiology is the follicular microenvironment theory.[17] Within the basement membrane each follicle creates its own unique microenvironment. Many studies suggest that follicles that create a microenvironment rich in FSH and estradiol are the follicles most likely to grow rapidly and ovulate. This is not surprising since FSH and estradiol are potent stimulators of granulosa cell mitosis. Follicles that contain low concentrations of FSH and estra-

diol grow poorly and die. The factors that regulate the development of the microenvironment have not been fully delineated. However, follicles that capture a large percentage of total ovarian blood flow appear to be at an advantage in the race to produce a microenvironment rich in FSH. Although each follicle is exposed to the same circulating concentration of FSH, the follicle with the greatest total blood flow receives the largest flux of FSH.[17]

Follicle Selection and Dominance

At the beginning of the follicular phase of the cycle (day 1 of menses), there are four antral follicles 4 mm in diameter in the ovaries. By day 12 of the cycle there is only *one* large antral follicle 20 mm in diameter in the ovaries. The process by which the four small antral follicles are "winnowed" to one large, preovulatory antral follicle is called the process of *selection*. The mechanisms underlying the process of selection are not fully understood. However, the status of the follicular microenvironment is probably crucial to the process of selection. The small antral follicle that is able to create a microenvironment which is optimally conducive to growth will achieve dominance and go on to ovulate. At day 4 of the follicular phase, no one follicle has achieved dominance. By day 8 of a normal 14-day follicular phase a dominant follicle can always be identified. Once a dominant follicle is established, no new large antral follicles can appear until that dominant structure undergoes atresia at the end of the luteal phase. The dominant follicle prevents the growth of other new structures by steroid (estrogen, progesterone) and protein (inhibin, follicle-regulatory protein) secretions. Surgical removal of the dominant follicle is followed by the growth of a new cohort of small antral follicles that compete to become dominant. The processes of selection and dominance help ensure that, on the average, only one egg is ovulated each cycle.[18]

Ovulatory Events

The timing of ovulation is determined by the dominant ovarian follicle. The dominant follicle, not the hypothalamic-pituitary unit, is the gatekeeper for the timing of ovulation. When the dominant ovarian follicle produces enough estrogen to sustain a circulating estradiol concentration in the range of 300 pg/ml for 48 hours, the hypothalamic-pituitary unit responds by secreting a surge of LH.[19] The LH surge stimulates four events in the ovary that result in ovulation. The events initiated by the LH surge include: (1) an increase in intrafollicular proteolytic enzymes (plasmin), which destroy the basement membrane and allow follicular rupture; (2) luteinization of granulosa cells and theca resulting in increased progesterone production; (3) resumption of meiosis in the oocyte, preparing it for fertilization; and (4) an influx of blood vessels into the follicle, preparing it to become a corpus luteum. Both the granulosa cells and the theca contribute to the total mass of the corpus luteum. The beginning of the LH surge precedes ovulation by about 36 hours. The LH surge initiates an increase in follicle production of plasmin, collagenases, and prostaglandins that probably contribute to the disruption of the follicle wall and the extrusion of the oocyte. In addition the LH surge induces luteinization of the granulosa cells and allows the oocyte to reenter meiosis.

Luteal Phase

When the newly ruptured follicle completes the process of luteinization, corpus luteum function is established. Maximal corpus luteum activity (progesterone production) occurs 7 to 8 days after the LH peak. The progesterone produced by the corpus luteum stimulates changes in the endometrium, which prepare it for embryo implantation. If embryo implantation occurs, hCG secreted by the embryo increases the life span of the corpus luteum. If embryo implantation fails to occur, the corpus luteum will undergo its preprogrammed demise beginning 10 to 12 days after ovulation. The factors that regulate luteolysis are not well understood. Of clinical importance is the fact that the large amounts of progesterone (25 mg/d) produced by the corpus luteum cause the thermoregulatory center of the hypothalamus to increase body temperature by approximately 0.3°C. Therefore, the clinician can use the daily measurement of basal body temperature to monitor corpus luteum function.

Transition from Luteal to Follicular Phase

Approximately 12 days after ovulation, luteolysis begins. The factors that cause luteolysis are not clearly identified. As estradiol and progesterone production begins to decline, the endometrium becomes structurally unstable and menses ensues. The decrease in ovarian progesterone and estradiol is accompanied by an increase in FSH secretion. This in turn promotes the growth of a new cohort of follicles.

The Uterus

The uterus consists of an upper muscular portion called the corpus (or body) and a lower portion, the cervix. The endometrium is the inner epithelial lining of the uterine corpus. Functionally, the endometrium is divided into two zones. The zona functionalis is the upper zone of the endometrium. This zone undergoes cyclic changes in morphology during the menstrual cycle in response to estrogen (growth) and progesterone (differentiation). During the follicular phase, the functionalis layer grows from 0.5 mm to 3.5 mm in height. During menstruation the zona functionalis sloughs from the basal endometrium. The zona functionalis contains specially coiled blood vessels (spiral arteries) which contract and help limit the amount of blood loss during menses. The lower portion of the endometrium is the zona basalis. This zone remains relatively unchanged during the menstrual cycle. The zona basalis provides the stem cells for the regeneration of the zona functionalis at the end of menses.

The endometrium is composed of a supporting stroma and a glandular epithelium. The stroma contains nerves, blood vessels, and endometrial stromal cells. The stroma is separated from the overlying glandular epithelium by a basement membrane. No blood vessels cross the basement membrane, so that the stroma "filters" and "modulates" all the nutritional and endocrine signals delivered to the glandular epithelium. A growing body of evidence suggests that the stroma secretes paracrine protein factors that cross to the glandular epithelium and regulate the histology of the glands.

The major identified hormone regulators of the endometrium are the steroid hormones. The endometrium contains receptors for estradiol, progesterone, and testosterone. The endometrium responds to steroid stimulation with highly stereotyped responses. For example, estrogen produces growth of the endometrium in a dose- and time-dependent manner. Long-term stimulation of the endometrium with "unopposed" estrogen will often result in endometrial hyperplasia, and occasionally carcinoma. The follicular phase of the menstrual cycle is characterized by the ovarian production of large amounts of estrogen. The endometrium responds to this estrogen stimulus by growing. The endometrial counterpart of the ovarian "follicular" phase is therefore called the "proliferative phase." The term "proliferative" refers to the large number of mitoses present in the endometrial glands.

Estrogen-primed endometrium responds to progesterone by ceasing proliferation and undergoing differentiation which results in a secretory epithelium. Under the stimulus of estrogen and progesterone the endometrium epithelium secretes large amounts of proteins and carbohydrates into the glandular lumen. The endometrial counterpart of the ovarian luteal phase is, therefore, called the secretory phase. The endometrial response to estrogen and progesterone is so well understood that a histologic examination of the endometrium can be used to determine the menstrual cycle day within an accuracy of 2 days.[20]

Luteolysis commences approximately 12 days after ovulation. Loss of luteal function results in a marked decrease in progesterone and estrogen production. The luteal phase (secretory) endometrium responds to the decreasing concentration of circulating estrogen and progesterone with a group of responses culminating in menstruation. Vascular responses include endometrial vasospasm, endometrial ischemia, and loss of endometrial integrity. Endometrial intracellular responses include: (1) decrease in lysosomal stability, (2) increased release of phospholipase resulting in cleavage of phospholipids to arachidonic acid, and (3) increased conversion of arachidonic acid to prostaglandins.[21,22] Prostaglandins PGF_2 and PGE increase uterine contractility, augmenting endometrial ischemia and further disrupting endometrial integrity.

The cervical canal is lined by glandular elements which respond to high concentrations of estradiol by producing copious amounts of a clear mucus rich in sodium and chloride. This characteristic response of the cervical glands to estrogen allows the clinician to use the observation of the cervical mucus as an estrogen bioassay. Estrogen-stimulated cervical mucus production is characterized by: (1) a large volume of clear fluid, (2) spinnbarkeit, and (3) ferning. Spinnbarkeit refers to the elastic properties of the cervical mucus that allow it to be stretched without breaking. Estrogen-stimulated cervical mucus can often be stretched 10 cm to 15 cm without breaking. The high NaCl content of estrogen-stimulated cervical mucus causes the mucus to crystallize in a branching pattern like a fern (ferning) when it is dried. Ferning and spinnbarkeit are not present if the cervix is exposed to progesterone. Therefore, spinnbarkeit and ferning are only seen in the middle and late follicular phase prior to ovulation.

CONTROL OF THE MENSTRUAL CYCLE: LEVEL 2

The increase is estradiol production associated with the follicular phase of the menstrual cycle results in increases in the secretion of growth hormone,[23] prolactin,[24] ACTH,[25] and oxytocin.[26] These changes suggest that estrogen may have an effect on the neuroendocrine control of the hypothalamus and anterior and posterior pituitary function. As noted above, progesterone secretion in the luteal phase of the cycle increases hypothalamic endorphin tone, therefore implicating progesterone in the neuroendocrine control of hypothalamic function. In addition to estrogen and progesterone, secretions of the adrenal, thyroid, and pancreas also have important effects on the neuroendocrine control of the hypothalamus and pituitary. To further complicate this situation, special areas of the brain, such as the limbic system, also appear to modulate the neuroendocrine function of the hypothalamus. The control of the menstrual cycle by these secondary systems will be reviewed in greater detail in this section.

The Limbic System

In the rat, the limbic structures, especially the amygdala, have direct and reciprocal neural connections with the major hypothalamic nuclei controlling GnRH secretion: ventromedial, preoptic, and arcuate.[27] In women with seizure disorders arising from or involving the limbic system (temporal lobe epilepsy), anovulation is very common.[28,29] For example, Herzog and colleagues[29] reported that 60% of women with temporal lobe epilepsy were anovulatory, 20% had abnormally elevated concentrations of circulating LH, and 15% had abnormally low concentrations of circulating LH. These endocrine abnormalities imply that the regulation of GnRH pulse frequency and amplitude may be perturbed in these women. Of interest is the observation that animals with experimentally induced seizures of the amygdala[30] and women with temporal lobe epilepsy[31] have altered central nervous system (CNS) dopamine and homovanillic acid concentrations. Since dopamine is a major regulator of GnRH secretion, it is possible that abnormalities in limbic function impact GnRH secretion through catecholamine-dependent pathways. Limbic-hypothalamic intercommunication is a model system for how diverse CNS lesions can modulate hypothalamic function.

Corticotropin-Releasing Hormone (CRH)

Multiple epidemiologic studies suggest that stress may inhibit GnRH secretion and result in anovulation. Evidence is accumulating that CRH is a mediator of the inhibitory effect of stress on GnRH secretion. In the rat[32] and the monkey[33] CRH administration decreases gonadotropin secretion, and this effect can be blocked by the administration of a CRH antagonist.[32] In both the rat and the monkey, the inhibitory effect of CRH on GnRH secretion is mediated by opioid peptides.[34,35] The hypothesized cascade of events—stress→increased CRH secretion→increased hypothalamic opioid tone→decreased GnRH secretion→anovulation—provides a fertile arena for future research.

The Adrenal

Genetic disorders in enzymes of adrenal steroidogenesis can result in anovulation. Defects in the 21-hydroxylase, 11-hydroxylase, and 3-beta-hydroxysteroid dehydrogenase-isomerase genes have all been implicated as causes of anovulation and oligomenorrhea.[36,37] Numerous genetic defects that cause 21-hydroxylase deficiency have been described and include point mutations, gene deletions, and gene conversion. A basic principle of genetics is that if a specific gene defect or marker segregates with a phenotype over many generations, then it is statistically likely that the gene defect causes the phenotype. A basic challenge for reproductive endocrinologists is to describe in detail how a mutation in the 21-hydroxylase gene can result in anovulation and oligomenorrhea.

The Thyroid

Clinically, hypothyroidism is known to be associated with anovulation and irregular menstrual cycles. The exact mechanisms by which hypothyroidism disrupts GnRH secretion are unknown. However, hypothyroidism may produce alterations in hypothalamic catecholamine turnover, which may in turn disrupt GnRH secretion.[38]

The Pancreas

Women who are underweight or too lean[39] and women of normal body composition with low caloric intake[40] may develop anovulation due to low GnRH secretion.[41] The mechanisms by which the hypothalamus monitors body composition and nutritional intake and integrates this data into the global control of GnRH secretion are poorly defined. Insulin may be a hormone of central metabolism that participates in the control of GnRH secretion. In diabetics with poor glucose control due to deficient insulin secretion, anovulation and oligomenorrhea are common. In a recent study of college women, 24-hour insulin secretion as determined by urinary C-peptide measurements was significantly lower in oligomenorrheic as compared to eumenorrheic women, even though the women were matched for height, weight, body fat, caloric intake, psychosocial stress, exercise, and 24-hour urinary cortisol secretion.[42] This study suggests that hypoinsulinemia may be associated with decreased GnRH secretion. Of interest is the observation that women with the polycystic ovary syndrome often are hyperinsulinemic[43] and have increased GnRH pulse frequency.[12]

Women with normal ovulatory cycles who are placed on an experimental eucaloric diet low in fat (20% of calories) often develop oligomenorrhea.[40] This effect was most marked if saturated fats were replaced by polyunsaturated fats. This study suggests that the hypothalamus not only monitors total caloric intake but also saturated fat intake, and this information is used to modulate GnRH secretion.

CONTROL OF THE MENSTRUAL CYCLE: LEVEL 3

In the elucidation of the mechanisms causing PMS, a central question is, "How can cyclic changes in estradiol and progesterone produce the PMS phenotype in susceptible women?" Since many of the symptoms of PMS are mediated through the CNS, this question is a component of a more general problem in reproductive biology, "How do estradiol and progesterone modulate CNS and hypothalamic function?" There is little doubt that estradiol and progesterone modulate CNS and hypothalamic function. For example, estrogen plus progesterone stimulate an increase in hypothalamic endorphin production.[5] It is likely that only a fraction of the CNS effects of estrogen and progesterone have been discovered, and that many additional CNS effects of these hormones will be described in the near future. The remainder of this review focuses on the CNS effects of progesterone that have already been reported.

For many decades it was known that progesterone can modulate CNS function. For example, in humans progesterone increases basal temperatures approximately 0.3°C during the luteal phase of the menstrual cycle. This effect is probably mediated, in part, by direct effects of progesterone on hypothalamic centers that control temperature. In addition, progesterone and other sex steroids clearly play a role in modulating reproductive behaviors, territorial behaviors, mood, and affect in animals.[44] Progesterone probably modulates CNS function by two separate mechanisms: by direct effects on neuron membrane ion channels and by binding to nuclear progesterone receptors. The interaction of metabolites of progesterone with neural ion channels is an exciting and rapidly developing area of research that deserves special focus.

Progesterone and metabolites of progesterone can act as sedatives and clearly modulate the potency of many anesthetic agents.[45,46] Progesterones appear to have properties similar to those of short-acting barbiturates.[47] A major advance was made by Majewski and colleagues[48] with the discovery that 3-alpha-hydroxy derivatives of progesterone interact with sites on the GABA receptor. The GABA receptor, also known as the GABA-benzodiazepine receptor-chloride ionophore complex (GBRC), modulates neuronal excitability by allowing chloride ions to flow down their electrochemical gradient, hyperpolarizing the cells and rendering the neuron less prone to excitation.[49] GBRC contains at least three drug binding sites that modulate the function of the GBRC. The GBRC contains benzodiazepine and barbiturate recognition sites. Both barbiturates and benzodiazepine stabilize the GBRC in an open state allowing for chloride ion flux, hyperpolarization, and decreased excitability of the neuron. Certain steroids, especially 3-alpha-hydroxy, 5-alpha reduced metabolites of progesterone and deoxycorticosterone, also potentiate chloride ion conductance through the GBRC at nanomolar concentrations.[49] These neurally active steroids do not exert their effects through the barbiturate or benzodiazepine recognition sites on the GBRC.[49]

The pharmacology of one metabolite of progesterone, 3-alpha-hydroxy, 5-alpha dihydroprogesterone (3-OH-DHP), has been studied in detail. This metabolite suppresses penicillin-induced seizures[50] and metrazol-induced seizures.[49] In rats, sensitivity to electroshock seizures is high when 3-OH-DHP concentrations are low.[51,52] In rats, 3-OH-DHP circulates at a concentration similar to the concentration required to produce effects in vitro.[51] In women with epilepsy, medroxyprogesterone acetate administration may reduce the frequency of seizures.[53] Of special interest is the observation that there is a marked variation in the concentration of metabolites of progesterone between women, and that low levels of circulating metabolites of progesterone may be associated with increased seizure activity around the time of menses.[54]

The "progestin hypothesis" deserves additional study as a possible etiologic explanation for PMS. It is possible that women who produce low amounts of the most neurally active metabolites of progesterone are at increased risk of developing PMS.

SUMMARY

Basic science and clinical researchers hope to identify those factors that trigger PMS in susceptible women. Thorough knowledge of the physiology of the normal menstrual cycle is the springboard for this research. Unfortunately, even today our understanding of the control mechanisms for the menstrual cycle is incomplete. We are only just beginning to identify the biologic variables that contribute to PMS.

REFERENCES

1. Treolar AE, Boynton RE, Behn BG, et al. Variations of the human menstrual cycle through reproductive life. *Int J Fertil.* 1967;12:77.
2. Landren BM, Unden AL, Diczfalusy E. Hormonal profile of the cycle in 68 normally menstruating women. *Acta Endocrinol.* 1980;94:89.
3. Halberg L, Nilsson L. Determination of menstrual blood loss. *Scand J Clin Lab Invest.* 1964;16:244.
4. King JL, Anthony ELP, Fitzgerald DM, et al. Luteinizing hormone releasing hormone neurons in the human: differential intraneuronal localization of immunoreactive forms. *J Clin Endocrinol Metab.* 1985;60:88.
5. Ferin M. A role for the endogenous opioid peptides in the regulation of gonadotropin secretion in the primate. *Hormone Res.* 1988;28:119.
6. Heritage AS, Stumpf WE, Sar M, et al. Brain stem catecholamine neurons are target sites for sex steroid hormones. *Science.* 1980; 207:1377.
7. Ropert JF, Quigley ME, Yen SCC. The dopaminergic inhibition of LH secretion during the menstrual cycle. *Life Sci.* 1984;34:2067.
8. Knobil E. The neuroendocrine control of the menstrual cycle. *Recent Prog Hormone Res.* 1980;36:53.
9. Santoro N, Wierman ME, Filicori M, et al. Intravenous administration of pulsatile gonadotropin releasing hormone in hypothalamic amenorrhea: effect of dosage. *J Clin Endocrinol Metab.* 1986;62:109.
10. Crowley WF, Filicori, Spratt DI, et al. The physiology of gonadotropin-releasing hormone secretion in men and women. *Recent Prog Hormone Res.* 1985;41:473.
11. Ropert JF, Quigley ME, Yen SCC. Endogenous opiates modulate pulsatile LH release in humans. *J Clin Endocrinol Metab.* 1981; 52:583.
12. Waldstreicher J, Santoro NF, Hall JE, et al. Hyperfunction of the hypothalamic-pituitary axis in women with polycystic ovarian disease—indirect evidence for partial gonadotroph desensitization. *J Clin Endocrinol Metab.* 1988;66:165.
13. Wang CF, Lasley BL, Lein A, et al. The functional changes of the pituitary gonadotrophs during the menstrual cycle. *J Clin Endocrinol Metab.* 1976;42:718.
14. Parsons TF, Peirce JG. Glycoprotein hormones: structure and function. *Ann Rev Biochem.* 1981;50:465.
15. Gosden RG. *Biology of Menopause.* London: Academic Press; 1985.
16. McNatty KP, Makris A, DeGrazia C, et al. The production of progesterone, androgens, and estrogens by granulosa cells, theca tissue, and stromal tissue from human ovaries in vitro. *J Clin Endocrinol Metab.* 1979;49:687.
17. McNatty KP, Moore-Smith D, Makris A, et al. The microenvi-

ronment of the human antral follicle. *J Clin Endocrinol Metab.* 1979;49:851.

18. Goodman AL, Hodgen GD. The ovarian triad of the primate menstrual cycle. *Recent Prog Hormone Res.* 1983;39:1.

19. Liv JH, Yen SCC. Induction of midcycle gonadotropin surge by ovarian steroids in women: a critical evaluation. *J Clin Endocrinol Metab.* 1983;57:797.

20. Noyes RW, Hertig AT, Rock J. Dating the endometrial biopsy. *Fertil Steril.* 1950;1:3.

21. Henzl MR, Smith RE, Boost G, et al. Lysomal concept of menstrual bleeding in humans. *J Clin Endocrinol Metab.* 1972;34:860.

22. Turksoy RN, Safaii HS. Immediate effect of prostaglandin during the luteal phase of the menstrual cycle. *Fertil Steril.* 1975;26:634.

23. Yen SCC, Vela P, Rankin J, et al. Hormonal relationships during the menstrual cycle. *JAMA.* 1970;211:1513.

24. Vekemans M, Delvoye P, L'Hermite M, et al. Serum prolactin levels during the menstrual cycle. *J Clin Endocrinol Metab.* 1977;44:989.

25. Genazzi AR, Lemarchand-Beraud TH, Aubert ML, et al. Patterns of plasma ACTH, hGH, and cortisol during the menstrual cycle. *J Clin Endocrinol Metab.* 1975;41:431.

26. Amico JA, Seif SM, Robinson AG. Elevation of oxytocin and the oxytocin-associated neuroplupin in the plasma of normal women during midcycle. *J Clin Endocrinol Metab.* 1981;53:1229.

27. Renaud LP. Influence of amygdala stimulation on the activity of identified tuberoinfundibular neurons in the rat hypothalamus. *J Physiol.* 1976;260:237.

28. Herzog AG, Russell V, Vaitukaitis JL. Neuroendocrine dysfunction in temporal lobe epilepsy. *Arch Neurol.* 1982;39:133.

29. Herzog AG, Seibel MM, Schomer DL, et al. Reproductive endocrine disorders in women with partial seizures of temporal lobe origin. *Arch Neurol.* 1986;43:341.

30. Sato M, Nakashima T, Kindling. Secondary epileptogenesis, sleep, and catecholamines. *Can J Neurol Sci.* 1975;2:439.

31. Papeschi R, Molina-Negro P, Sourkes TL. The concentration of homovanillic and 5-hydroxy-indoleacetic acid in ventricular and lumbar CSF. *Neurology.* 1972;22:1151.

32. Rivier C, Rivier J, Vale W. Stress-induced inhibition of reproductive function: role of endogenous corticotropin-releasing factor. *Science.* 1986;231:607.

33. Olster DH, Ferin M. Corticotropin releasing hormone inhibits gonadotropin secretion in the ovariectomized Rhesus monkey. *J Clin Endocrinol Metab.* 1987;65:262.

34. Gindoff PR, Ferin M. Endogenous opioid peptides modulate the effect of corticotropin releasing factor on gonadotropin release in the primate. *Endocrinology.* 1987;121:837.

35. Petraglia F, Vale W, Rivier C. Opioids act centrally to modulate stress-induced decrease in LH in the rat. *Endocrinology.* 1986;119:2445.

36. Siegel SF, Finegold DN, Lanes R, et al. ACTH stimulation tests and plasma DHEAS levels in women with hirsutism. *N Engl J Med.* 1990;323:849.

37. Eldar-Geva T, Hurwitz A, Vecsei P, et al. Secondary biosynthetic defects in women with late onset congenital adrenal hyperplasia. *N Engl J Med.* 1990;323:855.

38. Contreras P, Generini G, Michelson H, et al. Hyperprolactinemia and galactorrhea: spontaneous versus iatrogenic hypothyroidism. *J Clin Endocrinol Metab.* 1981;53:1036.

39. Frisch RE, Wyshak G, Vincent L. Delayed menarche and amenorrhea of ballet dancers. *N Engl J Med.* 1980;303:17.

40. Jones DY, Judd JT, Taylor PR, et al. Influence of dietary fat on menstrual cycles and menses length. *Hum Nutr Clin Nutr.* 1987;41:341.

41. Vigersky RA, Anderson AE, Thompson RH. Hypothalamic dysfunction in secondary amenorrhea associated with simple weight loss. *N Engl J Med.* 1977;297:1141.

42. Snow RC, Schneider J, Barbieri RL. High dietary fiber and low saturated fat intact among oligomenorrheic undergraduates. *Fertil Steril.* 1990;54:632.

43. Barbieri, RL, Ryan KJ. Hyperandrogenism, insulin resistance, acanthosis nigricans: a common endocrinopathy with unique pathophysiologic features. *Am J Obstet Gynecol.* 1983;147:90.

44. Pfaff DW, McEwan BS. Action of estrogen and progestins on nerve cells. *Science.* 1983;219:808.

45. Seyle H. The antagonism between anesthetic steroid hormones and penta-methylenetetrazol. *J Lab Clin Med.* 1942;27:1051.

46. Datta S, Migliozzi RP, Flanagan HL, et al. Chronically administered progesterone decreases halothane requirements in rabbits. *Anesth Analg Reanim.* 1989;68:46.

47. Bellville JW, Howland WS, Bogan CP. Comparisons of the electroencephalographic patterns during steroid and barbiturate narcosis. *Br J Anesth.* 1956;28:50.

48. Majewski MD, Harrison NL, Schwartz RD, et al. Steroid hormone metabolites are barbiturate like modulators of the GABA receptor. *Science.* 1987;232:1004.

49. Gee, KW. Steroid modulation of the GABA/benzodiazepine receptor-linked chloride ionophore. *Mol Neurobiol.* 1988;2:291.

50. Backstrom T, Bixo M, Hammarback S. Ovarian steroid hormones: effects on mood, behavior, and brain excitability. *Acta Obstet Gynecol Scand.* 1985;130(suppl):19.

51. Holzbauer M. Physiological aspects of steroid with anesthetic properties. *Med Biol.* 1976;54:227.

52. Wooley DE, Timiras PS. The gonad-brain relationship: effects of female sex hormones on electroshock convulsions in the rat. *Endocrinology.* 1962;70:196.

53. Mattson RH, Kramer JA, Caldwell BV, et al. Treatment of seizures with medroxyprogesterone (abstract 63). Epilepsy International Symposium. Washington, DC; 1983.

54. Rosciszewska D, Butner B, Guz I, et al. Ovarian hormones, anticonvulsant drugs, and seizures during the menstrual cycle in women with epilepsy. *J Neurol Neurosurg Psych.* 1986;49:47.

CHAPTER 5

Etiology of Premenstrual Syndrome

Steven J. Sondheimer

In reproductive-age women, cyclic changes including premenstrual changes are normal. The relationship between these known physiologic events and the symptoms popularly known as premenstrual syndrome (PMS) continues to be elusive. Whether those women who have premenstrual symptoms affecting the quality of their life have greater hormonal changes or a greater central response to the hormonal change, or a difference in psychosocial makeup, is still unknown. Further, surveys of large numbers of women presenting with premenstrual complaints suggest that a large proportion suffer exacerbations of affective symptoms that are present throughout the cycle.[1]

It is therefore unlikely that a single etiology will be found for the variety of somatic and affective changes occurring prior to menses.

NORMAL EVENTS

In primitive societies ovulation is a relatively rare event, and consequently cyclic changes are less frequent as well. Menarche may not occur until age 17 or 18 because of poor nutrition; pregnancy typically occurs shortly after menarche and is followed by lactation with suppression of ovulation, which is followed by another pregnancy. Furthermore, as many as 10% of women may eventually die during childbirth.

Premenstrual syndrome by definition requires a menstrual cycle, and 13 menstrual cycles per year over 40 reproductive years provide those cycles. We therefore begin by discussing those changes that occur during a menstrual cycle. The questions include whether these changes cause symptoms, and whether those women who have symptoms severe enough to affect their quality of life differ from those who do not perceive such severe changes?

It is unlikely that there is a single etiology of all symptoms of PMS. Factor analysis suggests there is some tendency toward clustering of symptoms in a number of categories.[2] Table I lists potential clusters as determined by factor analysis. Nonetheless, there is quite a bit of individual variation. Further confusion relates to separating dysmenorrhea from PMS. Many patients have both premenstrual symptoms and dysmenorrhea. Some premenstrual symptoms are related to cramping and may be a variation on dysmenorrhea. That notwithstanding, there does seem to be a separation between these two categories of symptoms.

46

Table I
PMS Symptoms Grouped by Factor Analysis

Emotional
Nervous tension
Irritability
Mood swings
Depression
Cognitive physical
Poor coordination
Aches
Confusion
Fatigue
Food craving
Insomnia
Physical symptoms
Swelling
Breast tenderness
Headache
Cramps

PATHOPHYSIOLOGIC THEORIES OF PMS

Prostaglandin Etiology

Dysmenorrhea has been fairly well categorized in terms of its prostaglandin etiology. Prostaglandin F_2 (PGF_α) stimulates uterine and other smooth muscle contractions and is responsible for dysmenorrhea and gastrointestinal side effects. Endometrial production of PGF_α is higher in women with dysmenorrhea compared to asymptomatic women.[3] Prostaglandin synthetase inhibitors are relatively successful in the treatment of dysmenorrhea but are not uniformly successful in treating premenstrual symptoms.[4]

Prostaglandins seem to be responsible for at least some symptoms of PMS. A number of studies have shown luteal phase use of inhibitors of prostaglandin synthesis relieves premenstrual cramps, backache, headache, and gastrointestinal symptoms. It is unlikely that these medications are better than placebo in long-term relief of affective symptoms. In one study in which luteal phase blood was taken from women with PMS and then returned to them at a later follicular phase, these women experienced their luteal symptoms in the follicular phase.[5] Though no substance was isolated as the culprit, it seems likely that it was a prostaglandin that recreated the luteal phase symptoms. At least prostaglandin seems to be an internal, patient-perceived signal of the luteal phase. Oral contraceptive pills, which

are very good at suppressing ovulation and relieving dysmenorrhea, are less likely to help PMS. Approximately one-third of women are helped, one third worsened, and one-third unchanged of their affective PMS symptoms. Some patients complain of PMS-like symptoms after starting oral contraceptive pills.[6,7]

Gonadal Steroids

The temporal relationship between gonadal steroid changes, particularly progesterone and the psychological symptoms of PMS, suggests a causal link. However, most studies find that gonadal steroid levels in peripheral blood are the same in PMS sufferers and controls.[8]

During the midfollicular phase when estrogen levels are rising, many PMS sufferers feel their best, but some women complain of periovulatory symptoms when estrogen is highest or during the 24- to 48-hour estrogen nadir at midcycle.[9] Estrogen levels change during the cycle: during the early follicular phase when the initial follicles are recruited, estrogen levels are relatively low. In the earliest days of the follicular phase, estrogen levels may be as low as those seen in menopausal women. In fact, some patients may note PMS symptoms peaking at that time.[10] In the days before ovulation, estrogen levels rise very quickly. The rise in estrogen reflects the growth of the dominant follicle and is responsible for the increase in cervical mucus and the increase in pituitary sensitivity responsible for the LH surge. Women who have ovulation artificially induced with human menopausal gonadotropins reach much higher levels of midcycle estrogen than do normally ovulating individuals. Though women with artificially induced cycles often complain of more bloating or more awareness of their ovary, in general there is not an increase in other somatic or affective symptoms. This is in contrast to the use of clomiphene citrate for ovulation induction. Although clomiphene citrate is only used for 5 days early in the cycle, many women complain of affective symptoms during those days.

In general, older women and perimenopausal women have estrogen levels that are lower than younger women, probably because fewer oocytes remain and fewer follicles are recruited. Vasomotor instability, the so-called "hot flushes," can occur even in the premenopause when estrogen levels are low. Hot flushes are peripheral vasodilatory events apparently related to central release of norepinephrine uninhibited by estrogen. Episodes occur more frequently at night, and can be a cause of sleep disturbance. However, studies suggest that menopausal estrogen deprivation is only weakly related to menopausal mood disturbances.[11,12]

Acute declines in serum estrogen may occur during therapy with clomiphene citrate, during the midcycle luteinizing hormone (LH) surge, and in the late luteal phase; declining estrogen levels may trigger affective symptoms in some patients.

The gonadal steroid effect may be related to changes within the central nervous system not measured by peripheral hormone levels. The brain contains specific receptors for steroids. In the rat, some areas of the brain have many estrogen receptors while other areas have none. Although estrogen receptors are scattered throughout the brain, they are concentrated in the hypothalamus, the preoptic area, and more laterally in the amygdala. In the brain, as well as in other tissues, estrogen has two general effects. Estrogen and its receptor complex bind to DNA and regulate activation or suppression of specific messenger RNA and subsequent protein synthesis affecting brain structure, cognitive function, and neurochemical function. Estrogens, as well as progestogens and glucocorticoids, also affect neurotransmission events.[13,14]

Progesterone

The luteal phase is dominated by the corpus luteum formed from the dominant follicle after ovulation. It is a well-vascularized organ, a steroid factory, producing large amounts of progesterone and estrogen. Some studies of PMS patients have demonstrated lower progesterone levels in the luteal phase; other studies have found no difference, and one study demonstrated an increased level. In those patients who do demonstrate reduced luteal phase progesterone levels, the "stress" of PMS may be causing reduced progesterone secretion. Inadequate luteal function or anovulation has been demonstrated to occur in a variety of clinical "stress" models.[15] It is doubtful that progesterone deficiency causes PMS.

In the rat model, the central effect of estrogen is a stimulatory "antidepressant" effect. Progesterone demonstrates a suppressant or "sedative" effect. However, this generalization does not take into account differences in specific areas of the brain and differences between rodents and primates. For example, the midcycle surge in LH and FSH occurs in primates even with absence of the hypothalamic feedback, probably because of an increase in gonadotropin releasing hormone (GnRH) receptors in the anterior pituitary. In the rodent, positive feedback is due to hypothalamic stimulation by the high levels of estrogen. Primates may have

a redundancy of controls, since high midcycle estrogen does increase the frequency of GnRH pulses.

Since there is a temporal relationship between PMS and peripheral serum progesterone changes, and since peripheral hormone levels may not reflect levels within the CNS or their central receptor population, ovarian hormones may still be central to PMS.

A recent study suggests that the hormonal changes of the late luteal phase do not appear to be the cause of PMS. The use of an antiprogestational agent, mifepristone (RU486), in the midluteal phase caused luteolysis, with a fall in estrogen and progesterone to follicular phase levels, and menstruation without relieving symptoms of PMS such as sadness, anxiety, and bloating.[16] The blockage of progesterone action with mifepristone also did not cause symptoms of PMS in normal unaffected women.[17] The symptoms of PMS may be triggered by hormonal changes at other times in the cycle since medical or surgical castration causes remission of symptoms.[18,19] Furthermore, there is still much evidence linking hormonal shifts and mood changes, at least for some PMS patients. The creation of a medical menopause with a gonadotropin releasing hormone agonist with addition of various combinations of estrogen and/or progesterone is a powerful tool to investigate hormonal influence on symptoms.[20,21]

Progesterone and progestational agents have sedative effects and are occasionally associated with negative mood changes. Clinically, these events appear more commonly with the more potent progestational agents than progesterone itself. Progesterone or one of its metabolites bind to the GABAnergic receptor complex in the brain.[22] The sedative effect may be related to this mechanism or to the stimulation of endogenous opiate activity. This opiate activity would seem contradictory to reports describing a beneficial effect of progesterone in the treatment of PMS. However, no controlled clinical trials have found progesterone vaginal suppositories better than placebo. Interestingly, in one study more patients preferred placebo over progesterone, possibly because of progestational negative effects on feelings of well-being.[23]

Benzodiazepine drugs and phenobarbitol bind to different areas of the γ-aminobutyric acid (GABA) receptor complex involving a chloride channel. Recent evidence suggests that this complex also has a unique site for progestin and progesterone binding. Binding at these sites is usually associated with anxiolytic, sedative, or cognitive neuromotor impairment. Although progesterone and progestins have sedative effects, they are not as potent as the benzodiazepine drugs. Even though large doses of progesterone may result in high serum levels of progesterone, sedation is not uniformly observed.[24]

Progesterone is metabolized to a number of compounds; 20-alpha hydroxyprogesterone is the most abundant but appears to be inactive. In localized areas of the brain enzymes form 3-alpha-5-alpha dihydroprogesterone and 3-alpha-5-alpha tetrahydrodeoxycorticosterone, which bind to the GABA receptor complex.[25,26] Progesterone metabolites may therefore potentiate the effects of some benzodiazepine medications.

The central noradrenergic system is important in anxiety symptoms, particularly outflow from the locus ceruleus region, the so-called "alarm center." Normally norepinephine release suppresses its own release via alpha-2-adrenegic receptor binding back to its own cell body. In addition, GABA also suppresses the locus ceruleus output. Benzodiazepines augment this effect of GABA.[19]

PMS Is a Form of Depression?

A recent review reevaluates current thinking on depression.[27] The etiology of depression, although far from complete, involves the interaction of various components such as thinking patterns and chronic stress with activation of the locus ceruleus. Increased locus ceruleus firing occurs due to the lack of inhibition of the alpha-2-adrenergic receptors located on the dendrites and/or cell bodies of neurons in the locus ceruleus. Major depression is therefore associated with increased postsynaptic stimulation, rather than decreased stimulation. Antidepressants such as monoamine oxidase (MAO) inhibitors and the classic tricyclics could then be understood as suppressing locus ceruleus firing.

Alterations in norepinephrine and other neurotransmitters may be involved in depression. Patients with depression may have increased acetycholine action. GABA, one of the main inhibitory agents in the brain, decreases firing of the locus ceruleus and tends to be at low levels in depressed patients. Low serotonin transmission may also be present in depression.

This new understanding of depression may lead to insight into PMS as depression or an anxiety illness due to increased locus ceruleus firing premenstrually. Locus ceruleus pathways exist to the hypothalamus. These pathways probably account for the alterations in hypothalamic function seen in major depression. The most consistent neuroendocrine abnormality noted in depression is increased peripheral blood cortisol, which is also increased in anorexia nervosa.[28,29] If PMS is a variation on depression this same cortisol abnormality might

exist. However, at least one study in PMS patients has found cortisol secretory patterns to be more like controls than depressed patients, even during the luteal phase.[30] On the other hand, a milder or more transient illness like PMS might be associated with more subtle and less consistent abnormalities of the hypothalamic pituitary adrenal axis. Patients with melancholic depression and anorexia nervosa often have hypersecretion of corticotropin releasing hormone (CRH) and a blunted adrenocorticotropic hormone (ACTH) response to exogenous CRH. Alprazolam, the benzodiazepine drug that helps the affective symptoms of PMS, can suppress CRH.[31,32] However CRH testing during either the follicular phase or luteal phase in PMS patients did not show a pattern at all similar to depression or anorexia nervosa. Rather, the PMS patients studied had an increased response to CRH. It was suggested that PMS might be a condition with an intermittent increase in CRH release.[33] In any event the classic dexamethasome suppression test as used in diagnosis of depression has not been useful in PMS diagnosis.[27,34]

The lack of a modulating effect by estrogen and progesterone on ACTH response to synthetic CRH does not rule out estrogen and progesterone acting at the hypothalamus or higher levels to influence behavior.[35]

Endogenous Opiate Abnormalities

Although many peptides may act as neurotransmitters and neuromodulators, the endogenous opiate peptides (EOP), particularly β-endorphin, appear to be regulated in part by changes in gonadal sex steroids. The brain and hypothalamus are important sources of endorphins. Although the pituitary also secretes endorphins, peripheral endogenous levels probably do not reflect central, nonpituitary secretion. At the level of the hypothalamus, endorphins influence temperature, cardiovascular and respiratory function, central pain perception, and mood.[36]

High levels of estrogen and progesterone act centrally to reduce GnRH pulse frequency. Progesterone and estrogen appear to act synergistically to increase central levels of endorphins. The opiate receptor antagonist naloxone reverses the midluteal slowing of LH secretory activity normally resulting from progesterone inhibition of GnRH pulses.[37] LH release in response to naloxone occurs during the luteal phase but not during the follicular phase. β-endorphin-mediated suppression of LH pulses may be due to inhibition of central norepinephrine activity because alpha-adrenergic receptor blockers of norepinephrine synthesis inhibit naloxone-induced LH secretions.[38]

The relationship between β-endorphin and decreased LH release during the luteal phase has led to a β-endorphin theory of PMS.[39] The hypothesis presumes that the fall in gonadal steroids, with concomitant central decrease in β-endorphins, leads to a narcotic withdrawal-like syndrome. For example, narcotic withdrawal often is associated with emotional lability, headaches, constipation, and feelings of bloating and general malaise. β-endorphin theories of PMS assume both increased β-endorphin activity and withdrawal of opiate activity.

The problem with confirming this hypothesis is that peripherally measured plasma β-endorphin arises from pituitary pro-opiomelanocortin (POMC), the parent hormone for both ACTH and β-endorphin, and is secreted in parallel with ACTH during stressful stimuli. β-endorphin in the hypothalamic portal circulation arises from median eminence secretion, and may not parallel pituitary secretion. Some studies have found luteal phase levels of plasma β-endorphins to be lower in PMS sufferers than in controls.[40] Putting this all together in a coherent dogma is difficult. Treatment approaches recognizing a possible endorphin role in PMS have had some success but have not yet been duplicated in larger studies. For example, the central alpha-2-adrenergic agonist clonidine was better than placebo in a small study in PMS patients.[41] Clonidine probably acts at the locus ceruleus to suppress norepinephrine, which is increased during narcotic withdrawal. In another study, the oral narcotic antagonist naltrexone was more effective than placebo in reducing PMS symptoms when it was started prior to the midluteal phase increase in gonadal steroids. In addition, high doses of naloxone were found to elicit symptoms similar to PMS in normal controls.[42]

Weight loss and stress-induced amenorrhea are associated with increased β-endorphin levels peripherally, and some patients with these disorders may ovulate when given naloxone.[30] Most likely, peripheral β-endorphins respond to exercise or stressors while changes in central β-endorphins correlate with changes in gonadal steroids. These central changes are among the signals that apparently make cycling women aware of their cyclicity; however, it is unknown whether changes in β-endorphins are central to PMS. Furthermore, after ovariectomy in monkeys, hypothalamus-pituitary portal blood demonstrates undetectable levels of endorphins; with replacement of progesterone and estradiol portal blood endorphins increase. Endorphin administration is associated with increased serum prolactin, presumably by suppressing dopamine activity. However, several studies have shown that PMS patients have normal serum prolactin levels, and patients with hyperprolactinemia do not necessarily have premenstrual-like symptoms.[8,34,43]

Thyroid Dysfunction

The role of subtle changes in thyroid function on affective symptoms is controversial. Nonetheless, thyroid hypofunction, even subclinical hypofunction, does not appear to be a cause of PMS. Well-designed studies comparing normal subjects to PMS sufferers found no significant difference between baseline TSH or thyrotropin-releasing hormone (TRH) stimulated TSH concentrations. A small but well-designed study found no difference in relief of PMS symptoms between placebo and thyroid replacement therapy (54% of treated patients and 68% of placebo had at least partial relief).[44]

Although screening of baseline T4 and TSH is probably useful in those presenting with PMS, this is to eliminate thyroid dysfunction from the differential diagnosis and not because of its role in PMS.[45,46]

Fluid Retention

The feeling of "bloatedness" premenstrually may be caused by redistribution of body fluid into the abdomen or in the wall of the gut. However, it may actually be due to gaseous distention of the large bowel secondary to the smooth muscle relaxant effect of progesterone during the luteal phase. Smooth muscle relaxation in pregnancy due to progesterone causes dilation of the ureters, slowing of gastrointestinal motility and constipation, and possibly decreased peripheral vascular resistance. The premenstrual sensation of bloating may be a manifestation of distention due to the decrease in gastrointestinal motility.[47]

Progesterone binds to the mineralocorticoid receptor and is a mineralocorticoid antagonist, eliciting a diureticlike effect. However progesterone also is converted into the potent mineralocorticoid deoxycorticosterone (DOC) and peripheral DOC levels are elevated in parallel to progesterone during the cycle. The circulatory DOC arises from peripheral conversion of progesterone in tissues such as the kidney and aorta.[48]

Individual patients display marked fluctuations in weight during the cycle, but no study has shown a relationship between weight changes and other premenstrual symptoms. Rather there is a relationship between the subjective feeling of "water retention" and "bloatedness" and other premenstrual symptoms.

Premenstrually, patients subjectively describe increased bloatedness despite an absence of measurable increases in body weight, waist, or abdominal girth. In spite of this, patients with bloatedness complain of tight fitting clothing.[49]

Idiopathic edema, a condition seen more frequently in women, has been suggested to be caused by decreased dopaminergic tone acting on the adrenal, causing diminished orthostatic excretion of sodium.[50] A luteal phase decrease in vascular osmotic pressure causing increased interstitial space fluid has also been demonstrated.[51] It is unknown whether these latter changes are important determinants of bloatedness. It is difficult to demonstrate that patients who complain of premenstrual symptoms have different changes than those who are asymptomatic. For example, although there is a luteal phase increase in aldosterone there is no difference between controls and women with PMS.[52]

In a group of women who did not complain of any premenstrual symptoms but who were followed on a daily basis (without knowledge of the purpose of the study), the only symptom to reach statistical significance premenstrually was a feeling of water retention; no affective symptoms demonstrated significant cyclic variation.[53] It seems likely that women respond differently to this feeling of water retention, bloatedness, or not feeling comfortable in their clothes.[45]

Hormonal changes of the menstrual cycle result in other clinically apparent bodily changes, notably cyclic changes of the breast, vagina, endocervix (cervical mucus), and body temperature. Cyclic breast changes, for example, are often clearly perceived and at times premenstrual breast changes are disturbing.[54] During menstruation estrogen and progesterone levels are low and the breasts tend to be smaller and flattened laterally. As estrogen levels rise the nipples and areolae become more prominent, and there is rounding of the lateral aspects of the breast. The luteal phase rise in progesterone is associated with an exaggerated venous pattern of the breast surface, prominence of the Montgomery tubercles of the areola, and the breasts are fully rounded. Breast tenderness and swelling are common symptoms of PMS. The dopamine agonist bromocriptine or the androgen danazol often helps breast symptoms.

Allergy

A patient with cyclic premenstrual rashes was noted to have a possible IgG antibody with binding to progesterone and 17-hydroxyprogesterone.[55] Another patient had recurrent severe anaphylatic reactions that appeared to be related to estrogen or progesterone, and was relieved by GnRH agonist therapy, lactation, and oophorectomy.[56] Neither of these patients was described as having premenstrual somatic or affective symptoms. Furthermore, classic allergic reactions are not usually described in PMS patients. It is likely that progesterone allergy is the cause of only classic allergic symptoms in PMS.

Nutritional Theories

It is unlikely that dietary inadequacy is the cause of premenstrual changes or that dietary changes "cure" PMS. Rather, the patient who is sensitive to hormonal fluctuations—body awareness and emotional changes—may also be sensitive to the stimulatory effects of caffeine, the catecholamine rush secondary to the rise in insulin that occurs after the ingestion of sugar, and/or the effects of alcohol. Therefore, good nutrition, along with the avoidance of alcohol, caffeine, and free sugars, may result in improvement of symptoms.

Glucose Intolerance

Human placental lactogen is primarily responsible for the glucose intolerance observed during pregnancy. However, the high levels of progesterone in pregnancy also contribute to insulin resistance by decreasing cellular insulin receptors. This suggests that relative glucose intolerance might occur during the luteal phase.[57] If so, increased serum insulin concentration might explain the craving for carbohydrates or chocolates that many women experience. A recent study failed to demonstrate glucose intolerance during the luteal phase in normal women.[58] In addition, no differences in glucose tolerance were demonstrated between PMS subjects and normal women. Undoubtedly, food cravings are a normal part of many women's premenstrual phase; what relationship they have to PMS is unknown.

Pyridoxine Deficiency

Vitamin B$_6$ (pyridoxine) is a cofactor in the synthesis of serotonin, dopamine, and prostaglandins. Stress can cause hepatic breakdown of glycogen and depletion of hepatic vitamin B$_6$. Estrogen, by stimulating protein synthesis in the liver, may also deplete pyridoxine, and vitamin B$_6$ replacement has helped the depression of some women on oral contraceptives. However, recent studies have failed to find pyridoxine more effective than placebo in the treatment of PMS.[59] Sensory neuropathy has also been reported in patients treated with vitamin B$_6$.[60]

Magnesium Deficiency

Differences in serum magnesium between PMS patients and patients without PMS have been reported. Magnesium has a sedative effect on neuromuscular excitability. One study reported a reduced content of monocyte magnesium in the premenstrual phase of PMS patients. However, the range of data from PMS patients overlapped significantly with controls, and there was no evidence of differences in nutritional intake between PMS subjects and controls.[61] Another recent report noted that the zinc to copper ratio in the blood of PMS patients was decreased compared to controls; however, there was much overlap in data.[62] The results of these two studies are interesting, but must be taken as phenomena associated with PMS, not causally linked phenomena.

Serotonin Deficiency

Reducing serotonin activity in monkeys is associated with irritability and withdrawal from social activity. In one human study, whole blood serotonin levels were lower in a group of well-selected PMS sufferers.[63] Decreased luteal phase peripheral serotonin levels and decreased platelet uptake of serotonin have also been noted in PMS patients.[64] Fluoxetine, a serotonin reuptake blocker, is more effective than placebo in PMS.[65,66] However, administration of pyridoxine, a cofactor in serotonin synthesis, is generally ineffective for PMS.[59] Decreased serotonin activity may also contribute to the carbohydrate craving observed in PMS patients.[67] Moreover, d-fenfluramine, a medication that enhances central serotonin activity, significantly reduces carbohydrate craving and depression in PMS patients.[68] The relationship between serotonin and PMS clearly warrants investigation, both to document its existence and to confirm that serotonin changes are not due to depression or chronic anxiety.

Circadian Rhythm Disturbance

A central neural oscillator regulates circadian rhythms of rapid eye movement sleep, temperature, cortisol, and melatonin levels. Some patients with depression have disturbances in this pattern. Some animal studies found estrogen and progesterone to have opposing effects on the timing of these rhythms. One small study of melatonin, looking only at PMS patients with predominant premenstrual depressive symptoms, found differences in melatonin pattern and total release rates compared to normal controls.[69]

Preliminary studies also found that treatments that affect circadian physiology, such as sleep deprivation or bright light therapy, help some women with premenstrual syndrome. This preliminary information suggests that certain PMS patients may have an abnormal circadian pattern.[69]

Learned Event

There is no doubt that chemical and physical changes occur over the menstrual cycle which women perceive to be cyclic. Even among women not complaining of PMS symptoms, a statistically significant increase in feelings of premenstrual water retention occurs. This sensation may be due to changes in fluid retention or even to a decrease in gastrointestinal motility. Undoubtedly, most women are aware of premenstrual changes distinct from prostaglandin-mediated menstrual cramps and gastrointestinal symptoms. For some patients, affective symptoms may be related to distress over physical changes. For example, women who are very sensitive to their body image, or who have poor self-esteem, are more likely to be distressed by the feeling of bloating or swelling. Furthermore, the cues of the menstrual cycle and the experiences of previous cycles are learned events that can lead women to complain of physical symptoms such as water retention.[70] There is little doubt that premenstrual affective symptoms are modified by concomitant emotional stress.

In a recent study a small amount of the antiprogestational agent mifepristone was administered in the midluteal phase to induce menses in PMS subjects, while serum progesterone levels were maintained with exogenous HCG injections. The induction of menstruation did not relieve the subjects' PMS symptoms. This suggests that an early menstrual flow is not sufficient for removing PMS symptoms.[16]

SUMMARY

More than 100 symptoms are described as part of the premenstrual syndrome, illustrating the variety of cyclic hormonal events. The pulsatility of GnRH, the changes of midcycle LH, and most importantly the fluctuation in gonadal steroids cause a multitude of multisystem changes. These so-called normal changes may interact with other underlying psychological, social, or medical problems of an individual woman to produce the symptoms of what we call PMS. The observation that major affective diseases may worsen during the premenstrual phase, and situational stress can exaggerate premenstrual complaints, underlies the difficulty in pinpointing a precise etiology. Rather, premenstrual syndrome is a complex interaction of the above. Changes in gonadal steroids may be more important than the actual level of steroids. Affective and physical symptoms are likely related to central and peripheral effects of these hormonal fluctuations.

REFERENCES

1. Roy-Byrne PP, Hoban MC, Rubinow DR. The relationship of menstrually related mood disorders to psychiatric disorders. *Clin Obstet Gynecol*. 1987;30:386.
2. York R, Freeman E, Lowery B, et al. Characterization of premenstrual syndrome. *Obstet Gynecol*. 1989;73:601.
3. Rickels V, Hall W, Best F, et al. Prostaglandins in endometrium and menstrual fluid from normal and dysmenorrheic subjects. *Br J Obstet Gynaecol*. 1965;72:185.
4. Smith S, Schiff I. The premenstrual syndrome—diagnosis and management. *Fertil Steril*. 1989;52:527.
5. Irwin J, Morse G, Riddick D. Dysmenorrhea induced by autologous transfusion. *Obstet Gynecol*. 1981;58:286.
6. Andersch B, Hahn L. Premenstrual complaints. II. Influence of oral contraceptives. *Acta Obstet Gynecol Scand*. 1981;60:579.
7. Herzberg B, Coppen A. Changes in psychological symptoms in women taking oral contraceptives. *Br J Psychiatry*. 1970;116:161.
8. Rubinow Dr, Hoban MC, Grover GN, et al. Changes in plasma hormones across the menstrual cycle in patients with menstrually related mood disorder and in control subjects. *Am J Obstet Gynecol*. 1988;158:5.
9. Reid RL. Premenstrual syndrome (editorial). *N Engl J Med*. 1991;324:1208.
10. Freeman EW, Sondheimer S, Weinbaum PJ, et al. Evaluating premenstrual symptoms in medical practice. *Obstet Gynecol*. 1985;65:500.
11. Sherwin B, Gelfand M. Differential symptoms response to parenteral and/or androgen administration in the surgical menopause. *Am J Obstet Gynecol*. 1985;152:153.
12. Schiff I, Regestein Q, Tulchinsky D, et al. Effects of estrogens on sleep and psychological state of hypogonadal women. *JAMA*. 1979;242:2405.
13. Gorski J. Welshons WV, Sakai D, et al. Evolution of a model of estrogen action. *Rec Prog Hor Res*. 1986;42:297.
14. Mcewen BS. Actions of sex hormones on the brain: organization and activation in relation to functional teratology. *Prog Brain Res*. 1988;73:121.
15. Villanueva AL, Schlosser C, Hopper B, et al. Increased cortisol production in women runners. *J Clin Endocrinol Metab*. 1986;63:133.
16. Schmidt PJ, Neiman LK, Grover GN, et al. Lack of effect of induced menses on symptoms in women with premenstrual syndrome. *N Engl J Med*. 1991;324:1174.
17. Li TC, Dockery P, Thomas P, et al. The effects of progesterone receptor blockage in the luteal phase of normal fertile women. *Fertil Steril*. 1988;50:732.
18. Muse KN, Cetal NS, Futterman LA, et al. The premenstrual syndrome: effects of "medical ovariectomy." *N Engl J Med*. 1984;311:1345.
19. Casson P, Hahn PM, VanVogt DA, et al. Lasting response to ovariectomy in severe intractable premenstrual syndrome. *Am J Obstet Gynecol*. 1990;162:99.
20. Mortola JF, Girton L, Fischer L. Successful treatment of severe premenstrual syndrome by combined use of gonadotropin-releasing hormone agonist and estrogen/progestin. *J Clin Endo Metab*. 1991;72:252A.
21. DeVane GW. Editorial: Premenstrual syndrome. *J Clin Endo Metab*. 1991;72:250.
22. ElSayed AS, Hargrove JT, Maxson WS, et al. Sedative and hypnotic effects of oral administration of micronized progesterone may be mediated through its metabolites. *Am J Obstet Gynecol*. 1988;159:1203.
23. Freeman EW, Rickels K, Sondheimer SJ, et al. Ineffectiveness of progesterone suppository treatment for premenstrual syndrome. *JAMA*. 1990;264:249.
24. Freeman EF, Weinstock L, Rickels K, et al. A placebo-controlled study of effects of oral progesterone on performance and mood. Submitted for publication.
25. Majewska MD, Harrison NL, Schwartz RD, et al. Steroid hormone metabolites are barbituate-like mediators of the GABA receptor. *Science*. 1986;232:1004.
26. Smith SS, Waterhouse BD, Chapin JK, et al. Progesterone alters GABA and glutamate responsiveness: a possible mechanism for its anxiolytic action. *Brain Res*. 1987;400:353.
27. Gold PW, Goodwin FK, Chrousos GP. Clinical and biochemical manifestations of depression: relation to the neurobiology of stress. *N Engl J Med*. 1988;319:348, 413.
28. Gold PW, Gwirtsman H, Avergerinos PC, et al. Abnormal hypothalamic-pituitary-adrenal function in anorexia nervosa. *N Engl J Med*. 1986;314:1335.
29. Gold PW, Loriaux L, Roy A, et al. Responses to corticotropin-releasing hormone in the hypercortisolism of depression and Cushing's disease. *N Engl J Med*. 1986;314:1329.
30. Mortola JF, Girton L, Yen SSC. Depressive episodes in premenstrual syndrome. *Am J Obstet Gynecol*. 1989;161:1682.
31. Kalogeras KT, Calogero AE, Kuribayiashi T, et al. In vitro and in vivo effects of the triazolobenzodiazepine alprazolam on hypothalamic-pituitary-adrenal function: pharmacologic and clinical implications. *J Clin Endocrinol Metab*. 1990;70:1462.
32. Smith S, Rinehart JS, Ruddock VE, et al. Treatment of premenstrual syndrome with alprazolam: results of a double-blind, placebo-controlled, randomized crossover clinical trial. *Obstet Gynecol*. 1987;70:37.
33. Rabin DS, Schmidt PJ, Campbell G, et al. Hypothalamic-pituitary-adrenal function in patients with the premenstrual syndrome. *J Clin Endocrinol Metab*. 1990;71:1158.
34. Sondheimer SJ, Freeman EW, Scharlop B, et al. Hormonal changes in premenstrual syndrome. *Psychosomatics*. 1985;26:10.
35. Liu JH, Rasmussen DD, Rivier J, et al. Pituitary responses to synthetic CRH: absence of modulating effect by estrogen and progestin. *Am J Obstet Gynecol*. 1987;157:1387.
36. Seifer DB, Collins RL. Current concepts of β-endorphin physiology in female reproductive dysfunction. *Fertil Steril*. 1990;54:757.
37. Quigley ME, Yen SSC. The role of endogenous opiates on LH secretion during the menstrual cycle. *J Clin Endocrinol Metab*. 1980;51:179.
38. Kalra SP, Simpkins JW. Evidence for noradrenergic mediation of opioid effects on luteinizing hormone secretion. *Endocrinology*. 1981;109:776.
39. Reid RL, Yen SSC. Premenstrual syndrome. *Am J Obstet Gynecol*. 1981;139:85.
40. Chuong CJ, Coulam CB, Kao PC, et al. Neuropeptide levels in premenstrual syndrome. *Fertil Steril*. 1985;44:760.
41. Giannini AJ, Sullivan B, Sarachene J, et al. Clonidine in the treatment of premenstrual syndrome: a sub-group study. *J Clin Psychiatry*. 1988;49:62.
42. Choung CJ, Coulam CB, Bergstralh EJ, et al. Clinical trial of naltrexone in premenstrual syndrome. *Obstet Gynecol*. 1988;72:332.
43. Steiner M, Haskett RF, Carroll BJ, et al. Plasma prolactin and

severe premenstrual tension. *Psychoneuroendocrinology.* 1984;9: 29.

44. Nikolai TF, Mulligan GM, Gribble RK, et al. Thyroid function and treatment in premenstrual syndrome. *J Clin Endocrinol Metab.* 1990;70:1108.

45. Roy-Byrne PP, Rubinow DR, Hoban MC, et al. TSH and prolactin responses to TRH in patients with premenstrual syndrome. *Am J Psychiatry.* 1987;144:480.

46. Casper RF, Patel-Christopher H, Powel AM. Thyrotropin and prolactin responses to TRH in PMS. *J Clin Endocrinol Metab.* 1989;68:608.

47. Wald A, Vanthiel D, Hoechstetter O, et al. Gastrointestinal treatment: the effect of the menstrual cycle. *Gastroenterology.* 1981; 80:1497.

48. Antonipillai I, Moghissi E, Howks D, et al. The origin of plasma deoxycorticosterone in men and in women during the menstrual cycle. *J Clin Endocrinol Metab.* 1983;56:93.

49. Farratian B, Gaspar A, O'Brien PMS, et al. Premenstrual syndrome: weight, abdominal swelling and perceived body image. *Am J Obstet Gynecol.* 1984;150:200.

50. Sowers J, Beck F, Berg G. Altered dopaminergic modulation of 18-hydroxycorticosterone secretion in idiopathic edema: therapeutic effect of bromocriptine. *J Clin Endocrinol Metab.* 1982;55: 749.

51. Qian P, Tollan A, Fadnes HO, et al. Transcapillary fluid dynamics during the menstrual cycle. *Am J Obstet Gynecol.* 1987;156: 952.

52. O'Brien PMS, Craven D, Selby D, et al. Treatment of premenstrual syndrome by spironolactone. *Br J Obstet Gynecol.* 1979;86: 142.

53. Laymeyer HW, Miller M, DeLeon-Jones F. Anxiety and mood fluctuation during the normal menstrual cycle. *Psychosom Med.* 1982;44:183.

54. Bates GW, Garza D, Garza M. Clinical manifestation of hormonal changes in the menstrual cycle. *Obstet Gynecol Clin North Am.* 1990;17:299.

55. Cheesman K, Gaynor L, Chatterton R, et al. Identification of a 17-hydroxyprogesterone binding immunoglobulin in the serum of a woman with periodic rashes. *J Clin Endocrinol Metab.* 1982;55: 597.

56. Meggs WJ, Pescouitx OH, Metcalfe D, et al. Progesterone sensi-tivity as a cause of recurrent anaphylaxis. *N Engl J Med.* 1984; 311:1236.

57. DePirro R, Fusco H, Bertoli A, et al. Insulin receptors during the menstrual cycle in normal women. *J Clin Endocrinol Metab.* 1978;47:1387.

58. Spellacy WN, Ellingson AB, Keith G, et al. Plasma glucose and insulin levels during the menstrual cycles of normal women and premenstrual syndrome patients. *J Reprod Med.* 1990;35:508.

59. Kleijnen J, Riet GT, Knipschild P. Vitamin B6 in the treatment of the premenstrual syndrome. *Br J Obstet Gynaecol.* 1990;97: 847.

60. Schaumberg H, Kaplan J, Windebank A, et al. Sensory neuropathy from pyridoxine abuse: a new megavitamin syndrome. *N Engl J Med.* 1983;309:445.

61. Facchinetti F, Borella P, Fioroni L, et al. Reduction of monocyte magnesium in patients affected by premenstrual syndrome. *Psychosom Obstet Gynecol.* 1990;11:221.

62. Choung CJ, Dawson EB, Smith ER. Zinc levels in premenstrual syndrome. Program of the 46th Annual Meeting of the American Fertility Society, October 13–18, 1990, Washington, DC.

63. Rapkin A, Edelmuth E, Chang LC, et al. Whole blood serotonin in premenstrual syndrome. *Obstet Gynecol.* 1987;70:533.

64. Taylor DL, Matthew RJ, Beng TH, et al. Serotonin levels and platelets uptake during premenstrual tension. *Neuropsychobiolgoy.* 1984;12:16.

65. Rickels K, Freeman E, Sondheimer S, et al. Fluoxetine in the treatment of premenstrual syndrome. *Curr Ther Res* 1990;48:161.

66. Wood SH, Mortola J, Chan Y, et al. Treatment of premenstrual syndrome with fluoxetine: a double-blind, placebo-controlled, crossover study. *Obstet Gynecol.* 1992;80:339.

67. Wurtman RJ, Wurtman JJ. Carbohydrates and depression. *Sci Am.* 1989;260:68.

68. Brzezinski AA, Wurtman JJ, Wurtman RJ, et al. D-Fenfluramine suppresses the increased calorie and carbohydrate intakes and improves the mood of women with premenstrual depression. *Obstet Gynecol.* 1990;76:296.

69. Parry BL, Berga SL, Kripke DF, et al. Altered waveform of plasma nocturnal melatonin secretion in premenstrual depression. *Arch Gen Psychiatry.* 1990;47:1139.

70. Ruble DN. Premenstrual symptoms: a reinterpretation. *Science.* 1977;197:291.

CHAPTER 6

Brain Neurochemistry and Mood

David L. Keefe and Frederick Naftolin

Elucidation of the neurobiological basis of mood holds great promise for millions of people who suffer from disorders of its regulation, yet presents a formidable challenge to basic and clinical neuroscientists. The sensitivity of mood to psychological and social forces has led some investigators to question whether mood has its origin within the mind or the brain. While the debate over "soft" vs "hard-wiring" of mood remains unsettled, since the time of Hippocrates investigators have invoked physiological theories to explain the etiology and pathophysiology of mood disorders.[1] Freud, himself trained as a neurologist, initially sought a physical mechanism to explain psychiatric disorder,[2] but not until recently has experimental evidence accumulated in support of the idea that "twisted molecules" underlie "twisted moods." This chapter reviews the major neurobiological theories of mood disorder and explores the role ovarian steroids might play in each.

BIOLOGIC BASIS OF MOOD

Most research on the biological basis of mood has involved subjects suffering from major affective disorders.[3] The major affective disorders include major depression and bipolar mood disorder. Major depressive illness in humans is characterized by episodes of sadness, feelings of helplessness, pervasive loss of inter-

est or pleasure, sleep disturbances with hypersomnia, insomnia or early awakening, motor retardation, feelings of guilt or worthlessness, and thoughts of death or suicide. The other major affective disorder, bipolar disorder, differs from major depression only by whether the patient also has experienced a manic episode, characterized by elevated mood, grandiosity, excessive involvement in activities with a high potential for painful consequences, decreased sleep, increased activity, pressured speech, talkativeness, and flight of ideas. The neurobiological basis of premenstrual mood disorders has been much less studied. However, since symptoms of mood disorder respond to ovarian steroids,[4] some patients suffer premenstrual exacerbation of their symptoms, and women with premenstrual syndrome have a high prevalence of mood disorder; the two conditions may involve related neurobiological mechanisms.[5]

Research on the neurobiological basis of mood disorders has uncovered disorders of: (1) neurotransmission, (2) receptor function, (3) intracellular signal transduction, (4) psychophysiology, including sleep architecture, (5) biological rhythms, and (6) brain structure, especially hemispheric dominance. Although clinical study of the effects of ovarian steroids on these parameters has been limited, basic research shows that ovarian steroids can influence practically every one of these systems. In addition, recent studies on the neurobiological basis of steroid action within the central nervous system have uncovered a number of steroid-sensitive brain mechanisms that could underlie sex steroid modulation of mood, and possibly elucidate the biological basis of premenstrual syndrome and sex differences in the incidence of mood disorders.

Limbic Brain Structures Regulate Mood

Identification of specific areas of the brain that regulate mood has proven critical to the development of modern neurobiological theories of mood disorders. The role of limbic brain structures in the regulation of mood has gained the most attention[6] (Fig. 1). The limbic system includes the amygdala, hippocampus, and parahippocampal gyrus (which form part of the temporal lobes), hypothalamus, thalamus, mammillary bodies, septum pellucidum, cingulate cortex, and cingulum. These evolutionarily primitive brain structures regulate many physiological systems affected by mood disorder, including sleep, circadian rhythms, appetite, libido, and neuroendocrine activity. Stimulation or lesioning of these structures, either by disease or experimental manipulation, influences mood, as well as autonomic functioning in humans and in most animal species. Perhaps the most convincing demonstration of the importance of limbic structures in mood emerged from the experiments of the neurosurgeon W. Penfield, who elicited specific emotions, such as fear and joy, by stimulating specific areas of the medial temporal cortex at the time of surgery.[7] Clinical observations of patients with tumors or cerebrovascular accidents affecting the temporal lobe who show altered emotionality provided further evidence of the importance of these structures in the regulation of mood. Experimental lesions or stimulation of homologous areas in animals produce changes in behavior that are consistent with altered emotionality. Humans with temporal lobe epilepsy, who presumably experience chronic temporal lobe stimulation from their epileptic focus, often present with altered mood and behavior.[8] As will be discussed below, receptors for ovarian steroid hormone are abundant in the limbic structures of the brain.

Mechanisms of Action of Steroid Hormones

The ubiquitous effects of ovarian steroids on the central nervous system (CNS) and on mood should come as no surprise, since these molecules and their receptors are widely distributed throughout the brain, with the highest concentrations in the phylogenetically ancient limbic system.[9,10,11] Studies in experimental animals, including nonhuman primates and humans, have identi-

Fig. 1   This schematic representation of the limbic system shows how structures from the cerebral hemispheres and diencephalon form a neural circuit. This neural circuit, which is highly conserved among vertebrate species, is thought to underlie many aspects of emotion. Stimulation or lesions of components of the circuit either experimentally or by disease processes alters emotionality, sexuality, and aggression. (Adapted from Kolb B, Whishaw IQ. *Fundamentals of Human Neuropsychology,* 3rd ed. San Francisco: Freeman; 1980, 1985, and 1990, with permission.)

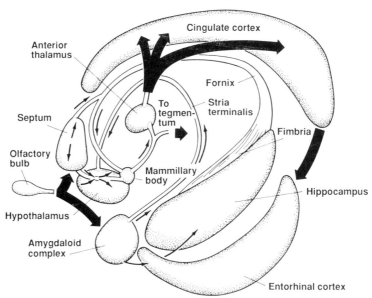

fied estrogen and progesterone receptors in the brain by a variety of methods, including competitive binding assays, immunohistochemistry, and in situ hybridization. Studies combining autoradiography to detect steroid receptors with neuroanatomical tract tracing reveal that steroid-concentrating cells send axons to many other parts of the brain. Thus, steroids may influence not only neurons bearing their specific receptors, but also a broad spectrum of neurons synapsing with steroid receptor-containing neurons.

The identification and characterization of cDNAs encoding all of the known steroid hormone receptors revealed that estrogen and progesterone receptors are members of the steroid receptor superfamily.[12,13,14] Steroid receptors function as ligand-dependent transcription factors; that is when hormone binds to unoccupied receptor, the receptor undergoes change in its conformation which allows the complex to bind to specific DNA sequences, called hormone response elements (HREs), upstream of steroid-sensitive genes. HREs then regulate transcription of steroid-sensitive genes. Some of these steroid-sensitive genes in turn may regulate the transcription of other genes, whose protein products themselves regulate transcription (eg, adenylate cyclase and the proto-oncogenes c-*myc*, c-*fos*-, and c-*jun*), so that the steroid–receptor complex can initiate a cascade of regulatory events within the cell.[15] While many of these mechanisms originally were elucidated in nonneural systems, steroid receptors within the CNS probably act in a similar manner.

Clearly, the transcriptional regulatory activity of the steroid hormone–receptor complex provides the most complete model of steroid hormone action, yet a growing body of data suggests that steroid hormones also can act independently of their receptors. Some steroid actions appear so rapidly after administration of the hormone that transcriptional regulation becomes unlikely, such as when estrogen exerts immediate effects on neuronal firing,[16] while transcription of early-response genes begins only minutes to hours later.[15] Other evidence supports the existence of specific binding sites for estrogen and progesterone within cell membranes, a part of the cell that has never been shown by immunohistochemistry to contain steroid receptors. Membrane localization of steroid binding sites may explain how progesterone, covalently bound to bovine serum albumin to prevent its binding to nuclear receptor, does not eliminate its effect on some neurons within the central nervous system.[17] Similarly, glial cells that do not contain detectable levels of steroid receptors by competitive binding assay,[18] immunohistochemistry or in situ hybridization,[10] do bind fluorescein-conjugated

estradiol in an extranuclear site.[19] Finally, steroid hormones may act in vitro in a reconstituted system lacking steroid receptors. For example, estrogen influences the activity of an enzyme, protein disulfide isomerase (PDI), in an vitro assay system.[20] Interestingly, the primary structure of PDI contains a region homologous with the estrogen-binding domain of the estrogen receptor, suggesting that the phylogenetically ancient steroid binding motif may have emerged in genes otherwise not related to the steroid receptor superfamily.

Cellular Organization of the Central Nervous System

Function within the CNS depends on cellular structure. The basic structural units within the brain consist of two broad classes of cells called neurons and glia. While neurons vary in size and shape, the prototypical neuron consists of a cell body and a number of projections called dendrites and axons (Fig. 2). The membrane of neurons contains a number of ion pumps, exchangers, and channels that maintain an electrical potential across the cell membrane.[21] Neurons transmit electrical signals as waves of membrane depolarization that propagate across dendrites to axons. Communication takes place between neurons when electrical impulses in the axon terminal induce release of neurotransmitters into the synaptic cleft. Neurotransmitters travel across the synaptic cleft and bind to highly selective receptors located on the postsynaptic neurons. Receptors on the presynaptic terminal, called autoreceptors, also bind neurotransmitters, and regulate the rate of presynaptic release of neurotransmitters. Binding of excitatory neurotransmitters to their receptors depolarize, and thereby activate the receiving neuron, while inhibitory neurotransmitters hyperpolarize, and thereby inhibit the receiving neuron. Some receptors directly influence the permeability of ion channels located on the neuronal membranes, while others interact with one or more intracellular signal transduction pathways. Specific transporters take up unbound neurotransmitter remaining in the synaptic cleft, then enzymes located on the pre or postsynaptic synapse or in neighboring glia metabolize the neurotransmitter molecules. The cDNAs for many of the molecules involved in these processes have been cloned and sequenced, enabling ever more precise understanding of the workings of the brain.[22] As will be discussed below, mood disorders may arise from abnormalities in one or a number of these steps in neurotransmission. Ovarian steroids influence many of the same neural networks

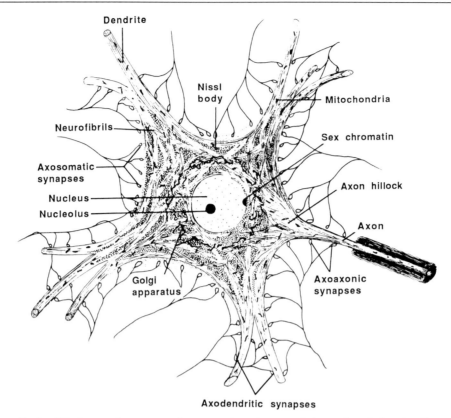

Fig. 2   This diagram of a representative neuron shows how morphology reflects its function. The cytoskeleton stabilizes its polarized shape, enabling axons to project to and synapse with distant neurons. The neuron itself also receives many synapses, thus enabling a high level of intercellular communication. (Reprinted from Barr ML. *The Human Nervous System,* 2nd ed. New York: Harper and Row; 1974, with permission.)

implicated in mood disorders by altering neurotransmitter synthesis and release, membrane depolarization, channel activity, receptor number, neurotransmitter uptake, and metabolism. Such neural actions of ovarian steroids may explain in part the reported sex differences in the incidence of mood disorders and effects of ovarian sex steroids on mood.

A second group of cells called glia carry out many structural and homeostatic functions in support of neurons.[23] Glial cells include astrocytes, oligodendrocytes, and microglia (Fig. 3). Processes from astrocytes ensheath synapses and neurons, and contribute to the blood–brain barrier. Equipped with a rich supply of metabolic enzymes, they buffer the neuronal and synaptic environments by taking up potassium and hydrogen ions, as well as neurotransmitters such as glutamate. Oligodendrocytes surround and insulate axons, and microglia, derivatives of macrophages, mediate the inflammatory response within the brain. While most studies of steroid action within the CNS have focused on

neurons, recent studies demonstrate that steroids can alter the morphology of, and induce enzymes in glia.[19] Some glia even themselves synthesize steroid hormones.[24] The physiological role of such "neurosteroids" and their relationship to other steroid metabolic enzymes within the brain remain incompletely understood.

Molecular and Cellular Basis of Steroid Action on Behavior

Just how steroid-induced changes in cellular activity translate into changes in behavior for the most part remains poorly understood, possibly with the exception of reproductive behavior in rodents.[25] During the ovarian cycle in many species the sequential secretion of estrogen and progesterone from the ovary activates a stereotypical behavior in females characterized by receptivity to the male (lordosis). High doses of estra-

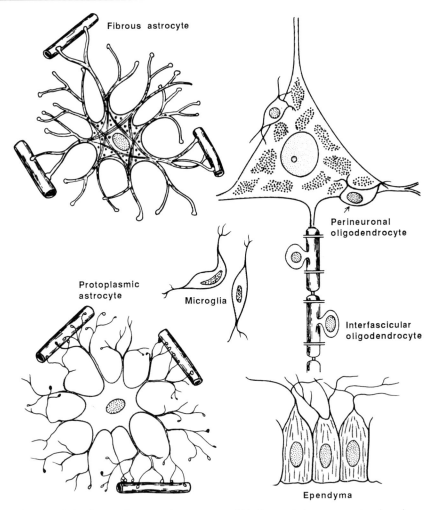

Fig. 3 Glial cells actually outnumber neurons within the central nervous system by a large margin. Previously thought to serve only support functions, glial cells are shown in recent studies to carry out many important physiologic functions, including regulating neuronal migration and synaptogenesis during development, uptake of neurotransmitters, and regulation of ion and pH homeostasis. Glia include astrocytes, which may be fibrous or protoplasmic, microglia, oligodendrocytes, and ependyma. (Reprinted from Barr ML. *The Human Nervous System,* 2nd ed. New York: Harper and Row; 1974, with permission.)

diol activate this same response in ovariectomized rats, but progesterone administered 24 to 48 hours after estradiol (E2) has a synergistic effect with increased intensity of the lordotic response and decreased requirement for E2. During other phases of the ovarian cycle the female refuses the male, and in some species becomes increasingly aggressive. Such behavioral actions of gonadal steroids serve important functions in the reproductive strategies of many species in that they increase the probability of mating during the periovulatory phase. Essentially the entire circuitry necessary for this behavior in rodents, from

brain to pelvic muscles, has been elucidated using techniques of experimental neuroanatomy and neurophysiology, such as lesioning, autoradiography, tract-tracing, and electrical stimulation. These studies show that specific areas of the diencephalon (the ventromedial nucleus and the medial preoptic area) play important roles in regulating female sexual behavior. Both of these areas contain high levels of estrogen and progesterone receptors.[26] Furthermore, estrogen induces progesterone receptors in these areas, which may explain in part the synergistic effects of the hormones in lordosis itself. At this time it is not clear whether steroid-induced behavioral and mood changes in humans involve analogous neural mechanisms.

Methodologic Issues in Neurobiologic Studies of Mood

While rapid advances in basic neurobiology hold great promise for expanding our understanding of the neurobiologic basis of psychiatric disease, the inaccessibility of the living human brain to study by molecular and cell biological methods has prompted clinical investigators to employ a number of indirect methods. One of the most fruitful approaches to the clinical investigation of mood has been to measure neurotransmitter metabolites and/or the enzymes involved in neurotransmitter metabolism in a number of bodily fluids. After a neurotransmitter is metabolized, it is excreted into cerebrospinal fluid (CSF), blood, or urine.[27] Measurements of these metabolites can then be compared between normal controls and affected subjects or in individual subjects in their normal versus affected states. A second approach studies the pharmacological actions of drugs known to influence mood disorders. By determining which mechanisms are shared by such drugs, one can infer about possible mechanisms involved in the regulation of mood. A third approach studies receptor number and sensitivity in human autopsy material, circulating platelets, or animal models, reasoning that mood disorders may involve widespread abnormalities in receptor function. Still other approaches employ neuroendocrine testing,[28] since mood disorders frequently are associated with endocrinopathies (eg, thyroid, Cushings, and Addison's diseases) and/or hormone therapies (eg, ACTH, glucocorticoid therapy), and peptide hypothalamic releasing hormones are themselves regulated by neurotransmitters in the CNS, suggesting they may serve as markers of CNS neurotransmitter function. Psychophysiological studies employ polysomnography to evaluate sleep and other biological rhythms in patients with mood disorder.[29] An approach still in its infancy uses recent advances in brain imaging, such as positron emission tomography (PET)[30,31] and magnetic resonance spectroscopy,[32] to study neurochemistry and metabolism in living subjects. Many radioactive receptor ligands currently in development may enable direct measurement of receptor function and neurotransmitter turnover in specific areas of the brain in vivo. Other imaging systems, such as computed axial tomography (CT) and magnetic resonance imaging, measure brain structures in living subjects with great accuracy, enabling studies of morphologic correlates of affective disease. A final avenue of research on human mood disorders employs animal and in vitro models to mimic components of mood disorders.[33] Applications of such experimental models include evaluation of drug therapies, and isolation of individual behaviors that are too complex for experimental analysis in humans, such as disruption of attachment bonds in nonhuman primates, which produces many behavioral changes associated with human depression, and pharmacologic models in rodent and primate species, which reproduce some neurochemical changes seen in human depression.

NEUROBIOLOGIC THEORIES OF MOOD DISORDER

The various approaches to clinical investigation of mood disturbance have generated a large number of theories about its etiology and pathophysiology. Some theories of mood disorder propose abnormalities in the function of classical neurotransmitters, which include serotonin, acetylcholine, and the catecholamines (norepinephrine, epinephrine, and dopamine). Other theories propose abnormalities in neuropeptide function, sleep, circadian organization, or brain structure, especially hemispheric dominance.

Catecholamine Theory of Affective Disorder

The catecholamine theory of affective disorder, while still quite speculative, has been studied most extensively.[34] This hypothesis states that depression results from deficiency, while mania results from excess of norephinephrine at central receptors. A variation of this theory proposes that dysfunction of the catecholamine receptor underlies affective disorder.

The catecholamine hypothesis arose out of observations on the effects of various monoamine oxidase inhibitors (MAOIs) (eg, iproniazid) on mood when these drugs were first administered for treatment of tuberculosis. Other studies demonstrated the capacity of MAOIs to increase brain amine levels. Subsequent studies showed that many drugs that deplete brain catecholamines, such as the antihypertensive agent reserpine, can produce depressive episodes which are clinically indistinguishable from major depressive disorder. Administration of these pharmacologic agents to animals produces behavioral changes that mimic many aspects of depression in humans. Administration of l-dopa, a precursor of catecholamine biosynthesis, reverses reserpine-induced symptoms in animals. This hypothesis received further support from findings that structurally diverse drugs which have antidepressant activity share the ability to block reuptake of norepinephrine, and therefore increase the availability of this catecholamine at the synapse. Many of these drugs, such as tricyclic antidepressants (TCAs) and MAOIs, even trigger mania in predisposed individuals. Other drugs that produce depression as a side effect also affect catecholamine function, although these drugs tend to reduce noradrenergic activity by a variety of mechanisms; for example, reserpine depletes synaptic NE, methyldopa replaces catecholamine with a false neurotransmitter, and propranolol blocks beta-adrenergic receptors.

These chemical and pharmacologic findings led to clinical investigation of the metabolites of norepinephrine in depressed individuals.[35] While norepinephrine and epinephrine do not readily cross the blood–brain barrier, their major metabolite in the brain, 3-methoxy-4-hydroxyphenylglycol (MHPG), appears in the circulation of urine and CSF in its free form. Cross-sectional studies show a subset of depressed patients who have decreased levels of urinary MHPG compared to controls. Longitudinal studies of urinary MHPG in patients with bipolar affective disorder demonstrate that during depressive episodes urinary MHPG levels drop compared to levels measured during manic phases or after recovery from depression. Urinary MHPG values may also predict the response of the depressive episode to specific antidepressants.

Interpretation of these results has been limited because only 20% to 65% of circulating MHPG derives from the brain, MHPG itself may be further metabolized, and MHPG levels measured in CSF may represent metabolites from spinal cord rather than brain neurons. Further difficulty with the catecholamine hypothesis of mood disorders arises from the finding that some agents that inhibit catecholamine reuptake function poorly as antidepressants, such as cocaine, while other agents with no effect on catecholamine uptake (eg, iprandole) function well as antidepressants. Furthermore, while blockade of catecholamine reuptake appears immediately after administration of antidepressants, their antidepressant effects require several weeks of continuous administration.

Clinical data, coupled with studies from basic pharmacology showing that release of neurotransmitters from axon terminals is in part controlled by autoreceptors, led to studies of long-term changes in receptor number and sensitivity of receptors to agonist and antagonists. Autoreceptors, also known as alpha-2-adrenergic

receptors, reside on the presynaptic component of the synapse.[36] Binding of neurotransmitter to alpha-2 receptors inhibits the rate of norepinephrine synthesis and release by the presynaptic bouton, and thus provides a feedback loop that regulates synaptic firing. The autoreceptor hypothesis proposes that depression results from supersensitivity of this receptor, which results in decreased catecholamine release into the synapse. In support of this hypothesis are the findings that antidepressants decrease sensitivity of autoreceptors in vitro, and that they do so only after 2 to 3 weeks of continuous treatment in vivo, the same duration required for clinical improvement to become apparent. Chronic administration of any of a number of structurally diverse antidepressants (heterocyclic antidepressants and MAOIs) also attenuates the suppression of noradrenergic neuron firing rate and MHPG levels that occur after administration of an alpha-2 agonist, such as clonidine. Chronic treatment with the MAOI clorgyline also decreases binding of [3H]clonidine to alpha-2 receptors. Changes in alpha-2 receptor sensitivity appear in some drug-free depressed patients who have decreased urine MHPG levels and increased suppression of plasma MHPG in response to clonidine.

Alpha-2 receptors appear not only in neurons, but also in circulating platelets, where they can be more readily measured. Some depressed patients have higher levels of platelet alpha-2 receptors, and antidepressant therapy decreases platelet alpha-2 receptor number. Labeling of alpha-2 receptors with the alpha-2 antagonist [3-H]yohimbine also reveals increased alpha-2 receptors in depressed patients compared to normal controls.

Ovarian Steroid Effects on Catecholamines and Their Receptors

Ovarian steroids influence catecholamine function at a number of steps including synthesis, release, uptake, metabolism, and receptor activation. Some neurons in the diencephalon contain estrogen and progestin receptors, as well as tyrosine hydroxylase, the rate-limiting enzyme in the synthesis of catecholamines.[37] Such colocalization suggests that gonadal steroids play a role in the activity of these neurons. Estradiol decreases MAO[38] and tyrosine hydroxylase[39] activity in some diencephalic nuclei, which suggests that it can differentially regulate catecholamine synthesis and degradation. Estrogen-induced increases in norepinephrine turnover and content reported in some diencephalic nuclei, and blockade of labeled norepinephrine uptake into synaptosomes also suggest an overall stimulation of norepinephrine activity by estrogen.

Estrogen has effects on adrenergic receptors as well. In general, estrogen increases the number of beta- and alpha-1-adrenergic receptors, although some differences exist in different regions of the brain, since it also decreases beta-adrenergic receptors in cortex.[40] Such estrogen-induced effects on adrenergic receptors may explain how estrogen increases the number of neurons responding to norepinephrine, as measured by electrophysiological recording.

The metabolism of estrogen produces 2- and 4-hydroxy estrogens, also called catechol estrogens, which share enough structural features with catecholamines[41] so that they compete with catecholamines in serving as substrates for catechol-o-methyl transferase, an enzyme involved in the degradation of catecholamines, and thus indirectly influence catecholaminergic activity. Interestingly, formation of some catechol estrogens from estrogens is catalyzed by peroxidases,[42] and peroxidase activity itself is induced by estrogen in parts of the diencephalon.[19,43] Since formation of catechol estrogens forms toxic free radical intermediates, such a positive feedback loop could explain formation of neuropathologic lesions observed in some areas of rodent brain after high doses and/or prolonged administration of unopposed estrogen.[19,43] Dopamine also may influence directly the activity of some steroid receptors, perhaps by second messenger-induced phosphorylation of the steroid receptor, demonstrating that "cross-talk" between amine and steroid receptors may take place within cells.[44]

Serotonin and Mood Disorders

A growing body of evidence suggests that altered serotonergic activity may underlie mood disorders in some patients.[45] Both hypofunction and hyperfunction of serotonin neurotransmission have been proposed to underlie depression. Tryptophan, the precursor to serotonin (5-hydroxytryptamine or 5-HT), as well as the principal metabolite of serotonin, 5-hydroxyindolacetic acid (5-HIAA) are reduced in the CSF of some depressed individuals, and in the brains of postmortem suicide victims with a history of depression. Antidepressants increase 5-HT receptor sensitivity and neurotransmission as determined by neuroendocrine challenge tests and electrophysiological recording studies. Drugs that deplete 5-HT induce depression in humans and a depression-like syndrome in animals.

Findings supportive of 5-HT hyperfunction include decreased binding of [3H]imipramine to the regulatory site of the serotonin transporter, and decreased [3H]5HT reuptake in platelets and in autopsied brain

specimens, defects that would tend to increase the availability of 5-HT for its receptor.[46]

Other studies suggest dysfunction of the serotonin receptor in mood disorder. Serotonin receptor number may be increased in depressed compared to normal individuals, since the number of binding sites for a marker of the postsynaptic 5-HT serotonin receptor, [3H]ketanserin, is increased in the brains of suicide victims and depressed individuals obtained postmortem and in platelets from depressed individuals.

PET imaging of serotonin receptors have been carried out in vivo using the ligand N-([11C)methylspiperone, but these studies must be interpreted with caution, since this ligand also labels D2 receptors. Another problem with all PET scanning studies arises from heterogeneity of neurotransmitter receptors themselves. Radioligand binding analyses have shown at least six serotonin receptor subtypes in the brain, and the cDNAs for at least three of these receptors have been cloned. The affinity of these various receptors for 5-HT, and the effect of 5-HT on neurotransmission after binding to the receptors differs significantly. Progress in this field will depend on the development of safe ligands that are highly specific for each of the receptor subtypes.

Many clinically effective antidepressants act on the serotonergic system; for example, chronic antidepressant therapy normalizes [3H]ketanserin and [3H]imipramine binding, and some of the newer antidepressants have relative selectivity for the serotonin receptor in vitro, lending further support of a role for serotonin in affective disorder.

Ovarian Steroid Effects on Serotonin and Its Receptors

Estrogen regulates the action of serotonin and the activity of its receptors in many sensitive parts of the brain. In vitro electrophysiological recording from hypothalamic slices demonstrates that estrogen increases the response of some neurons to serotonin.[47] Estrogen enhances serotonin-mediated electrophysiologic responses in slices of rat hippocampus, an effect that appears to arise from an action on adenylate cyclase.[48] Estrogen also increases the number of serotonin receptors in brain, a finding that may explain the reported sex differences in serotonin receptor binding reported in many brain areas.[49] Estradiol or progesterone administered separately or in combination potentiates, and ovariectomy abrogates the effects of the antidepressant imipramine on serotonin receptor binding in rat cortex and hippocampus.[50]

Perturbation of serotonin neurotransmission in animals produces a characteristic behavioral syndrome that mimics some aspects of premenstrual mood disorders.[51] Administration of the MAOI drug pargyline combined with the 5-HT precursor l-tryptophan to rodents produces a state of 5-HT excess characterized by resting tremor, hyperactivity, hypersensitivity to touch, rigidity, head weaving, and salivation. Although both male and female rats develop this syndrome, the threshold for induction of the syndrome in females is much lower than in males, and this difference arises from gonadal hormones. Androgens acting via androgen receptors also play a role in this syndrome.

Cholinergic System in Mood Disorders

The cholinergic system has been implicated in the pathophysiology of mood disorders by clinical observations of an association between centrally acting cholinergic agents and depression in some individuals.[52] Also, cholinergic agents administered to animals produce a syndrome consisting of decreased motor activity, self-stimulation, and lethargy that resembles human depression. Physostigmine, a central-acting cholinesterase inhibitor, reduces elation, pressured speech, and hyperactivity in manic patients, although the effects are short lived. Neither placebo nor neostigmine, a cholinesterase inhibitor that does not cross the blood–brain barrier, influences mood in control experiments. Acetylcholine precursors, such as choline and lecithin, depress mood. Cholinergic drugs influence mood in normal individuals as well, although patients with mood disorders appear to be more sensitive than unaffected individuals to cholinergic drugs. Many of the adrenergic drugs that influence mood, such as clonidine, methyldopa, and reserpine, also have cholinomimetic properties. Central-acting anticholinergic agents can elevate mood, and may switch some depressed bipolar patients into mania. Most clinically effective antidepressants have potent anticholinergic activity, although this activity does not correlate with antidepressant activity.

Cholinergic receptors also may be altered in mood disorder. Muscarinic cholinergic receptors are increased in fibroblasts cultured from patients with affective disorder as compared to controls. One study of muscarinic binding sites in the frontal cortex of suicide victims showed increased binding as compared to age-matched brains, but another study with similar design failed to confirm this finding.

Cholinergic neurons enervate some peptidergic neurons that control the release of pituitary peptide hormones. Neuroendocrine testing has shown that some adult patients with major depression have hyposecre-

tion of growth hormone during the insulin tolerance test, a deficit that has been interpreted to reflect altered cholinergic (as well as serotonergic) function.

A variant of the cholinergic hypothesis of mood disorder proposes that imbalance between cholinergic and adrenergic activity underlies mood disorder.[53] According to this hypothesis, depression arises from cholinergic dominance and mania from adrenergic dominance.

Effects of Ovarian Steroids on Acetylcholine and Its Receptors

Sex steroids have a number of effects on acetylcholine and its receptors. Estradiol increases the number of muscarinic cholinergic receptors in the medial basal and ventromedial hypothalamus,[54] and decreases the number of these receptors in the medial preoptic area of ovariectomized rats.[55] Estrogen increases the electrical firing of neurons in slices of hypothalamus after administration of acetylcholine,[56] and heightens the behavioral response to intracerebral injection of muscarinic cholinergic agonists.[57] The acetylcholine synthesis inhibitor hemicholinium reduces the lordotic behavior response to steroid hormone administration.

Hypothalamic–Pituitary–Adrenal Axis in Mood Disorders

Dysfunction of the hypothalamic–pituitary–adrenal axis (HPAA) has been implicated in the pathophysiology, if not the etiology, of affective disorder by a large number of basic and clinical studies.[58] Psychological or physical stress, which often precedes the onset of affective disorder, induces activation of the HPAA. Patients with pathological activation of the HPAA from Cushing's disease or Cushing's syndrome, or who receive exogenous glucocorticoids or ACTH commonly develop significant affective symptoms.[28] Depressed patients consistently display elevated concentrations of plasma and urinary cortisol and its metabolites, disruption of the normal circadian rhythm of cortisol secretion, elevated plasma ACTH, and nonsuppression in the low-dose dexamethasone suppression test.[28,58–60]

Elevation of cortisol not only may serve as a marker for depression, but also may play a role in its pathophysiology. Elevation of glucocorticoid levels through chronic stress or pharmacologic administration induces pathologic changes in the hippocampus of rodents, an area of the brain that is critical for cognitive function in humans.[61,62] These changes include glial activation and alterations in the morphology of dendritic spines. Both morphologic findings have been implicated in synaptic plasticity.

Some patients with depression have elevated levels of corticotropin releasing hormone (CRH) in their cerebrospinal fluid and abnormal, "pseudo-Cushing"-like changes on the CRH stimulation test.[63] CRH produces a characteristic behavioral syndrome when injected into the CNS of rats that mimics anxiety and depression in humans. CRH neurons send axons to and receive reciprocal innervation from catecholaminergic neurons in the brain stem, and therefore may be involved in the regulation of neurovegetative function and behavior. Cholinergic and serotoninergic neurons also regulate CRH secretion from the within the CNS. Thus, the abnormalities of noradrenergic, cholinergic, serotonergic, and CRH activity may be related.

Effects of Ovarian Steroids on the HPAA

Estrogen may influence the secretion of CRH within the brain, since the levels of mRNA for CRH within the paraventricular nucleus of the hypothalamus vary across the estrous cycle in rats.[64] Interestingly, some PMS patients, like depressed patients, have disturbances in their HPAA axis, although they are mild and transient.[65]

Endorphins and Mood Disorders

Endogenous opiates, or endorphins, are peptides produced in the brain, pituitary, and other tissues that have narcotic-like activity and compete with narcotics for specific receptors.[66] Even before the discovery of endorphins, the psychiatric effects of opioids were well known; for example, tincture of opium was sporadically used to treat depression for decades. Intravenous administration of morphine suppresses cortisol secretion, and patients with depression have defective opioid regulation of the HPAA. Some studies report low, while other studies report normal CSF opioid activity in depressed patients.[67] However, plasma β-endorphin immunoreactivity probably does not differ between patients with major depression and controls.[68] Some of the inconsistencies in these studies may be attributed to the measurement of β-endorphin, which is dependent on assays which lack specificity, are responsive to stress, and probably do not reflect CNS β-endorphin.

Effect of Ovarian Steroids on Endorphins

Many studies have demonstrated the sensitivity of the hypothalamic and circulating endogenous opioid peptides to gonadal steroids.[69,70] For the most part, these studies have examined the effect of gonadal steroids on endorphin modulation of gonadotropin regulation and reproductive behavior. Estrogen decreases endorphin levels in the mediobasal hypothalamus of rats,[71] an effect that may be mediated by a subset of neurons in the hypothalamus which contain estrogen receptors and synthesize β-endorphin.[72]

GABA and Mood Disorders

Gamma amino butyric acid (GABA) is an amino acid that serves as a ubiquitous inhibitory neurotransmitter within the CNS. The widespread distribution of this neurotransmitter within the CNS makes pharmacologic perturbation of GABA or its receptor in humans difficult because of the high incidence of toxic side effects. Thus, clinical studies of GABA function in mood disorder have been limited. A number of studies have shown low levels of GABA in blood and CSF, while other studies show low levels of glutamic acid decarboxylase (GAD), the rate-limiting enzyme in the synthesis of GABA. Most clinically effective antidepressants increase binding of GABA to the GABA-B receptor, and drugs that enhance GABA often improve symptoms of depression.

Rapid progress in understanding the mechanism of action of GABA has followed the cloning of the cDNA for its receptor. The GABA receptor is coupled to a chloride channel, and has binding sites for benzodiazepines, barbiturates, and progestins. Benzodiazepines and barbiturates presumably exert their anxiolytic action by altering the permeability of the chloride channel and thereby the excitability of the neuron.

Effects of Gonadal Steroids on GABA and Its Receptor

Naturally produced A ring reduced metabolites of progesterone bind to the GABA receptor complex at a site that is distinct from the benzodiazepine or barbiturate binding site, as determined by recombinant DNA studies, that engineered GABA-A receptors with specific combinations of its subunits.[73] Yet, the potency of progestin actions on GABA receptors equals or exceeds that of antianxiety drugs. Long known to possess antianxiety activity, progestins induce a response, called operant behavior, that serves as an animal model of antianxiety action. In humans, progestins administered in high doses induce hypnosis comparable to that observed with administration of the barbiturates and benzodiazepines. Indeed, at one time parenteral progesterone was used as an anesthetic agent. The dose of progestins needed to induce an anxiolytic response is comparable to that which induces estrus behavior in animals, suggesting that this behavioral effect of progestins may have a physiological role, at least in rodents. Interestingly, alprazolam, a benzodiazepine that also has some antidepressant properties, is effective in reducing premenstrual symptoms in some patients.[74]

Physiologic levels of estrogen increase binding of [3H]labeled GABA agonists in various areas of the CNS of rats in a dose-dependent manner.[75] Estrogen-induced upregulation of GABA receptors can be blocked by the estrogen receptor antagonist tamoxifen, and requires an intact transcriptional system, suggesting a genomic effect of estrogen.[76] Furthermore, estradiol decreases glutamic acid decarboxylase activity in the hypothalamus.[77]

Glutamate and the Excitotoxicity Theory of Psychiatric Disease

Glutamate is an excitatory neurotransmitter found widely throughout the CNS. Glutamate can bind to a number of receptor subtypes, which can be distinguished by their selective binding of pharmacologic ligands and by their distinctive neurophysiologic profile on stimulation.[78] One type of glutamate receptor, which binds N-methyl-D-aspartic acid (NMDA) with high affinity, plays a central role in the physiology of learning,[78] neural plasticity underlying the establishment of binocular vision[79] and structural damage within the hippocampus that often arises in association with epilepsy and ischemia. The NMDA receptor is associated with an ion channel and thus regulates intracellular calcium levels. After activation of the NMDA receptor, the neuron develops increased sensitivity to subsequent stimulation. This heightened sensitivity to stimulation may be prolonged, and thus provides a molecular mechanism for long-term alterations of neural behavior. Interestingly, excessive stimulation of the NMDA receptor, as well as other glutamate receptors, can lead to profound alterations in the neuron structure and function, ranging from subtle alterations in the morphology of dendritic spines, to profound disruptions in cellular metabolism and neuronal death.[80] While little clinical research has examined the role of glutamate excitotoxicity in the pathophysiology of mood disorders, it provides an attractive hypothesis for future studies, since it provides a molecular mechanism which explains how learning-based processes could lead to long-term changes in brain function and structure.

Structural Changes in the Brain Cytoskeleton

Dendritic spines may play an important role in synaptic plasticity. Their small size makes their conductance sensitive to even small changes in diameter. Under electrophysiologic conditions known to activate NMDA receptors and induce synaptic plasticity, calpain, a calcium-activated protease, cleaves the cytoskeletal component spectrin, and thereby alters the shape and conductance of spines within hippocampal neurons.[81] As discussed above, chronic exposure to glucocorticoids, either from administration or from chronic stress, also induces changes in the morphology of hippocampal neurons.

Ovarian Steroid Effects on Cytoskeleton

Spine density in hippocampal neurons examined from Golgi-impregnated tissue removed at various times fluctuates across the estrous cycle.[82] This finding suggests that steroid-sensitive dendritic plasticity occurs within the hippocampus with each ovarian cycle. Such effects on cytoskeleton could also underlie the reported changes in arcuate hypothalamic synapses across the estrous cycle of rats.[83]

Gonadal steroids influence cytoskeleton in glial cells as well as neurons. In rat hippocampus, estrogen alters the distribution of the astrocyte-specific intermediate filament, glial fibrillary acidic protein (GFAP).[84] In rats and monkeys, the apical surface of estrogen receptor-negative glial cells lining the wall of the third ventricle, called tanycytes, exhibit sexual dimorphism in the number of microvilli and bulbous projections.[85] The pattern of these membrane specializations also varies across the ovarian cycle. In the preovulatory monkey, tanycyte apical surfaces have many bulbous projections, while after ovulation microvilli predominate. In tanycytes from proestrus rats microvilli predominate, while during diestrus the ventricle surfaces become smooth and devoid of membrane specializations. Tanycytes from sexually immature rats and humans also exhibit the smooth apical surfaces of the diestrus rat. Despite the existence of sexual dimorphism and sensitivity to the estrus cycle, tanycytes have never been found to contain detectable levels of estrogen receptors by a variety of sensitive methods. The functional significance of these changes in glial morphology remains unknown, although presumably changes in the cytoskeleton of astrocytes could alter nearby synapses, and changes in tanocytes could alter the blood–brain barrier.

Hemispheric Symmetry and Mood

Studies in animals, as well as in normal and neurologically impaired humans, reveal considerable asymmetry in the morphology and function of the two sides of the brain.[86] Asymmetries also exist in the distribution and concentration of most neurotransmitters (a fact many studies neglect). While the left hemisphere plays a dominant role in speech, the right hemisphere is critical for emotional gesturing, speech inflection, comprehension of facial affects, and the emotional nuances of speech (prosody). Intracarotid sodium amytol injected unilaterally into the left side produces depressed mood, while right-sided injection causes euphoria. This same pattern appears in patients with unilateral neurological lesions. Similarly, patients with an epileptigenic focus in the right temporal lobe tend to develop increased emotionality, whereas those with a left-sided focus tend to develop heightened obsession with abstract ideas. A number of investigators have attempted to compare symmetry of brain structure and function in patients with mood disorders versus normal controls using the various imaging technologies discussed above, although as yet no definitive conclusions can be reached.

Sex Differences in Hemispheric Symmetry

Marked sex differences exist in hemispheric morphology and dominance in animals and humans.[87] Boys have greater morphologic asymmetry than girls, especially in the temporal lobes. The anterior commissure and the corpus collosum, which connect the two sides of the brain, are larger in women than men, suggesting that women have less hemispheric asymmetry. It is not known when sexual differentiation of these structures occurs, or to what extent these differences arise from genomic versus hormonal effects in humans. Furthermore, we do not know to what extent these sex differences underlie reported differences between men and women in cognitive skills (whereby women generally perform better on verbal tests and men in spatial and mathematical skills), and in the predisposition of boys to developmental language disorders, such as dyslexia, stuttering, and delayed speech acquisition, and women to develop mood disorders.[88,89] Finally, we do not know whether such morphologic sex differences become fixed during a critical period of development, or fluctuate in concert with changing gonadal hormone levels. As discussed above, at least one steroid-sensitive area of the hypothalamus undergoes alterations in the number of synapses throughout the ovarian cycle of the rat, suggesting that morphologic sex differences may

remain plastic in response to fluctuating sex hormone levels, even outside the "critical period" of development of the hypothalamus.[83]

Sleep and Mood Disorder

Polysomnography distinguishes two major sleep states: rapid eye movement (REM) sleep, characterized by low-voltage EEG, rapid eye movements, inhibition of skeletal muscle tone, cardiorespiratory irregularity, diminished hypothalamic regulation of body temperature, and dreaming; and nonrapid eye movement (NREM) sleep, characterized by high-voltage, slow EEG activity, absence of rapid eye movements, cardiorespiratory regularity, and minimal or absent dreaming.[29] After 70 to 90 minutes of NREM sleep, the healthy adult first enters REM sleep. The time from the onset of sleep until the first REM period is defined as REM latency. Sleep then cycles between NREM and REM phases. The percentage of time in REM sleep increases in the latter half of sleep. The circadian system and some factors that accumulate during sleep deprivation interact to regulate the timing and duration of sleep. Serotonin and acetylcholine, neurotransmitters which have been implicated in the regulation of mood, also regulate sleep.

A number of studies have demonstrated that patients with mood disorders tend to have disrupted sleep, including increased sleep latency, multiple awakenings, and shortened REM latency.[90,91] Antidepressants alleviate sleep symptoms, frequently well before other antidepressant effects become apparent.

Effect of Ovarian Steroids on Sleep

Estrogen has a number of effects on sleep architecture when administered to hypoestrogenic women, including decreased sleep latency, reduction of waking episodes, and prolongation of REM sleep.[92] The beneficial effect of estrogens on sleep may arise in part from cessation of hot flushes, but estrogen probably also has a direct effect on sleep because many estrogen-sensitive waking episodes occur independently of hot flushes. Progestins, especially A-ring reduced metabolites of progesterone, have potent sedative activity, although their effect on sleep architecture has been much less studied.

Circadian Rhythms and Mood Disorders

A great deal of evidence has accumulated in support of the hypothesis that a disruption of the circadian organization of humans may be involved in the pathophysiology of mood disorders.[93] Even the earliest descriptions of depressed patients describe diurnal variation in mood and disruption of sleep and activity rhythms.

All eukaryotic organisms exhibit approximately 24-hour (circadian) rhythms in physiology and behavior that permit the organisms to adapt to 24-hour cyclic changes in the environment. Circadian rhythms are endogenous, so that even if rhythmic environmental time cues are eliminated by placing the organism in constant environmental conditions, the rhythms persist, although their period usually differs slightly from 24 hours. Under physiologic conditions, the rhythms are entrained to external time cues (eg, work schedules and/or light and dark cycles). These time cues synchronize the endogenous biological rhythms, so that the time cues and the rhythms have a stable phase relationship. The stability of circadian oscillators is very important for the organism's adaptation to its environment, and is reflected in the resistance of circadian rhythms to fluctuations in the internal milieu.

Studies of circadian rhythms in patients with mood disorders have led some investigators to suggest that some mood disorders involve specific abnormalities of circadian organization, such as a phase advance of certain circadian rhythms relative to others, abnormal amplitude of circadian rhythms, and/or disorder in entrainment of these rhythms to the day/night cycle.[94] Evidence in support of this hypothesis comes from clinical studies of depressed patients showing abnormal temporal distribution of REM sleep relative to non-REM sleep. While in normal subjects REM sleep reaches a maximum near dawn, REM is phase advanced in depressives. This would explain the shorter REM latency (time from sleep onset to REM sleep onset) and long first REM episodes reported in sleep studies of depressed patients (see above). The circadian rhythm of cortisol also may be phase advanced in some patients with major depression. Thus, the circadian rhythms of REM sleep and cortisol seen early in the night in depressed patients resemble those of normal subjects later in the night, as if the oscillator controlling these rhythms were shifted to an earlier time.

Experimental phase shifts of the sleep/wake cycle in normal human subjects can mimic the pattern of REM–nonREM sleep described in depressives. Similar changes have been reported in shift workers and transcontinental travelers, and these phase shifts may be associated with mild mood changes. Phase shifts in activity and temperature rhythms have been reported as individual patients with bipolar affective disorder shift from mania to depression and vice versa. Acute 6-hour phase shifts of the sleep/wake cycle were found to temporarily correct the disordered circadian rhythms and lead to brief remission of symtpoms in some depressed patients. In the patients who experienced remission, the sleep phase advance led to more normal synchronization between the circadian rhythm of REM propensity and the sleep/wake cycle.

Interestingly, in the best available animal model for grief- and loss-related depression, the mother-infant separation paradigm in monkeys, the circadian rhythms of heart rate and body temperature were abnormally phased relative to other rhythms. Normal synchronization of rhythms was attained following the reuniting of mother and infant.

Lithium, the most effective antimanic pharmacologic agent available today, can change the period of certain pacemakers in man and rodents. Lithium slows the period of several rhythms in many animal species and man, promotes entrainment, and delays the phase position of the sleep-wake cycle in normal subjects. Thus, one would expect that lithium might promote synchronization of pathologically slow circadian rhythms.

Ovarian Steroid Effects on the Circadian System

A large number of studies carried out in a variety of animal species and in man suggest that gonadal steroids can influence the circadian pacemaker.[95] The circadian rhythm of locomotor activity, the most commonly measured output of the circadian clock in animal studies, shifts with changing levels of gonadal steroids throughout the estrous cycle. Administration of estradiol to ovariectomized rodents shortens the period of the circadian rhythm of locomotor activity, while progesterone lengthens the period and can block estrogen-induced shortening of the period. Recent studies of the circadian rhythm of body temperature carried out in humans kept in environmental isolation demonstrate a fluctuation in the underlying period throughout the menstrual cycle, although other studies of the circadian system, such as those that studied the circadian rhythm of cortisol, do not show changes over the menstrual cycle. Little is known about the circadian system in patients with PMS.[96,97] The mechanism by which gonadal hormones affect the circadian pacemaker remains incompletely understood. The suprachiasmatic nuclei (SCN), the site of the circadian clock in mammals, itself does not bind estrogen by autoradiography[9] or contain mRNA for the estrogen receptor by in situ hybridization.[10] On the other hand, estrogen alters the firing rate of neurons within the SCN in response to acetylcholine.

SUMMARY

A variety of theories have been proposed to explain the neurobiological basis of mood disorders, including abnormalities in the functioning of classic neurotransmitters, neuropeptides, sleep, circadian rhythms, and hemispheric dominance. Expanding knowledge of molecular and cellular neurobiology promises to further refine existing theories and give rise to others. Ovarian steroid hormones exert remarkably diverse actions on the CNS, including effects on many of the neural networks implicated in the pathophysiology of mood disorders. Future studies are needed to test the clinical relevance of these effects.

REFERENCES

1. Hippocrates. *The Medical Works of Hippocrates.* Oxford: Blackwell; 1950.
2. Freud S. Project for a scientific psychology. In: *The Complete Psychological Works of Sigmund Freud,* Vol. I. London: Hogarth Press; 1974:281.
3. American Psychiatric Association. *Diagnostic and Statistical Manuel,* 3rd edition. Washington: APA Press; 1977.
4. Klaiber EL, Broverman DM, Vogel W, et al. Estrogen therapy for severe persistent depressions in women. *Archiv Gen Psychiatr.* 1979;36:550.
5. DeJong R, Rubinow DR, Roy-Byrne P, et al. Premenstrual mood disorder and psychiatric illness. *Am J Psychiatr.* 1985;142:1359.
6. Papez JW. A proposed mechanism of emotion. *Arch Neurol Psychiatr.* 1937;38:725.
7. Penfield W, Rasmussen T. *The Cerebral Cortex of Man: A Clinical Study of Localization of Function.* New York: Macmillan; 1950.
8. Bear D. The temporal lobes: an approach to the study of organic behavioral changes. In: Gazzaniga MS, ed. *Handbook of Behavioral Neurobiology,* Vol II. New York: Plenum Press; 1979:75.
9. Pfaff DW, Keiner M. Atlas of estradiol-concentrating cells in the central nervous system of the female rat. *J Comp Neurol.* 1973; 151:121.
10. Simerly RB, Chang C, Muramatsu M, et al. Distribution of androgen and estrogen receptor mRNA-containing cells in the rat brain—an in situ hybridization study. *J Comp Neurol.* 1990;294:76.
11. MacLusky NJ, Liederberg I, Krey LC, et al. Progesterone receptors in the brain and pituitary of a primate, the bonnet monkey (*Macaca radiata*). *Endocrinol.* 1980;106:185.
12. Evans, RM. The steroid and thyroid receptor superfamily. *Science.* 1988;240:889.
13. O'Malley, BW. Steroid hormone action in eurkaryotic cells. *J Clin Invest.* 1984;74:307.
14. Carson-Jurica MA, Schrader WT, O'Malley BW. Steroid receptor family: structure and function. *Endocr Rev.* 1990;11:201.
15. Spelsberg TC, Fink K, Rories C, et al. Role of proto-oncogenes as

16. Pfaff DW. Impact of estrogens on hypothalamic nerve cells: ultrastructural, chemical, and electrical effects. *Rec Prog Horm Res.* 1983;39:127.
17. Dluzen DE, Ramirez VD. Progesterone effects on dopamine release from the corpus stratium of female rats. II. Evidence for a membrane site of action and the role of albumin. *Brain Res.* 1989;476:338.
18. Brown TJ, MacLusky NJ, Toran-Allerand D, et al. Characterization of 11B-methoxy-16a-(125I) iodoestradiol binding: neuronal localization of estrogen-bound sites in the developing rat brain. *Endocrinol.* 1990;124:2074.
19. Keefe DL, Michelson D, Lee SH, et al. Astrocytes within the hypothalamic arcuate nucleus contain estrogen-sensitive peroxidase, bind fluorescein-conjugated estradiol, and may mediate synaptic plasticity in the rat. *Am J Obstet Gynecol.* 1991;164:959.
20. Tsibris JCM, Schwardt RA, Eggold DL, et al. Estrogen and protein disulfide isomerase. In: Hochberg RB, Naftolin F, eds. *The New Biology of Steroid Hormones.* New York: Raven;1991;235.
21. Kandel ER. Brain and behavior. In: Kandel EF, Schwartz JH, eds. *Principles of Neural Science.* New York: Elsevier; 1985:3.
22. Pacholczyk T, Blakely RD, Amara SG. Expression and cloning of a cocaine- and antidepressant-sensitive human noradrenaline transporter. *Nature.* 1991;350:350.
23. Jessen KR, Mirsky R. Introduction: neurobiology of glia. *Sem Neurosci.* 1990;2:421.
24. Jung-Testas I, Hu Z, Baulieu E, et al. Steroid synthesis in rat brain cell cultures. *J Steroid Biochem.* 1989:34:511.
25. Pfaff DW, Schwartz-Giblin S. Cellular mechanisms of female reproductive behaviors. In Knobil E, Neill J, eds. *The Physiology of Reproduction.* New York: Raven Press;1988:1487.
26. Parsons B, Rainbow TC, MacLusky N, et al. Progestin receptor levels in rat hypothalamic and limbic nuclei. *J Neurosci.* 1982;2:1446.
27. Maas J, Dekirmijian H, Jones F. The identification of depressed patients who have a disorder of norepinephrine metabolism and/or disposition. In: Usdin E, Snyder SH, eds. *Frontiers in Catecholamine Research.* Oxford: Pergamon:1973;1081.
28. Carroll BJ, Curtis GC, Mendels J. Neuroendocrine regulation in depression. *Arch Gen Psychiatr.* 1976;33:1051.
29. Kupfer DJ. The sleep EEG in diagnosis and treatment of depression. In: Rush AJ, Altshuler KZ, eds. *Depression, Basic Mechanisms, Diagnosis and Treatment.* New York: Guilford; 1986; 102.
30. Fidia Research Foundation. PET: A method for combined structural and functional assessment of the brain. *Neurosci Facts.* 1991;2:1.
31. Council on Scientific Affairs, AMA. Instrumentation in positron emission tomography. *JAMA.* 1988;259:1531.
32. Moonen CTW, van Zijl PCM, Frank JA, et al. Functional magnetic resonance imaging in medicine and physiology. *Science.* 1990;250:53.
33. McKinney, WT. Interdisciplinary animal research and its relevance to psychiatry. In: Kaplan HI, Sadock G, eds. *Comprehensive Textbook of Psychiatry,* Vol. 5. Baltimore: Williams & Wilkins; 1988;326.
34. Maas JW, Leckman JF. Relationships between central nervous system noradrenergic function and plasma and urinary MHPG and other norepinephrine metabolites. In: Maas JW, ed. *MHPG: Basic Mechanisms and Psychopathology.* New York: Academic Press; 1983:33.
35. Maas JW. Norepinephrine and depression. In: Rush AJ, Altshuler KZ, eds. *Depression.* New York: Guilford Press;1986:72.
36. Charney DS, Menkes DB, Heninger GR. Receptor sensitivity and the mechanism of action of antidepressant drugs. *Arch Gen Psych.* 1981;38:1160.
37. Kaplan HI, Saddock BJ. Neurochemistry of behavior. In: Kaplan

HI, Freedman AM, Saddock BJ. *Comprehensive Textbook of Psychiatry/III.* Baltimore: Williams & Wilkins; 1980:177.

38. Luine VN, Rhodes JC. Gonadal hormone regulation of MAO and other enzymes in hypothalamic areas. *Neuroendocrinol.* 1983;36: 235.

39. Luine VN, McEwen BS, Black IB. Effect of 17B-estradiol on hypothalamic tyrosine hydroxylase activity. *Brain Res.* 1977;120: 188.

40. Biegon A, Reches A, Snyder L, et al. Serotonergic and noradrenergic receptors in the rat brain: modulation by chronic exposure to ovarian hormones. *Life Sci.* 1982;32:2015.

41. MacLusky NJ, Natolin F, Krey LC, et al. The catechol estrogens. *J Steroid Biochem.* 1981;15:111.

42. Jellinck PH, Bradlow HL. Peroxidase-catalyzed displacement of tritium from regiospecifically labelled estradiol and 2-hydroxyestradiol. *J Steroid Biochem.* 1990;35:705.

43. Schipper H, Lechan RM, Reichlin S. Glial peroxidase activity in the hypothalamic arcuate nucleus: effects of estradiol valerate persistent estrus. *Brain Res.* 1990;500:200.

44. Power R, Lydon JP, Conneely O, et al. Dopamine activation of an orphan of the steroid receptor superfamily. *Science.* 1991;252: 1546.

45. Maas JW. Biogenic amines and depression: biochemical and pharmacological separation of two types of depression. *Arch Gen Psychiatr.* 1975;32:1357.

46. Brown S-L, Bleich A, VanPraag HM. The monoamine hypothesis of depression. In: Brown S-L, VanPraag HM, eds. *The Role of Serotonin in Psychiatric Disorders.* New York: Brunner/Mazel; 1991:91.

47. Kow LM, Pfaff D. Estrogen effects on neuronal responsiveness to electrical and neurotransmitter stimulation: an in vitro study on the ventromedial nucleus of the hypothalamus. *Brain Res.* 1985; 347:1.

48. Fischette CT, Biegon A, McEwen BS. Sex differences in serotinin 1 receptor binding in rat brain. *Science.* 1983;222:333.

49. Clarke WP, Maayani S. Estrogen effects on 5-HT1A receptors in hippocampal membranes from ovariectomized rats: functional and binding studies. *Brain Res.* 1990;518:287.

50. Kendall DA, Stancel GM, Enna SJ. Imipramine: effect of ovarian steroids on modifications in serotonin receptor binding. *Science.* 1981;211:1183.

51. Fischette CT, Biegon A, McEwen BS. Sex steroid modulation of the serotonin behavioral syndrome. *Life Sci.* 1984;35:1197.

52. Carroll BJ, Frazer A, Schless A, et al. Cholinergic reversal of manic symptoms. *Lancet.* 1973;1:427.

53. Janowsky DS, El-Yousef MK, Davis JM, et al. A cholinergic-adrenergic hypothesis of mania and depression. *Lancet.* 1972;2: 6732.

54. Dohanich GP, Witcher JA, Weaver DR, et al. Alteration of muscarinic binding in specific brain areas following estrogen treatment. *Brain Res.* 1982;241:347.

55. Rainbow TC, DeGroff V, Luine VN, et al. Estradiol-17B increases the number of muscarinic receptors in hypothalamic nuclei. *Brain Res.* 1980;198:239.

56. Kow L-M, Pfaff DW. Suprachiasmatic neurons in tissue slices from ovariectomized rats: electrophysiological and neuropharmacological characterization and the effects of estrogen treatment. *Brain Res.* 1984;297:275.

57. Clemens L, Dohanich G, Barr P. Cholinergic regulation of feminine sexual behavior in laboratory rats. In: Balthazart E, Prove E, Gilles R, eds. *Hormones and Behavior in Higher Vertebrates.* Berlin: Springer; 1983:56.

58. Gold PW, Goodwin FK, Chrousos GP. Clinical and biochemical manifestations of depression. Relation to the neurobiology of stress (2 parts). *N Engl J Med.* 1988;319:348.

59. Sachar EJ. Disorders of feeling: affective diseases. In: Kandel ER, Schwartz JH, eds. *Principles of Neural Science.* New York: Elsevier; 1985:717.

60. Cohen MR, Pickar D, Extein I, et al. Plasma cortisol and β-endor-

phin immunoreactivity in nonmajor and major depression. *Am J Psychiatr.* 1984;141:628.

61. Landfield PW, Waymire JC, Lynch G. Hippocampal aging and adrenocorticoids. *Science.* 1978;202:1098.

62. Salpolsky RM, Uno H, Rebert CS, et al. Hippocampal damage associated with prolonged glucocorticoid exposure in primates. *J Neurosci.* 1990;10:2897.

63. Holsboer F, von Bardeleben U, Gerken A, et al. Blunted corticotropin and normal cortisol response to human corticotropin-releasing factor in depression. *New Engl J Med.* 1984;311:1127.

64. Bohler HC, Zoeller RT, King JC, et al. Corticotropin releasing hormone mRNA is elevated on the afternoon of proestrus in the parvocellular paraventricular nuclei of the female rat. *Molec Brain Res.* 1990;8:259.

65. Rabin DS, Schmidt PJ, Campbell G, et al. Hypothalamic-pituitary-adrenal function in patients with premenstrual syndrome. *J Clin Endo Metab.* 1990;71:1158.

66. Verebey K, Volavka J, Clouet D. Endorphins in psychiatry. *Arch Gen Psychiatr.* 1978;35:877.

67. Bunney WE, Pert CB, Klee W, et al. Basic and clinical studies of endorphins. *Ann Int Med.* 1979;91:239.

68. Naber D, Pickar D, Post RM, et al. Endogenous opioid activity and β-endorphin immunoreactivity in CSF of psychiatric patients and normal volunteers. *Am J Psychiatr.* 1981;138:1457.

69. Casper RF, Bhanot R, Wilkinson M. Prolonged elevation of hypothalamic opioid peptide activity in women taking oral contraceptives. *J Clin Endocrinol Metab.* 1984;58:582.

70. Wilkinson M, Brawer JR, Wilkinson DA. Gonadal steroid-induced modifications of opiate binding sites in anterior hypothalamus of female rats. *Biol Reprod.* 1985;32:501.

71. Wardlaw SC, Thoron L, Frantz GA. Effects of sex steroids on brain beta endorphin. *Brain Res.* 1982;245:327.

72. Morrell J, McGinty JF, Pfaff D. A subset of β-endorphin or dynorphin containing neurons in the medial basal hypothalamus accumulate estradiol. *Neuroendocrinol.* 1985;41:417.

73. Majewska, MD. Steroid hormone metabolites are barbiturate-like modulators of the GABA receptor. *Science.* 1986;232:1004.

74. Smith S, Rinehart JS, Ruddock VE, et al. Treatment of premenstrual syndrome with alprazolam: results of a double-blind, placebo-controlled, randomized crossover clinical trial. *Obstet Gynecol.* 1987;70:37.

75. Maggi A, Perez C. Estrogen-induced up-regulation of gamma aminobutyric acid receptors in the CNS of rodents. *J Neurochem.* 1990;47:1793.

76. Perez J, Zucchi I, Maggi A. Estrogen modulation of the gamma aminobutyric acid receptor complex in the central nervous system of rat. *J Pharm Exp Ther.* 1990;244:1005.

77. Wallis GJ, Luttge WG. Influence of estrogen and progesterone on glutamate acid decarboxylase activity in discrete regions of the rat brain. *J Neurochem.* 1980;34:609.

78. Choi DW. Glutamate neurotoxicity and diseases of the nervous system. *Neuron.* 1988;1:623.

79. Cline HT, Debski EA, Contantine-Paton M. N-methyl-D-aspartate receptor antagonist desegregates eye-specific stripes. *Proc Natl Acad Sci USA.* 1987;84:4342.

80. Kennedy MB. Regulation of synaptic transmission in the central nervous system: long-term potentiation. *Cell.* 1989;59:777.

81. Lynch G, Baudry M. Brain spectrin, calpain and long-term changes in synaptic efficacy. *Brain Res Bull.* 1987;18:809.

82. Woolley CS, Gould E, Frankfurt M, et al. Naturally occurring fluctuation in dendritic spine density on adult hippocampal pyramidal neurons. *J Neurosci.* 1990;10:4035.

83. Naftolin F, Garcia-Segura M, Keefe D, et al. Estrogen effects on the synaptology and neural membranes of the rat hypothalamic arcuate nucleus. *Biol Reprod.* 1990;42:21.

84. Garcia-Segura LM, Torres-Aleman I, Naftolin F. Astrocytic shape and glial fibrillary acidic protein immunoreactivity are modified by estradiol in primary rat hypothalamic cultures. *Dev Brain Res.* 1989;47:298.

85. Brawer JR, Lin PS, Sonnenschein C. Morphologic plasticity in the wall of the third ventricle during the estrous cycle in the rat: a scanning electron microscopic study. *Anat Rec.* 1974;179:481.

86. Kupfermann I. Hemispheric asymmetries and the cortical localization of higher cognitive and affective functions. In: Kandel EF, Schwartz JH, eds. *Principles of Neural Science.* New York: Elsevier;1985:673.

87. deLaCoste MC, Adesanya T, Woodward DJ. Measures of gender differences in the human brain and their relationship to brain weight. *Biol Psychiatr.* 1990;28:931.

88. Hampson E. Estrogen-related variations in human spatial and articulatory-motor skills. *Psychoneuroendocrinol.* 1990;15:97.

89. Weissman M, Klerman G. Sex differences and the epidemiology of depression. *Arch Gen Psychiatr.* 1977;34:98.

90. Beersma DGM, Daan S, van den Hoofdakker RH. Sleep structure in depression. *Exp Brain Res, suppl 8.* 1984;285.

91. Borbely AA. Sleep regulation: outline of a model and its implications for depression. *Exp Brain Res, suppl 8.* 1984;272.

92. Schiff I, Regestein Q, Tulchinsky D, et al. Effects of estrogens on sleep and psychological state of hypogonadal women. *JAMA.* 1979;242:2405.

93. Rusak B. Assessment and significance of rhythm disruptions in affective illness. In: Brown GM et al, eds. *Neuroendocrinology and Psychiatric Disorder.* New York: Raven Press:1984;267.

94. Wehr TA, Wirz-Justice A, Goodwin FK, et al. Phase advance of the circadian sleep-wake cycle as an antidepressant. *Science.* 1979;206:710.

95. Keefe DL, Turek FW. Circadian time keeping processes in mammalian reproduction. *Oxford Rev Reprod Biol.* 1985;7:346.

96. Steiner M, Haskett RF, Carroll BJ, et al. Circadian hormone secretory profiles with severe premenstrual tension syndrome. *Br J Obstet Gynaecol.* 1984;91:466.

97. Parry BL, Wehr TA. Therapeutic effect of sleep deprivation in patients with premenstrual syndrome. *Am J Psychiatr.* 1987;144:808.

CHAPTER 7

Parallels Between Premenstrual Syndrome and Psychiatric Illness

Peter J. Schmidt and David R. Rubinow

Several parallels exist between premenstrual syndrome (PMS) and formal psychiatric illness. These similarities are particularly evident when the presenting symptoms, past psychiatric history, course, and, to some extent, biological markers and treatment response characteristics of PMS and affective disorders are compared. In fact, some investigators have suggested that PMS resembles atypical depression[1] and can best be understood as a recurrent affective state that is linked to or triggered by the luteal phase of the menstrual cycle.[2,3] Independent of a specific relationship between PMS and affective disorder, PMS may increase our understanding of the many ways in which the menstrual cycle may interact with or give rise to disturbances in mood and behavior.

In this chapter we first review findings that suggest an association between PMS and certain forms of psychiatric illness, particularly affective disorder. Next, we describe the variety of ways in which the menstrual cycle may influence coexisting disturbances in mood and behavior. Investigation of this linkage between mood and the menstrual cycle may further inform us about mechanisms relevant to the development and expression of symptoms observed in premenstrual syndrome.

PREMENSTRUAL SYNDROME AND PSYCHIATRIC DISORDERS

Improved diagnostic methods for both PMS and psychiatric illnesses have allowed for the selection of more homogeneous samples for research purposes. Therefore, more meaningful comparisons can be drawn between these diagnostic groups for each of the following variables: symptom profile, longitudinal course, family history, biologic characteristics, and treatment response.[4]

Symptom Profile

Evidence from both psychiatric and gynecologic practices and in both clinical and research settings suggests that premenstrual mood changes are the symptoms that most commonly lead women to seek treatment for PMS.[5–7] Freeman et al[6] reported that the five most frequent presenting symptoms in 241 women with (subsequently confirmed) PMS were depression (56%), irritability (48%), anxiety (36%), mood swings (26%), and headaches (23%). Similarly, in 100 consecutive women seeking treatment for PMS, Schinfeld et al[7] described the most frequent complaints as depression (55%), headache (42%), irritability (33%), fatigue (23%), and crying (19%). Furthermore, this prominence of affective and behavioral symptoms was observed in samples of women with PMS without past psychiatric illness. Thus, Mortola[8] reported that in a sample of 28 women with prospectively confirmed PMS, in whom coexisting medical conditions and coexisting or past psychiatric disturbances were excluded, the most common and consistent symptoms experienced during the luteal phase of the menstrual cycle were as follows (expressed as percentage of cycles studied): fatigue (92%), irritability (91%), bloating (90%), tension (89%), breast tenderness (85%), mood lability (81%), depression (80%), and food cravings (78%). The prominence and nature of these affective symptoms led several investigators to suggest that the symptoms of PMS closely resemble those of atypical depression[1]; that is, depressed mood accompanied by hypersomnia, increased appetite with carbohydrate cravings, and emotional reactivity.[9] Further support of this hypothesis is derived from studies observing disturbances of appetite and sleep in women with prospectively diagnosed PMS. Both-Orthman et al[10] observed a significant increase in appetite in patients with prospectively confirmed PMS as well as in controls, with a significantly greater premenstrual increase in appetite observed in the PMS patients. Furthermore, these investigators observed that the premenstrual increase in appetite was correlated with self-ratings of depression in the patient sample only. While anecdotal reports describe the prominence of carbohydrate cravings, a feature of atypical depression, in women with PMS, the existence of these cravings as well as their relationship to the observed increase in appetite in PMS are not yet documented. At least one investigation suggested that the pathophysiology of carbohydrate cravings and that of PMS may be linked.[11] Alternatively, the changes in appetite observed in women with PMS may equally represent a symptom of recurrent depression as reported by Frank et al.[12] Thus, these changes in appetite may be more a reflection of a woman's experience of depression than suggestive of a specific relationship between PMS and atypical depression.

In addition to changes in appetite, women with PMS are reported to experience prominent changes in sleep and daytime fatigue similar to those seen in atypical depression. Mauri et al[13] reported that a clinic sample of PMS patients could be distinguished from samples of women from the general population (with and without complaints of premenstrual symptoms) by the self-reporting of the following symptoms during the premenstrual phase: unpleasant dreams, frequent awakenings during sleep, failure to wake at the expected time, tiredness in the morning, and heightened mental activity during the night and on wakening. In contrast, when Jensvold et al[14] monitored symptoms of sleep disturbance longitudinally over at least two menstrual cycles, no significant differences were observed between patients with PMS and controls or between follicular and late luteal phases of the menstrual cycle in self-reports of sleep characteristics, hours of sleep, and number of sleep interruptions. However, these investigators did find significant increases in daytime fatigue and mood symptoms during the premenstrual compared with the postmenstrual phase of the menstrual cycle in patients, but not in controls. Additionally, measures of fatigue correlated with changes in mood in the patients. In a separate but related report from Mauri et al,[15] sleep studies performed in a small sample of women with PMS identified abnormalities in sleep architecture in those women with low premenstrual scores on the premenstrual tension syndrome rating scale.[16] There are presently no reports investigating in PMS the phenomenon of reverse diurnal variation observed in atypical depression. However, we found no evidence of diurnal variation in 20 women with PMS (unpublished observation). In summary, in addition to marked affective disturbances, women with PMS may also report the experience of prominent changes in sleep as well as in energy and appetite similar to those reported to occur in atypical depression.

Despite the apparent similarities, a number of prominent symptoms of PMS are distinct from those experienced in either atypical or typical affective disorders. For example, Mortola[8] observed that breast tenderness was the symptom that best distinguished the premenstrual from the postmenstrual phase of the cycle in women with prospectively diagnosed PMS. Furthermore, although objective evidence of bloating has not been observed,[17] the subjective experience of bloating is a prominent symptom in PMS, unlike traditional affective disorders in women. Finally, recent reports have observed the presence of severe hot flushes in a sample of women with PMS.[18] It is unclear whether these symptoms differentiate PMS and affective disorders or, alternatively, represent menstrual cycle symptoms unrelated to the diagnosis of PMS. Moreover, an association between PMS and major affective disorder cannot be inferred solely on the basis of symptom similarity. Further evidence supporting this putative relationship has emerged from studies of the longitudinal course of psychiatric illness in women with PMS.

Longitudinal Course

At least seven studies examining the prevalence of affective disorder in women reporting premenstrual mood changes have been performed and observed a higher than expected prevalence of a past history of affective disorder in women with PMS.[19–25] Mackenzie et al.[21] noted a 41% lifetime prevalence rate of major affective disorder in women reporting moderate to severe "premenstrual or menstrual difficulties." In four additional reports, the presence of PMS was prospectively confirmed as a study entry criterion. Halbreich and Endicott[22] observed a 60% lifetime prevalence of major depressive disorder in 10 women with prospectively confirmed "premenstrual full depressive syndrome," consistent with their observations in other samples diagnosed with solely retrospective methods. DeJong et al[23] observed a 45% lifetime prevalence of psychiatric illness and a 30% prevalence of major depressive disorder in patients with menstrually related mood disorders. Pearlstein et al[24] observed a 55% lifetime prevalence of major depressive disorder and a 75% prevalence of major or minor depression in 56 women with late luteal phase dysphoric disorder. Furthermore, these investigators found that among the parous subjects in this sample, 30% had a history of postpartum depression.[24] More recently, Freeman et al.[25] evaluated a larger sample of 168 women with prospectively confirmed PMS, participating in a treatment study of progesterone suppositories, and observed that 73% of the patients had a past history of mental illness and 56% had a past history of major depressive disorder. The observed lifetime prevalence rates of major depressive disorder in PMS are higher than those observed in women in general.[26] Further, the prevalence rate of postpartum depression reported by Pearlstein et al is approximately twice the reported lifetime prevalence rate of postpartum depression (10%–15%).[27] Although these reports suggest a higher lifetime prevalence rate of affective disorders in women with PMS, Johnson[28] cautioned that this observation may equally reflect a selection bias where women with both PMS and a past history of major depressive disorder are more likely to seek treatment than women with only PMS. This, then, would artificially elevate the lifetime prevalence rate for major depressive disorder observed in women with PMS seen at clinics. Further studies employing more rigorous epidemiologic methods, prospective confirmation of diagnoses, and appropriate control groups are necessary to establish the increased rate of co-occurrence of PMS and depressive disorders.

Schuckit et al[19] and Wetzel et al[20] described both an increased lifetime history of depression and an increased subsequent presentation with affective disorder in college women reporting PMS. However, preliminary results of a 5-year follow-up of women with PMS previously diagnosed at the National Institute of Mental Health show an apparent diagnostic stability rather than a progression to major affective disorders, suggesting some nosologic independence between premenstrual and major mood disorders (Schmidt et al, unpublished observation).

In addition to symptoms of depression, patients with PMS experience anxiety and occasional panic-like symptoms during the premenstrual period. A recent report[29] suggested an association between PMS and certain anxiety disorders, specifically panic disorder. Patients with panic disorder can be distinguished on a biological basis from patients with other forms of anxiety disorders and nonpsychiatrically ill controls by their increased vulnerability to develop panic attacks when challenged with sodium lactate infusions,[30] caffeine,[31] or inhalation of a 35% carbon dioxide (CO_2) mixture in oxygen.[32] Harrison et al[29] found that a 35% CO_2 mixture in oxygen induced a panic attack reaction in 9 of 14 women with premenstrual dysphoria, who had no history of panic disorder, compared to none of 12 controls. Further, they found neither patients nor controls experienced panic symptoms in response to the control stimulus of air inhalation. Panic reactions to CO_2 inhalation were not confined to the late luteal phase (symptomatic phase) in patients, suggesting a vulnerability or trait relationship to panic disorder rather than a state-related phenomenon. These findings are of interest given the anecdotal reports of caffeine-related exacerbation of symptoms in some women with PMS[33,34] and the reports of therapeutic effects of certain anxiolytic medications such as alprazolam in PMS.[35,36] Additionally, phenomenologic associations between PMS and other anxiety disorders, specifically posttraumatic stress disorder and obsessive compulsive disorder, have been described.[37]

Family History

No report to date has described the history of PMS in family members of patients with major depressive disorder. Obviously, the requirement for prospective confirmation of the diagnosis of PMS would allow only the current or future diagnosis of family members. Descriptions of the family psychiatric history of women with confirmed PMS have similarly been lacking, with the exception of two reports. In a preliminary study, Harrison et al[38] observed an increased prevalence of a history of major depression in first-degree relatives of women with confirmed PMS. More recently, Freeman et al[25] observed that 45% of their sample of 168 women with prospectively confirmed PMS reported a family history of mental illness (unspecified) and 40% reported a family history of alcoholism.

BIOLOGIC CHARACTERISTICS

Neuroendocrine Studies

Abnormalities of both the hypothalamic–pituitary–adrenal (HPA) and hypothalamic–pituitary–thyroid (HPT) axes have been extensively investigated in affective disorders. In the past, investigators have obtained both static (basal) measures and dynamic measures (stimulation or suppression tests) of the hormonal axes. Although single basal hormone measures are able to distinguish gross differences between diagnostic groups, frequent and repeated sampling over a prolonged period of time is necessary to evaluate circadian variability and the pulsatile pattern of peripheral hormone secretion. Alternatively, dynamic measures enable investigators to assess the regulation and responsivity of the endocrine system. Several neuroendocrine studies have been performed in patients with PMS, employing measures that have been observed to be abnormal in patients with primary affective disorder.

Hypothalamic-Pituitary-Adrenal Axis

BASAL STUDIES

Elevated basal plasma cortisol levels have been observed in many, but not all, patients with endogenous depression compared with controls. One study reported normal morning basal plasma cortisol levels in women with PMS compared with controls.[39] However, Rabin et al[40] recently reported decreased evening basal plasma cortisol levels in patients with prospectively confirmed PMS during both the follicular and luteal phases compared with controls. The decreased cortisol levels were, therefore, phase independent and unrelated to symptom appearance. Urinary assessments provide an integrated measure of HPA activity over time, and urinary free cortisol (UFC) was found to both correlate with other measures of HPA function and be elevated in patients with endogenous depression compared with controls.[41] Two studies found no difference in the 24-hour UFC

secretion during the follicular and luteal phases of the menstrual cycle in women with PMS[42] and compared with controls,[40] suggesting no increased HPA activity in PMS. Two studies employing frequent plasma sampling over a 24-hour period found no difference in the circadian pattern of cortisol secretion[43] and no difference in 24-hour mean levels, pulse amplitude, duration, and integrated area[44] during the luteal phase in women with PMS compared with controls.

DYNAMIC STUDIES

Despite the well-established increased incidence of cortisol nonsuppression following dexamethasone administration in some patients with affective illness, Haskett et al[42] and Roy-Byrne et al[45] observed normal cortisol suppression following dexamethasone administration in patients with PMS. Further evidence of normal HPA activity in women with prospectively confirmed PMS is provided by the findings of Rabin et al.[40] These investigators observed no difference between the plasma ACTH response to ovine corticotropin-releasing hormone (CRH) (1 µg/kg), during the follicular and luteal phases of the menstrual cycle, in women with PMS compared with controls. Although these investigators did observe a significantly greater cortisol response to ovine CRH throughout the menstrual cycle in the PMS sample, the exaggerated response was most likely due to the lower baseline plasma cortisol values observed in this group. Further, these findings were menstrual cycle phase independent, and therefore the relationship to PMS symptoms is unclear. As the ovine CRH stimulation test is a particularly sensitive measure of HPA activity and patients with depression are observed to exhibit an attenuated ACTH response to ovine CRH compared with controls,[46] these findings do not suggest abnormal HPA axis activity in PMS and do not support an association between PMS and major depressive disorder.

Hypothalamic–Pituitary–Thyroid Axis

Hypothalamic-pituitary-thyroid (HPT) axis dysfunction is associated with a variety of mood and behavioral changes.[47] It has long been recognized that overt hypothyroidism may present with a clinical picture indistinguishable from that of major depression. Further, it is now clear that less severe forms of thyroid dysfunction occur with greater than expected frequency in individuals with mood disturbances.[48]

BASAL STUDIES

Abnormalities in basal thyroid function have been reported in association with depressive illness. Gold et al[48] found either grade 1 (overt) or grade 2 (mild) hypothyroidism in 4% of 250 consecutive patients referred to a psychiatric hospital for evaluation and treatment of depression. Further, both Cowdry et al[49] and Bauer et al[50] reported high rates of grades 1 and 2 hypothyroidism in rapid cycling bipolar patients. Finally, Nemeroff et al[51] observed the presence of significant titers of antithyroid antibodies in 20% of a sample of depressed patients consecutively admitted to the hospital. Similarly, a higher than expected prevalence of abnormal baseline thyroid function was reported in women with PMS.[52,53] We evaluated basal thyroid function in 120 women with prospectively confirmed PMS. Our preliminary results show that 10% (12 women) showed evidence of either grade 1 or 2 hypothyroidism or hyperthyroidism. Further, we observed that 7 of 45 women with PMS (15%) showed evidence of abnormally elevated titers of either antithyroglobulin or antimicrosomal autoantibodies. This may merely reflect a high prevalence of thyroid illness in women of reproductive age. However, we have observed at least 1 patient with autoimmune thyroiditis presenting with a menstrual-related mood disorder that remitted with thyroid hormone replacement.[54] This suggests that thyroid disease may be associated with symptoms appearing only in the luteal phase.

DYNAMIC STUDIES

Abnormalities (both blunted and exaggerated) of the thyroid-stimulating hormone (TSH) response to thyroid-releasing hormone (TRH) stimulation have been identified in some,[52,53,55] but not all,[56,57] studies of women with PMS or major affective disorder.[49,50,58] Although abnormalities in the TSH response to TRH stimulation may occur with higher than expected frequency in women with a prospectively confirmed diagnosis of PMS, our group observed[53,55] that abnormalities were not confined to the late luteal (symptomatic) phase of the menstrual cycle. Thus the significance of an abnormal TRH stimulation test in PMS is unclear. Brayshaw and Brayshaw[52] reported that of 34 PMS patients treated in an open trial with L-thyroxine, all obtained complete relief from symptoms once the dose had been titrated. These data represent uncontrolled observations from a study with major methodologic flaws. Nikolai et al[56] studied 44 women with a diagnosis of PMS (based on 1 month of ratings prior to study entry) in a double-blind placebo-controlled parallel design and found no significant differences in efficacy between placebo and L-thyroxine (0.15 μg/kg). Similarly, preliminary results from a double-blind placebo-controlled crossover trial of L-thyroxine (100 μg/d) in women with prospectively confirmed diagnoses of PMS (during the 3 months prior to study entry) conducted at the NIMH have not demonstrated superior therapeutic efficacy of this medication compared with placebo. No relationship was observed between TSH response to TRH and clinical response to L-thyroxine administration.

Receptor Studies

Possible biologic similarity between PMS and depression is suggested by reports, albeit inconsistently, in both disorders of a reduction in platelet serotonin uptake[59,60] and whole blood serotonin.[61,62] Additionally, Halbreich[63,64] suggested a possible abnormality in alpha-2-adrenergic receptor activity in women with PMS, although preliminary evidence of similar growth hormone response to clonidine (an alpha-2 agonist) in women with PMS and controls would not support this hypothesis.[65] Further, reduced platelet serotonin uptake could reflect a common pathophysiology in PMS and major depression or represent a concomitant of the depressed mood present in both disorders.

Circadian Studies

Abnormalities of circadian rhythm, specifically the pattern of appearance of rapid eye movement sleep and of change in temperature and cortisol and melatonin levels, are reported in affective disorders.[66,67] Moreover, some successful treatments of affective disorders include interventions that manipulate the postulated abnormalities of circadian rhythmicity, including total or partial sleep deprivation[68] and light therapy.[69] Although no abnormalities in circadian cortisol secretion are identified in PMS,[43,44] a number of reports provide evidence of circadian rhythm abnormality in other variables. Parry et al[70] observed earlier nocturnal temperature minima throughout the menstrual cycle in women with PMS compared with controls, suggesting a phase-advance disturbance in PMS. Additionally, these investigators recently provided further evidence of a phase-advance abnormality in PMS by observing an earlier offset of melatonin secretion as well as a decreased area of the melatonin secretory curve throughout the menstrual cycle in women with prospectively confirmed diagnoses of PMS.[71] It is also of interest that partial sleep deprivation, an antidepressant treatment that corrects a putative phase-advance abnormality, is reported by Parry and Wehr[72] to be therapeutically effective in some patients with PMS. Moreover, evening light but not morning light exposure was observed to be an effective treatment in PMS,[73] further suggestive of a phase-advance abnormality in this condition. Although some of these findings (earlier offset of melatonin) but not all (decreased area under the melatonin curve) appear unique to PMS compared to other affective disorders, further study is necessary to clarify the relevance of these circadian rhythm abnormalities to the pathogenesis of PMS. Additionally, the menstrual cycle phase independence of these findings suggests the possible involvement of biological vulnerabilities or "trait" mechanisms in the development and expression of PMS.

TREATMENT RESPONSE

Similar treatment response characteristics of PMS and major depressive disorder might suggest a common pathophysiologic substrate. Unfortunately, few published studies exist regarding the efficacy of antidepressants in women with confirmed PMS. Two preliminary reports described the successful treatment of PMS with nortriptyline in an open trial[74] and fluoxetine in a double-blind placebo-controlled trial.[75] Early reports of the efficacy of lithium carbonate were refuted by subsequent double-blind placebo-controlled trials, although one study suggested that lithium was an effective treatment for PMS in women with a history of "subclinical affective disorder."[76] Efficacy has also been claimed in some controlled studies for both alprazolam,[35,36] a triazolo-benzodiazepine that is unique among benzodiazepines for its purported antidepressant effects in the treatment of depression,[77] and buspirone, a nonsedating, nonbenzodiazepine anxiolytic drug.[78] The efficacy of light treatment and partial sleep deprivation is described above. As more is learned about the relevant mechanisms of action of these treatments and their efficacy in PMS, more will be understood about the neurobiology of both affective disorders and PMS.

THE MENSTRUAL CYCLE AND PSYCHIATRIC DISORDERS

Just as improved diagnostic methods enable investigators to more effectively compare and contrast PMS

with psychiatric illness, these same techniques allow us to better appreciate the many ways in which the menstrual cycle may modulate mood and behavioral disturbances independent of the presence of PMS. Thus, the menstrual cycle may interact with or give rise to disturbances in mood and behavior as follows: (1) the menstrual cycle may modify the severity or appearance of certain psychiatric illnesses; (2) the menstrual cycle may trigger the recrudescence of a previously experienced psychiatric illness; and (3) the menstrual cycle may entrain an otherwise autonomous cyclic psychiatric disorder. In general, these phenomena may be readily distinguished from PMS during longitudinal confirmation of the diagnosis.

Menstrual Cycle-Related Events May Modulate Preexisting Psychopathology

In addition to the de novo production of mood and behavioral symptoms in a menstrual cycle phase-dependent fashion (eg, PMS), a series of observations suggest that normal menstrual cycle function could influence or alter the expression of concurrent psychiatric symptoms. First, menstrual cycle phase-related exacerbation of psychiatric symptoms was observed. Warnock,[79] Glick and Steward,[80] and Williams and Weekes[81] described psychiatric patients (manic or schizophrenic patients) whose symptoms increased in severity prior to menses, with improvement noted after menses. More recently, Malikian et al[82] reported the premenstrual worsening of the symptoms of depression in a sample of women with chronic depressive illness.

Second, the potential influence of the menstrual cycle phase on the expression of the symptoms of psychiatric illness was also inferred from numerous reports of the disproportionate occurrence of suicide attempts and/or psychiatric admissions during the premenstrual phase.[83–86] However, a postmortem study employing endometrial biopsies as a method of dating menstrual cycle phase in a sample of suicide victims found no increased proportion of suicides occurring during the premenstrual phase of the cycle.[87]

In contrast, the menstrual cycle may be associated with the episodic improvement of a coexisting psychiatric illness. Abraham[88] emphasized the importance of the postmenstrual euphoria experienced by some women with PMS. Further, we reported elsewhere[89] that women with PMS differ from controls not only in the severity of premenstrual dysphoria but also in the degree of postmenstrual euphoria (Fig. 1). Fig. 2 illustrates the pattern of dysphoric symptoms in a woman initially

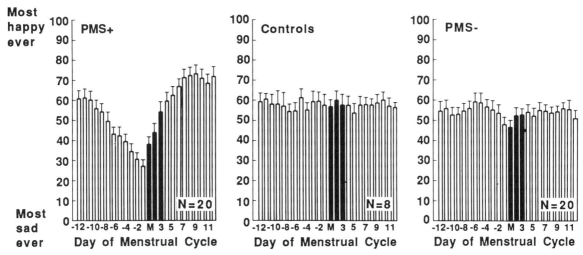

Fig. 1 Group mean daily AM ratings in relation to menses in three groups: prospectively confirmed women with PMS (PMS +), controls, women presenting with PMS but not meeting diagnostic criteria (PMS −). The solid histograms represent the first 3 days of menses. (Reprinted from Rubinow DR, et al. Premenstrual mood changes: characteristic patterns in women with and without premenstrual syndrome. *J Affect Dis.* 1986;10:85, with permission.)

presenting to our clinic with PMS and who had the diagnosis of PMS confirmed prospectively. Following the development of menstrual cycle irregularity, an alteration in the pattern and duration of depressive symptoms was observed, characterized by chronic dysphoria punctuated by symptom-free intervals during the menstrual and postmenstrual phases of the menstrual cycle. Thus, instead of PMS, it appeared that this patient experienced a follicular phase-triggered brief remission of the symptoms of a chronic affective disorder.

Menstrual cycle phase may influence the appearance (as opposed to the severity) of symptoms of a concurrent psychiatric disorder. Sutherland[90] noted that 99 of 162 women with mania characteristically experienced their mania during (88 women) or within 1 day to 1 week prior to (11 women) their menses. The occurrence

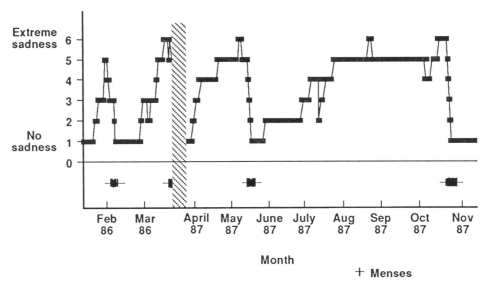

Fig. 2 Daily self-ratings of sadness in a woman with prospectively confirmed PMS. After the onset of menstrual cycle irregularity (hatched histogram), the patient's ostensible premenstrual dysphoria became a chronic dysphoria punctuated by symptom-free intervals during the menstrual and postmenstrual phases of the menstrual cycle.

of episodically experienced symptoms of psychiatric disorders (eg, bulimia and panic disorder) is anecdotally reported as disproportionately frequent during the premenstrual phase. While several authors note premenstrual increases in food cravings and appetite in normal women and women with PMS,[10,91–93] an absence of a menstrual cycle phase effect on bulimic episodes in patients with bulimia is found in some[94] but not all[95] investigations. Similarly, studies are unable to observe a menstrual cycle phase-related exacerbation or clustering of the symptoms of panic or anxiety in patients with panic disorder.[96–98]

Menstrual Cycle-Related Events May Trigger the Recrudescence of Previously Experienced Psychiatric Illness

The menstrual cycle is also described as influencing the reappearance of characteristic symptoms of a psychiatric disorder that otherwise appears to be in remission. In 1868 Ray stated that "in female patients, the menstrual period may produce an abnormal excitement after convalescence appeared to be firmly established."[99] Brockington et al[100] report this phenomenon in three cases of postpartum psychosis in which a remission was disturbed by a time-limited recrudescence of the original symptoms during the premenstrual phase of the menstrual cycle. This relationship between the menstrual cycle and postpartum illness is of particular interest given the reports of a higher than expected prevalence of a history of postpartum depression in some patients with PMS, suggesting that hormonal changes such as those seen during the postpartum period and the premenstrual phase of the normal menstrual cycle may trigger the recurrence of a previously experienced mood or behavioral disturbance. Thus, hormonal triggers (rather than hormonal causes) may be relevant to the onset and expression of symptoms of PMS.[2,3]

The Menstrual Cycle May Entrain an Otherwise Autonomous Cyclic Psychiatric Disorder

The menstrual cycle may entrain periodic psychiatric disorders by serving as a "zeitgeber," or synchronizer, such that the expression of the disorder is menstrual cycle phase dependent. Endo et al[101] described 7 patients with mental illness aligned with the menstrual cycle, with "complete remission" of symptoms observed during the intermenstrual phase. A case of temporal lobe epilepsy presenting as a premenstrual affective disorder

was reported by Price.[102] Hatotani et al[103] observed that of 47 women experiencing greater than three periodic psychiatric episodes, 23 (49%) repeatedly experienced their psychotic episodes during the middle or latter half of the menstrual cycle. Further, "the atypical psychoses"[103,104] and the "periodic psychoses of puberty"[105] both have as cardinal features the cyclic recurrence of psychotic symptoms during the late luteal and menstrual phases of the menstrual cycle. In some women with prospectively diagnosed PMS, the characteristic postmenstrual switch into euphoria is reminiscent of the mood state changes observed in bipolar illness.[76,89,106] Thus, some women with PMS may experience a menstrual cycle-entrained cyclic affective disorder that has become linked to but not caused by the menstrual cycle. Such women may have historical, biological, or treatment-response characteristics distinct from other women with PMS and may require different therapeutic modalities.

In addition to observations of menstrual cycle events triggering or synchronizing the timing of mood state changes, other evidence suggests that PMS is not caused by the late luteal phase of the menstrual cycle. For example, several reports suggest that the cyclical mood changes observed in some women with PMS may be independent of ovarian activity. Anecdotal case reports[107] describe characteristic premenstrual mood changes persisting after the natural or surgical menopause, when, by definition, ovarian function has ceased. These reports suggest that ovarian cyclicity is not necessary for the production of premenstrual mood symptoms in all women with PMS, and, in the patients described, the menstrual cycle may have entrained an autonomous cyclical mood disorder. Conversely, the dependence of the premenstrual mood state on menstrual endocrinology is suggested by descriptions of the remission of severe premenstrual mood changes following suppression of ovarian cyclicity with gonadotropin agonists or after a surgically induced menopause.[108–112]

We are currently examining the role of luteal phase endocrinology in PMS by altering the menstrual cycle with the antiprogestin RU 486. Seven days after the luteinizing hormone (LH) ovulatory surge, women with prospectively confirmed PMS are randomly administered placebo or RU 486, a progesterone receptor blocker that causes a sudden decrease in plasma progesterone and the onset of menses within 48 to 72 hours. Additionally, patients receive human chorionic gonadotropin (hCG) or placebo. Patients receiving hCG and RU 486 have menses within 48 to 72 hours; however, normal luteal phase progesterone levels are maintained due to the effects of hCG. Alternatively, patients receiving RU 486 and placebo enter the follicular phase after the RU 486-induced menses. Results demonstrate that some women with prospectively confirmed PMS experience their characteristic premenstrual mood state after RU 486-induced menses, at a time when the peripheral endocrine profile is that of the early follicular phase.[112]

Our observation that, as a group, women with prospectively confirmed PMS show no alteration of their symptoms despite the resetting of the menstrual cycle could support either of two possibilities. The symptoms of PMS may be triggered by hormonal events occurring prior to the late luteal phase of the menstrual cycle, consistent with reports that the suppression of ovulation results in a remission of PMS symptoms.[108-112] Alternatively, PMS may represent a cyclic disorder that is linked to but can be dissociated or desynchronized from the menstrual cycle. Our observations may be analogous to the "jet lag" phenomenon in travelers in which circadian rhythms temporarily become desynchronized or dissociated from the diurnal cues of the new time zone.

Post hoc analysis has revealed a past history of affective disorder in four of the five women experiencing the relative dissociation of their PMS from the late luteal phase of the menstrual cycle. Once again, this observation is consistent with either the "triggering" or "synchronization" mechanisms. Thus a hormonal event occurring prior to the late luteal phase of the menstrual cycle might trigger PMS symptoms in women whose past history of depression increased their vulnerability to the experience of mood disorders. Alternatively, the menstrual cycle may have acted to entrain an otherwise autonomous affective disorder in some of these women. Further, two women who received RU 486 alone did fail to evidence PMS symptoms when the menstrual cycle was reset, though these individual effects were obscured in group statistics. The possibility therefore exists that some patients with PMS may have an obligatory relationship between the premenstrual syndrome and the endocrine events of the late luteal phase.

In conclusion, our data suggest that, for some women, PMS may represent either a mood state disorder that is triggered by hormonal events occurring prior to the late luteal phase or an autonomous mood state disorder that is linked to but not caused by the menstrual cycle.

SUMMARY

While premenstrual syndrome shares similarities with major affective disorder, they are clearly distinguishable. Nonetheless, both PMS and major affective disorder represent mood state disorders, with the physiological factors responsible for regulating the entry into and exit from these states currently unidentified. As we learn more about the role of the reproductive endocrine system in PMS, we may be fortunate enough to uncover clues to more generalizable mechanisms of mood state regulation. By so doing, studies of PMS may significantly contribute to our search for the underlying pathophysiology of major affective disorder.

REFERENCES

1. Halbreich U, Endicott J, Nee J. Premenstrual depressive changes: value of differentiation. *Arch Gen Psych.* 1982;40:535.
2. Halbreich U, Endicott J, Goldstein S, et al. Premenstrual changes and changes in gonadal hormones. *Acta Psychiatr Scand.* 1986; 74:576.
3. Rubinow DR, Schmidt PJ. Models for the development and expression of symptoms in premenstrual syndrome. *Psych Clin North Am.* 1989;12:53.
4. Roy-Byrne PP, Hoban MC, Rubinow DR. The relationship of menstrually related mood disorders to psychiatric disorders. *Clin Obstet Gynecol.* 1987;30:386.
5. Endicott J, Halbreich U, Schacht S, et al. Premenstrual changes and affective disorders. *Psychosom Med.* 1981;43:519.
6. Freeman EW, Sondheimer S, Weinbaum PJ, et al. Evaluating premenstrual symptoms in medical practice. *Obstet Gynecol.* 1985;65:500.
7. Schinfeld JS, Cronin L, Parks-Truscs S. Presenting premenstrual symptoms: another look. In *International Symposium of Premenstrual Tension and Dysmenorrhoea*; Kiawah, SC; 1983.
8. Mortola JF. Premenstrual syndrome: past problems and new advances in the investigation of a model. In: Blumenthal S, Haseltine F, Rubinow DR, eds. *Late Luteal Phase Dysphoric Disorder: New Research Directions*, Washington, DC: American Psychiatric Press, Inc.; 1991.
9. Davidson JRT, Miller RD, Turnbull CD, et al. Atypical depression. *Arch Gen Psych.* 1982;39:527.
10. Both-Orthman B, Rubinow DR, Hoban MC, et al. Menstrual cycle phase-related changes in appetite in patients with premenstrual syndrome and in control subjects. *Am J Psych.* 1988;145: 628.
11. Wurtman JJ, Brzezinski A, Wurtman RJ, et al. Effect of nutrient intake on premenstrual depression. *Am J Obstet Gynecol.* 1989; 161:1228.
12. Frank E, Carpenter LL, Kupfer DJ. Sex differences in recurrent depression: are there any that are significant? *Am J Psych.* 1988; 145:41.
13. Mauri M, Reid RL, MacLean AW. Sleep in the premenstrual phase: a self-report study of PMS patients and normal controls. *Acta Psychiatr Scand.* 1988;78:82.
14. Jensvold MF, Muller KL, Rubinow DR. Sleep, fatigue and mood in premenstrual syndrome. In: Abstracts of the American Psychiatric Association 141st Annual Meeting, Montreal, Canada; 1988; New Research Abstract #185.
15. Mauri M, Reid RL, MacLean AW. Sleep disturbances in the premenstrual syndrome: the possible role of arousal. *Sleep Res Abstr.* 1986;15:196.
16. Steiner M, Haskett RF, Carroll BJ. Premenstrual tension syndrome: the development of research diagnostic criteria and new rating scales. *Acta Psychiatr Scand.* 1980;62:177.

17. Faratian B, Gaspar A, O'Brien PMS, et al. Premenstrual syndrome: weight, abdominal swelling, and perceived body image. *Am J Obstet Gynecol.* 1984;150:200.

18. Casper RF, Graves GR, Reid RL. Objective measurement of hot flushes associated with the premenstrual syndrome. *Fertil Steril.* 1987;47:341.

19. Schuckit MA, Daly V, Herrman G, et al. Premenstrual symptoms and depression in a university population. *Dis Nerv Syst.* 1975;36:516.

20. Wetzel RD, Reich T, McClure JM, et al. Premenstrual affective syndrome and affective disorder. *Br J Psych.* 1975;127:129.

21. Mackenzie TB, Wilcox K, Baron H. Lifetime prevalence of psychiatric disorders in women with perimenstrual difficulties. *J Affect Dis.* 1986;10:15.

22. Halbreich U, Endicott J. Relationship of dysphoric premenstrual changes to depressive disorders. *Acta Psychiatr Scand.* 1985;71:331.

23. DeJong R, Rubinow DR, Roy-Byrne P, et al. Premenstrual mood disorder and psychiatric illness. *Am J Psych.* 1985;142:1359.

24. Pearlstein TB, Thoft J, Rubinstein D, et al. Psychiatric diagnosis and luteal variation in PMS women. Abstracts of the American Psychiatric Association 141st Annual Meeting, Montreal, Canada; 1988: New Research Abstract #10.

25. Freeman E, Rickels K, Sondheimer SJ, et al. Ineffectiveness of progesterone suppository treatment for premenstrual syndrome. *JAMA.* 1990;264:349.

26. Baldessarini RJ. Risk rates for depression. *Arch Gen Psych.* 1984;41:103.

27. O'Hara MW. Postpartum "blues," depression, and psychosis: a review. *J Psychosom Obstet Gyn.* 1987;7:205.

28. Johnson SR. Epidemiology of premenstrual symptoms: study design issues and reproductive risk factors. In: Blumenthal S, Haseltine F, Rubinow DR, eds. *Late Luteal Phase Dysphoric Disorder: New Research Directions.* Washington, DC: American Psychiatric Press, Inc.; 1991.

29. Harrison WM, Sandberg D, Gorman JM, et al. Provocation of panic with carbon dioxide inhalation in patients with premenstrual dysphoria. *Psych Res.* 1989;27:183.

30. Liebowitz MF, Fyer AJ, Gorman JM, et al. Lactate provocation of panic attacks. I. Clinical and behavioral findings. *Arch Gen Psych.* 1984;41:764.

31. Uhde TW. Caffeine provocation of panic: a focus on biological mechanisms. In: Ballenger JC, ed. *Neurobiology of Panic Disorder.* New York, NY: Alan R. Liss, Inc.; 1990:219.

32. Gorman JM, Askanazi J, Liebowitz MR, et al. Response to hyperventilation in a group of patients with panic disorder. *Am J Psych.* 1984;141:857.

33. Rossignol AM. Caffeine-containing beverages and premenstrual syndrome in young women. *Am J Pub Health.* 1985;75:1335.

34. Steege JF, Rupp SL, Stout AL. Symptoms associated with caffeine consumption in women seeking treatment for premenstrual syndrome. In: Abstracts of the Second International Symposium on Premenstrual, Postpartum, and Menopause Related Mood Disorders, Kiawah Island, SC; 1987.

35. Smith S, Rinehart JS, Ruddock VE, et al. Treatment of premenstrual syndrome with alprazolam: results of a double-blind, placebo-controlled, randomized crossover clinical trial. *Obstet Gynecol.* 1987;70:37.

36. Harrison WM, Endicott J, Nee J. Treatment of premenstrual dysphoria with alprazolam: a controlled study. *Arch Gen Psych.* 1990;47:270.

37. Jensvold MF, Putnam F, Muller KL, et al. Abuse, dissociation, and PTSD in LLPDD patients. In: Abstracts of the 142nd Annual Meeting of the American Psychiatric Association; San Francisco, CA; 1989: New Research Abstract #41.

38. Harrison WM, Rabkin JG, Endicott J. Psychiatric evaluation of premenstrual changes. *Psychosomatics.* 1985;26:789.

39. Rubinow DR, Hoban MC, Grover GN, et al. Changes in plasma hormones across the menstrual cycle in patients with menstru-

40. Rabin DS, Schmidt PJ, Campbell G, et al. Hypothalamic-pituitary-adrenal function in patients with the premenstrual syndrome. *J Clin Endocrinol Metab.* 1990;71:1158.

41. Carroll BJ, Curtis GC, Davies BM, et al. Urinary free cortisol excretion in depression. *Psychol Med.* 1976;6:43.

42. Haskett RF, Steiner M, Carroll BJ. A psychoendocrine study of premenstrual tension syndrome: a model for endogenous depression? *J Affect Dis.* 1984;6:191.

43. Steiner M, Haskett RF, Carroll BJ. Circadian hormone secretory profiles in women with severe premenstrual tension syndrome. *Br J Obstet Gynaecol.* 1984;91:466.

44. Mortola J, Girton L, Yen SSC. Psychometric and hormonal assessments of depression in premenstrual syndrome. In: Abstracts of the Society for Gynecologic Investigation; Baltimore, MD; 1988: Abstract #428.

45. Roy-Byrne PP, Rubinow DR, Gwirtsman H, et al. Cortisol response to dexamethasone in women with premenstrual syndrome. *Neuropsychobiology.* 1986;16:61.

46. Gold PW, Loriaux DL, Roy A, et al. Responses to corticotropin-releasing hormone in the hypercortisolism of depression and Cushing's disease: pathophysiologic and diagnostic implications. *N Engl J Med.* 1986;314:1329.

47. Graves R. Clinical lectures. *Medical Classics.* 1940;5:25.

48. Gold MS, Pottash ALC, Extein I. Hypothyroidism and depression: evidence from complete thyroid function evaluation. *JAMA.* 1981;245:1919.

49. Cowdry RW, Wehr TA, Zis AP, et al. Thyroid abnormalities associated with rapid cycling bipolar illness. *Arch Gen Psych.* 1983;40:414.

50. Bauer MS, Whybrow PC, Winokur A. Rapid cycling bipolar affective disorder. I. Association with Grade I hypothyroidism. *Arch Gen Psych.* 1990;47:427.

51. Nemeroff CB, Simon JS, Haggerty JJ Jr, et al. Antithyroid antibodies in depressed patients. *Am J Psych.* 1985;142:840.

52. Brayshaw ND, Brayshaw DD. Premenstrual syndrome and thyroid dysfunction. *Integr Psych.* 1987;5:179.

53. Schmidt PJ, Khan RA, Rubinow DR. Thyroid function in premenstrual syndrome [letter]. *N Engl J Med.* 1987;317:1537.

54. Schmidt PJ, Rosenfeld D, Muller KL, et al. A case of autoimmune thyroiditis presenting as menstrual related mood disorder. *J Clin Psych.* 1990;51:434.

55. Roy-Byrne PP, Rubinow DR, Hoban MC, et al. TSH and prolactin responses to TRH in patients with premenstrual syndrome. *Am J Psych.* 1987;144:480.

56. Nikolai TF, Mulligan GM, Gribble RK, et al. Thyroid function and treatment in premenstrual syndrome. *J Clin Endocrinol Metab.* 1990;70:1108.

57. Casper RF, Patel-Christopher A, Powell AM. Thyrotropin and prolactin responses to thyrotropin-releasing hormone in premenstrual syndrome. *J Clin Endocrinol Metab.* 1989;68:608.

58. Loosen PT. The TRH induced TSH response in psychiatric patients: a possible neuroendocrine marker. *Psychoneuroendocrinology.* 1985;10:237.

59. Taylor DL, Mathew RJ, Ho BT, et al. Serotonin levels and platelet uptake during premenstrual tension. *Neuropsychobiology.* 1984;12:16.

60. Ashby CR Jr, Carr LA, Cook CL, et al. Alteration of platelet serotonergic mechanism and monoamine oxidase activity in premenstrual syndrome. *Biol Psych.* 1988;24:225.

61. Rapkin AJ, Edelmuth E, Chang LC, et al. Whole-blood serotonin in premenstrual syndrome. *Obstet Gynecol.* 1987;70:533.

62. Meltzer HY, Arora RC, Baber R, et al. Serotonin uptake in blood platelets of psychiatric patients. *Arch Gen Psych.* 1981;38:1322.

63. Halbreich U. Gonadal hormones and antihormones, serotonin and mood. *Psychopharmacol Bull.* 1990;26:291.

64. Halbreich U, Rojansky N, Barkai A, et al. Biological abnormali-

ties in premenstrual dysphoria. Abstracts of the American Psychiatric Association 142nd Annual Meeting; San Francisco, CA; 1989: New Research Abstract #199.

65. Jensvold M, Grover GN, Muller KL, et al. Growth hormone, cortisol and prolactin responses to intravenous clonidine in PMS patients and controls. In: Abstracts of 21st Congress of International Society of Psychoneuroendocrinology; Buffalo, NY; 1990: Abstract #144.

66. Kripke DF, Mullaney DJ, Atkinson M, et al. Circadian rhythm disorders in manic depressives. *Biol Psych.* 1978;13:335.

67. Wehr TA, Goodwin FK. Circadian rhythm desynchronization as a basis for manic-depressive cycles. *Psychopharmacol Bull.* 1980;16:19.

68. Gillin JC. The sleep therapies of depression. *Prog Neuro-Psychopharmacol Biol Psychiatry.* 1983;7:351.

69. Lewy AJ, Sack RL, Miller S, et al. Antidepressant and circadian phase-shifting effects of light. *Science.* 1987;235:352.

70. Parry BL, Mendelson WB, Duncan WB, et al. Longitudinal sleep EEG, temperature, and activity measurements across the menstrual cycle in patients with premenstrual depression and in age-matched controls. *Psych Res.* 1989;30:285.

71. Parry BL, Berga SL, Kripke DF, et al. Altered waveform of plasma nocturnal melatonin secretion in premenstrual syndrome. *Arch Gen Psych.* 1990;47:1139.

72. Parry BL, Wehr TA. Therapeutic effect of sleep deprivation in patients with premenstrual syndrome. *Am J Psych.* 1987;144: 808.

73. Parry BL, Berga SL, Mostofi N, et al. Morning versus evening bright light treatment of late luteal phase dysphoric disorders. *Am J Psych.* 1989;146:1215.

74. Harrison WM, Endicott J, Nee J. Treatment of premenstrual depression with nortriptyline: a pilot study. *J Clin Psych.* 1989; 50:136.

75. Stone AB, Pearlstein T, Brown W. Fluoxetine in the treatment of late luteal phase dysphoric disorder. *J Clin Psych.* 1991;52:7.

76. Steiner M, Haskett RF, Osmun JN, et al. Treatment of premenstrual tension with lithium carbonate. *Acta Psychiatr Scand.* 1980;61:96.

77. Rickels K, Feighner JP, Smith WT. Alprazolam, amitriptyline, doxepin and placebo in the treatment of depression. *Arch Gen Psych.* 1985;42:134.

78. Rickels K, Freeman E, Sondheimer S. Buspirone in treatment of premenstrual syndrome. *Lancet.* 1989;1:777.

79. Warnock J. On some of the relations between menstruation and insanity. *North Am Pract.* 1890;2:49.

80. Glick ID, Steward D. A new drug treatment for premenstrual exacerbation of schizophrenia. *Compr Psych.* 1980;21:281.

81. Williams EY, Weekes LR. Premenstrual tension associated with psychotic episodes. *J Nerv Ment Dis.* 1952;116:321.

82. Malikian JE, Hurt S, Endicott J, et al. Premenstrual dysphoric changes in depressed patients. In: Abstracts of the American Psychiatric Association 142nd Annual Meeting; San Francisco, CA; 1989:219.

83. Mandell AJ, Mandell MP. Suicide and the menstrual cycle. *JAMA.* 1967;200:792.

84. Tonks CM, Rack PH, Rose MJ. Attempted suicide in the menstrual cycle. *J Psychosom Res.* 1968;11:319.

85. Dalton K. Menstruation and acute psychiatric illnesses. *Br Med J.* 1959;1:148.

86. Janowsky DW, Gorney R, Castelnuovo-Tedesco P, et al. Premenstrual-menstrual increases in psychiatric admission rates. *Am J Obstet Gynecol.* 1969;103:189.

87. Vanezis P. Deaths in women of reproductive age and relationship with menstrual cycle phase. An autopsy study of cases reported to the coroner. *Forensic Sci Int.* 1990;47:39.

88. Abraham S. Premenstrual or postmenstrual syndrome? *Med J Aust.* 1984;327.

89. Rubinow DR, Roy-Byrne P, Hoban MC, et al. Premenstrual

mood changes: characteristic patterns in women with and without premenstrual syndrome. *J Affect Dis.* 1986;10:85.

90. Sutherland H. Menstruation and insanity. In: Tuke DH, ed. *A Dictionary of Psychological Medicine,* Philadelphia: P. Blakistone Son & Co.; 1892:801.

91. Smith SL, Sauder C. Food cravings, depression, and premenstrual problems. *Psychosom Med.* 1969;31:281.

92. Fankhauser M, Potter R, Shisslak C, et al. Eating behaviors during the menstrual cycle. In: Abstracts of the American Psychiatric Association 142nd Annual Meeting, San Francisco, CA; 1989:389.

93. Cohen IT, Sherwin BB, Fleming AS. Food cravings, mood, and the menstrual cycle. *Horm Behav.* 1987;21:457.

94. Leon GR, Phelan PW, Kelly JT, et al. The symptoms of bulimia and the menstrual cycle. *Psychosom Med.* 1986;48:415.

95. Gladis MM, Walsh BT. Premenstrual exacerbation of binge eating in bulimia. *Am J Psych.* 1987;144:1592.

96. Stein Mb, Schmidt PJ, Rubinow DR, et al. Panic disorder and the menstrual cycle: panic disorder patients, healthy control subjects, and patients with premenstrual syndrome. *Am J Psych.* 1989;146:1299.

97. Cook BL, Noyes R Jr, Garvey MJ, et al. Anxiety and the menstrual cycle in panic disorder. *J Affect Dis.* 1990;19:221.

98. Cameron OG, Kuttesch D, McPhee K, et al. Menstrual fluctuation in the symptoms of panic anxiety. *J Affect Dis.* 1988;15: 169.

99. Evans BD. Periodic insanity, in which the exciting cause appears to be the menstrual function: report of a typical case. *Medical News.* 1893;538.

100. Brockington IF, Kelly A, Hall P, et al. Premenstrual relapse of puerperal psychosis. *J Affect Dis.* 1988;14:287.

101. Endo M, Daiguji M, Asano Y, et al. Periodic psychosis recurring in association with menstrual cycle. *J Clin Psych.* 1978;39:456.

102. Price TRP. Temporal lobe epilepsy as a premenstrual behavioral syndrome. *Biol Psych.* 1980;15:957.

103. Hatotani N, Ishida C, Yura R, et al. Psychophysiological studies of atypical psychoses: endocrinological aspects of periodic psychoses. *Folia Psychiatr Neurol Jpn.* 1962;16:248.

104. Yamashita I, Shinohara S, Nakazawa A. Endocrinological studies of atypical psychosis. *Folia Psychiatr Neurol Jpn.* 1962;16: 293.

105. Altschule MD, Brem J. Periodic psychosis of puberty. *Am J Psychiatry.* 1963;119:1176.

106. Rubinow DR, Hoban MC, Grover GN. PMS: medical and psychiatric perspectives. In: Keye WR Jr, ed. *The Premenstrual Syndrome,* Philadelphia: W.B. Saunders Co.; 1988:27.

107. Dalton K. *The Premenstrual Syndrome and Progesterone Therapy.* London: William Heinemann; 1984.

108. Muse KN, Cetel NS, Futterman LA, et al. The premenstrual syndrome: effects of "medical ovariectomy." *N Engl J Med.* 1984;311:1345.

109. Hammarback S, Backstrom T. Induced anovulation as a treatment of premenstrual tension syndrome: a double-blind crossover study with GnRH-agonist versus placebo. *Acta Obstet Gynecol Scand.* 1988;67:159.

110. Casson P, Hahn PM, VanVugt DA, et al. Lasting response to ovariectomy in severe intractable premenstrual syndrome. *Am J Obstet Gynecol.* 1990;162:99.

111. Casper RF, Hearn MT. The effect of hysterectomy and bilateral oophorectomy in women with severe premenstrual syndrome. *Am J Obstet Gynecol.* 1990;162:105.

112. Mortola JF, Girton L, Fischer U. Successful treatment of severe premenstrual syndrome by combined use of gonadotropin-releasing hormone agonist and estrogen/progestin. *J Clin Endocrinol Metab.* 1991;7:252A.

113. Schmidt PJ, Nieman LK, Grover GN, et al. Lack of effect of induced menses on symptoms in women with premenstrual syndrome. *N Engl J Med.* 1991;324:1174.

C H A P T E R   8

Relationship of Medical Illness to the Menstrual Cycle

Keith Isaacson and Ashok Balasubramanyam

Many women experience a variety of physical signs and symptoms that occur with menstrual periodicity and are commonly attributed to premenstrual syndrome (PMS). However, there are no symptoms that are unique to and diagnostic of PMS.[1] Physicians who care for women in the reproductive years should be aware of a number of acute medical illnesses that recur or chronic diseases which intensify during particular phases of the menstrual cycle. The term "catamenial" (from the Greek "around the menses") was used originally to describe only a few striking illnesses such as catamenial epilepsy, pneumothorax, and migraine headaches, but the term may now be applied to many other well-described conditions as well (Table 1).

In this chapter we review the catamenial illnesses for which there is significant literature while omitting diseases with unclear associations to the menstrual cycle. The etiological theories concerning these disorders are sometimes well supported, often fanciful, and always interesting. In the words of Jeliffe (referring to catamenial migraine), "Naturally the endocrines cannot be neglected—various authors implicate now this, now that, and usually have three or four balls in the hypothetical endocrine air, and not all of them gonads."[2] We hope this chapter is a useful reference for the health care provider of patients who present with recurrent cyclical symptoms of unclear cause.

MEDICAL ILLNESS

Epilepsy

The occurrence of epilepsy with menstruation was noted by Gowers as early as 1885.[3] Subsequent observations have tended to confirm this association, although

Table 1
Medical Disorders Affected by the Menstrual Cycle

Epilepsy
Migraine headache
Neurologic disorders
Catamenial pneumothorax
Rheumatoid arthritis
Asthma
Diabetes mellitus
Porphyria
Hemostatic disorders
Appendicitis
Cholelithiasis
Hepatic diseases
Genital herpes
Recurrent urticaria and anaphylaxis
Glaucoma

uniformity is lacking and incidence estimates range from almost no association[4] to as high as 72% of epileptic women.[5] Laidlaw's is the largest survey (33,468 seizures in 939 patient years with 9293 menstrual cycles), with careful documentation of seizure dates and cycle days and strict definitions of cycle regularity and seizure type. Almost all women with catamenial influence had a significant reduction in seizure frequency during the postovulatory phase. There was a less regular increase in frequency immediately premenstrually and during the menses.[5] Similar associations are noted in numerous single-case studies or smaller series.[6,7] A more recent larger series[8] followed 69 women over 4 years and noted seizure exacerbation before and during menses in two-thirds, with nearly a doubling in frequency at the peak immediately premenstrually.

No particular type of seizure is more prone to catamenial exacerbation than any other, although many reports do not specify seizure type. Backstrom noted a catamenial periodicity in secondarily generalized seizures but not in partial seizures[9]; Helmchen et al noted the opposite in a single patient.[10]

Influence of Gonadal Hormones

The possible influence of sex hormones on epilepsy is underscored by the effects of the menarche. One study noted a statistical decrease in the frequency of preexisting generalized and partial seizures after menarche,[11] while another larger series observed an increase in seizure frequency or presentation of a new seizure type in two thirds of patients.[8] The case for onset of epilepsy at menarche is more striking. Lennox and Lennox noted that the first seizure occurred at menarche in 25% of young epileptic women, with the majority beginning within a month after menarche.[12] Onset shortly after menarche was also noted in over one-half of women with an established catamenial pattern of seizures.[6] The occurrence of any consistent, significant changes in seizure activity due to pregnancy or the menopause is more controversial.[13–17]

Laidlaw's observation that seizure frequency was lowest during the luteal phase and highest premenstrually and during the menses[5] raised the obvious hypothesis that low progesterone levels, high circulating estrogens, or a combination might be responsible for catamenial epilepsy. The observation is corroborated and the hypothesis refined in several subsequent studies correlating serial hormonal measurements with seizure frequency. In a small but carefully designed study, Backstrom found that secondary generalization of seizures increased with increasing estrogen/progesterone

ratio as measured through the menstrual cycle. The frequency of generalized seizures correlated positively with estradiol levels and negatively with progesterone levels; conversely, seizure frequency decreased with increasing progesterone levels. For partial seizure frequency, a positive correlation was noted to the estrogen/progesterone ratio alone. The study included three women with anovulatory cycles; in these women, with the effect of progesterone relatively absent, seizure frequency increased during days of high estrogen.[9] In a larger study measuring estrogen and progesterone metabolite excretion in groups of epileptic women with and without catamenial exacerbation and in normal controls, no relationship was seen between estrogen levels and seizures. However, a deficiency of progesterone relative to estradiol in the premenstrual period was marked in catamenial patients compared to the others.[18] Similar results were obtained in smaller studies.[19,20]

Animal experiments show that estrogen lowers and progesterone elevates the seizure threshold. In rats, Wooley and Timiras showed decreased electroshock seizure threshold when blood estrogens were elevated either endogenously (during estrus) or exogenously.[21,22] The decreased electroshock threshold was localized to areas in the dorsal hippocampus and medial amygdala, areas known to be directly affected by estrogen in the pathway governing reproductive behavior.[23] Logothetis and Harner demonstrated in rabbits that the epileptogenic potential of estrogens was greatest in the presence of a preexisting cortical lesion and disruption of the blood–brain barrier.[24] Estrogens also promote secondary generalization of seizures from discrete cortical foci.[25] The opposite, or protective effect of progesterone, was not uniformly seen in animal experiments except in very large doses.[26,27] The effect of sex steroids also appears to be different in male and female animals; in rats, estrogens are more epileptogenic in females than in males, and progesterone is protective in females but actually increases seizure severity in males.[28]

Human experiments involve electroencephalographic recordings either at "baseline" during various phases of the menstrual cycle or after infusions of sex steroids. Serial electroencephalograms (EEGs) in normal young women show an increase in alpha wave frequency and amplitude as well as increased paroxysms in the premenstrual period as compared to midcycle or follicular periods.[29,30] Rosciszewska performed serial EEGs on 41 women with catamenial exacerbations and noted that 24 had increased paroxysmal discharges on premenstrual days, while 17 had the same on days close to ovulation. In both groups, the lowest frequencies of paroxysmal discharges were noted in the early follicular and early luteal phases.[8] Logothetis et al infused large doses of Premarin into 16 epileptic women with premenstrual exacerbations and noted an activating effect in the EEG.[6]

To confirm that peripheral measurements of steroid levels are meaningful in interpreting central nervous system (CNS) effects, Backstrom's group correlated plasma estradiol and progesterone to cerebrospinal fluid (CSF) levels and confirmed that free serum estradiol equilibrates with the CSF.[31] Backstrom et al later infused progesterone into seven catamenial epileptics during the first week of the cycle to raise plasma progesterone to luteal phase levels. The four women with the lowest progesterone binding capacity showed a decrease in interictal spike frequency in the EEG during the infusion.[32] Despite the small sample size, this result is of interest because it indicates that the availability of free, unbound progesterone is important for the antiepileptic effect. It is significant that commonly used antiepileptic drugs elevate plasma cortisol binding globulin, which binds about 50% of circulating progesterone. In the study just mentioned, the smallest effect of progesterone was seen in women who were already on antiepileptic medications, despite high levels of total progesterone.

Given the complex interactions of hormones in the menstrual cycle, it is likely that an interplay of many factors—kinetics of rise and fall of estrogen and progesterone in addition to absolute levels of each, binding protein status, and higher modulating influences—create the milieu that leads to the classical late luteal phase exacerbation of seizures. This is underscored in a careful, controlled study by Rosciszewska et al addressing multiple variables in a large number of patients and controls. There was no correlation between estrogen levels and seizure frequency, and only an apparent relationship between low progesterone and increased seizures. The clearest difference between controls and epileptics was that in the former group the ratio of progesterone to estrogen increased premenstrually compared to the midfollicular phase, while in the latter this increase was not seen. Additionally, in the patient group, drug levels of phenytoin declined in the premenstrual period.[18]

The cellular biochemistry of CNS nuclei that underlies these phenomenological observations reveals some interesting points regarding neural regulation of sexual and reproductive function. CNS sites where sex hormones concentrate and which are known to influence mammalian reproductive behavior as well as ovulation include limbic forebrain structures in the medial amygdala, stria terminalis, septum, preoptic area, ventromedial hypothalamic nuclei and hippocampus. Two of these—the amygdala and the hippocampus—are known to be potentially epileptogenic. Seizure threshold in these areas is lowest when estrogen levels are elevated and is reversed when estrogen declines.[21] The same effect is seen in oophorectomized and hypophysectomized rats, suggesting a direct CNS effect of the exogenous estrogen.[22] The latency of this effect is short and cannot be explained by the well-known estrogen effect of triggering protein synthesis after binding to its intracellular receptor. Estradiol has been shown to have a rapid, direct effect on ionic conductance in the postsynaptic membrane of medial amygdala neuroma in rats.[33] Interestingly, the proportion of estrogen-responsive neurons was greater in females than in males.

The molecular basis for the anticonvulsive effect of progesterone may be found in recent observations linking the sedative-hypnotic effects of certain steroid molecules to their coupling with CNS receptors that regulate inhibitory signals. The γ-aminobutyric acid-agonist/benzodiazepine receptor-chloride ionophore (GBRC) complex is a receptor system that mediates the inhibitory effects of both γ-aminobutyric acid (GABA) and the therapeutic benzodiazepines. Steroids with sedative-hypnotic properties interact specifically with this complex and enhance by positive cooperativity the binding of GABA agonists and benzodiazepines to their respective recognition sites. The stringent structural requirements for activity at the GBRC are met by some naturally occurring metabolites of progesterone with significant potencies at physiological levels. It is likely that these steroids modulate brain excitability by potentiating the postsynaptic effects of GABA.[34]

Drug–hormone interactions are another mode by which sex hormones could influence seizure activity. There are several potentially significant interactions. The hepatic microsomal enzyme system is a common degradative pathway for progesterone and estrogens as well as several antiepileptic drugs. It is possible that lack of competition by the hormones during their premenstrual nadir might lead to greater metabolism of anticonvulsant drugs and thereby facilitate seizure activity.[35] Antiepileptics induce synthesis of sex hormone-binding globulin which leads to decreased levels of unbound, active estrogen.[36] Significant induction of the metabolism of synthetic progestogens can occur with anticonvulsants.[37]

The practical effect of these interactions on actual drug levels and on the clinical course of catamenial epilepsy is controversial. One study found no correlation between serum levels of phenytoin, carbamazepine, and phenobarbital and estrogen and progesterone levels,[38] while others found declines in phenytoin or carbamazepine levels in the late luteal phase.[18,39,40] Although in many patients luteal levels were significantly lower than at midcycle, in the majority this fall did not cause the serum level of the drug to fall below usually accepted "therapeutic" levels. On balance, it is likely that fluctuating antiepileptic levels play a peripheral role in the pathogenesis of catamenial epilepsy, perhaps provoking seizures in the presence of declining progesterone or on alteration in the estrogen/progesterone ratio. Nevertheless, this phenomenon is important to keep in mind when managing epileptic women in the reproductive period of their lives.

Therapy of Catamenial Epilepsy

Therapy of women with intractable catamenial exacerbations involves several manipulations to decrease the estrogen effect and enhance that of progesterone. Early drastic maneuvers such as ovariectomy were usually without success and have been abandoned.[41] Most success is obtained with various forms of progesterone, usually given in doses high enough to suppress menses. Earlier reports of single cases showed some dramatic results.[42–44] Mattson et al performed a controlled trial of medroxyprogesterone on 14 patients for an average of 13 months, monitoring antiepileptic drug levels. The 6 women who experienced secondary amenorrhea had more than 50% decrease in seizure frequency; five of the others discontinued the hormone because of continuous bleeding.[45,46] Similar results were noted using natural progesterone intermittently.[47] However, one placebo-controlled, double-blind study using norethisterone on 9 patients showed no benefit from the hormone.[48] Differences in results with different progestogens may be due to the specificity of structure required of progesterone metabolites to act at the GBRC complex, as discussed above. There is also a report of significant long-term success using the benzodiazepine clobazam for severe catamenial seizures.[49]

Effect of Seizures on Hormones

This discussion has focused on the effect of regular sex hormone variations on seizures rather than the converse relationship; however, the effect of seizures on hormone levels must always be borne in mind as a caveat when interpreting studies of catamenial epilepsy. Follicle-stimulating hormone, luteinizing hormone, and prolactin are significantly elevated by electroshock convulsions,[50,51] but the effect of seizures on cyclical estrogen and progesterone measurements is unknown.[52] In the case of complex partial structures, the effect on luteinizing hormone may be the result of temporal lobe discharges disrupting normal limbic modulation of pulsatile secretion of gonadotropin-releasing hormone (GnRH) discharges. Indeed, a significant correlation is noted between the incidence of polycystic ovarian disease (PCO) or hypogonadotropic hypogonadism (HH) and that of complex partial seizures, suggesting a coincident disruption of normal limbic region neuronal circuits and hypothalamic control of gonadotropin secretion. Adversely, the anovulatory cycles in PCO and HH could expose limbic structures to a constant high level of estrogen and potentiate epileptiform activity.[53]

Migraine

Although the clinical course of migraine has been known to be affected by the menstrual cycle for decades, studies on the association are less extensive than with catamenial epilepsy, and the correlation with particular hormonal variations is less clear. Up to 67% of women with migraines are noted to have frequent attacks related to menses,[54] although the proportion that have regular catamenial attacks is disputed, ranging from less than 10%[55] to over 50%.[56]

Lance and Anthony made the clinical observation in a large number of chronic migraine patients that pregnancy had a salutary effect on the frequency of attacks in a significant proportion, the percentage being highest in those whose pregravid migraine was catamenially exacerbated.[57] Epstein et al found a similar effect of pregnancy and noted that women with catamenial migraine were likely to have had onset of migraine at menarche and to relapse during the puerperium. These authors also measured sex hormone levels in migraine patients with and without catamenial attacks and in normals; they noted that both groups of migraine patients had higher estrogen and progesterone levels than the normal group, especially in the late luteal phase, but were indistinguishable from each other. Gonadotropin and prolactin levels in the migraine groups were not different from normal.[55] On the other hand, Murialdo et al noted lower than normal progesterone levels and low progesterone to estradiol ratios in the luteal and follicular phases of women with migraine.[58]

The few studies that have looked at progesterone or estrogen kinetics in relation to menstrual migraine fail to show any consistent patterns.[59–61] On balance, however, and in contradistinction to the situation with catamenial epilepsy, menstrual migraine is in some manner associated with decline in estrogen rather than changes in progesterone. In fact, Somerville used the term "estrogen-withdrawal migraine" to refer to this entity and noted that administration of exogenous estrogens for several days followed by abrupt withdrawal could induce attacks. However, migraine could not be delayed or prevented by prophylactic continuous estrogen treatment.[60]

Opioid Monoaminergic Activity

Recently, attention has been directed toward higher signaling pathways, especially those with cyclical variations in tone and those associated with central gonadotropin secretion. One system of obvious interest is the opioid pathway which, in addition to its involvement in pain perception, exerts a tonic influence on a number of hormonal releasing factors through receptors located in the hypothalamus.[62,63] Moreover, opioid activity in primates may fluctuate regularly through the menstrual cycle and peak in the midluteal phase.[64] Tonic opiate inhibition of GnRH secretion is inferred from the positive response of luteinizing hormone to the opiate antagonist naloxone.[64] Similarly, opioids negatively regulate secretion of proopiomelanocortin (POMC) peptides from the hypothalmus, and high doses of naloxone exert a parallel release of the POMC product beta-endorphin and ACTH in humans.[65] There is preliminary evidence that central opioid tone is abnormal in the luteal phase in patients with catamenial migraine, so that secretion of both gonadotropins and pain- and stress-related peptides are blunted basally and in response to naloxone.[66]

Abnormalities in central monoaminergic transmission are noted in cyclical migraine. Autonomic symptoms associated with migraine can be induced more frequently and intensely by the administration of dopamine agonists.[67] Murialdo et al found supersensitivity of postsynaptic dopaminergic neurons in the hypothalamus, suggesting a "transmitter-depleted" state in the presynaptic neurons. These data complement the opioid pathway observations because monoaminergic pathways mediate several opioid effects.[58] Taken together, the data suggest impairment of a hypothetical feedback loop in which cyclical ovarian hormones are unable to normally modulate central monoaminergic discharges, which in turn (tonically) affect gonadotropin secretion.

Endogenous opioid pathways, either independently or as part of the feedback, modulate monoaminergic hypothalamic tone; a net decrease in opioid action results in diminished release of POMC peptides that could attenuate pain and the stress response.

Other Neurological Syndromes

Compressive symptoms of meningiomas are noted to occur or worsen during periods of increased levels of reproductive hormones such as in pregnancy.[68] This observation of symptom exacerbation during pregnancy and the increased incidence of meningiomas in women with breast cancer[69] led to the discovery of putative estrogen and progesterone receptors in meningiomas and raised the hope of hormonal therapy.[70] However, using strict criteria for "receptor positivity" and further analyzing for competitive binding against a number of nonestrogenic or progestogenic steroid molecules, Schwartz et al concluded that the hormone binding proteins in meningiomas are unlikely to be specific steroid receptors.[71] The cause of the catamenial exacerbation of meningioma symptoms remains unclear.

A syndrome of hypersomnia associated with each menstruation, and clinically akin to the Kleine–Levin syndrome has been reported. The patients were successfully treated by suppressing menses with conjugated estrogen or a combination pill.[72,73]

There are well-documented case reports of catamenially exacerbated action myoclonus,[74] neuralgia paresthetica,[75] and paraparesis due to spinal cord vascular malformations.[76]

Catamenial Pneumothorax

In 1958, Maurer et al first reported a case of a woman with 15 documented episodes of spontaneous pneumothorax, all of which occurred during menstruation.[77] This clinical entity was subsequently referred to as catamenial pneumothorax by Lillington et al when they reported 5 patients with this disorder and compared them to the 15 patients previosly reported.[78] To date, more than 70 cases of catamenial pneumothorax have been described.

Catamenial pneumothorax is by definition a syndrome that affects only women. Characteristically, it presents as right-sided pneumothorax in more than 90% of affected women, has a close temporal relation to the onset of menstrual flow, an absence of symptoms between periods, rarely occurs during pregnancy or ovulation suppression, and is recurrent. These features contrast sharply with those of the commonly occurring spontaneous pneumothorax, which is 1.4 to 10 times more common in males than females[79,80] In addition, spontaneous pneumothorax occurs more frequently in the left lung and has only a 17% to 33% recurrence rate over 5 years.[81] Catamenial pneumothorax peaks within the third to fourth decade of life while spontaneous pneumothorax occurs most commonly between the ages of 16 to 25[78,79,81] and 55 to 65.[80]

If the air leak is minimal, the clinical presentation of spontaneous pneumothorax may be as mild as slight chest discomfort and cough. If, however, the air leak is large, profound dyspnea, pleuritic chest pain, shock, and death may occur. The physical findings of patients with catamenial pneumothorax include decreased chest movement and breath sounds on the affected side. The chest x-ray may demonstrate mediastinal shifting toward the unaffected side as well as air in the pleural space.

Various theories on the pathogenesis of catamenial pneumothorax exist. Maurer and others suggest that intraperitoneal air that enters via the genital tract at the time of menses may back into the pleural cavity through diaphragmatic defects.[77,82] This theory is supported by one case report of a woman with a 7-year history of catamenial pneumothorax that repeatedly developed following intercourse who was successfully treated by tubal ligation,[83] and another report of a women with spontaneous pneumoperitoneum occurring during postpartum exercises in the knee-chest position.[84] However, in Crutcher's series of 43 patients with catamenial pneumothorax, only 5 of 35 women who underwent thoracotomy demonstrated any diaphragmatic defect.[82] Therefore, it is unlikely that this theory is a major etiologic factor in the pathophysiology of catamenial pneumothorax.

Mayo demonstrated air leakage from an apical parenchymal bleb and concluded that intrapleural air originates in the lung of all patients with catamenial pneumothorax.[85] Pulmonary blebs do not explain why the disease occurs in only women and only during menstruation. Moreover, pulmonary blebs are found in only one-third of patients undergoing thoracotomy.[81]

Rossi and Goplerad suggested that the increased serum levels of prostaglandin F_2 during menstruation may be responsible for catamenial pneumothorax.[86] Prostaglandin F_2 has bronchoconstrictive properties and bronchospasm could lead to air trapping and alveolar rupture with resultant pneumothorax. Interestingly, Vernon et al demonstrated that endometriotic tissue does secrete $PGF_{2\alpha}$;[87] the presence of these lesions within the lung parenchyma could be a significant source of local prostaglandins. However, no one has demonstrated increased serum or tissue concentrations of prostaglandin or prostaglandin activity in patients with catamenial pneumothorax versus control populations. Therefore, this theory remains conjectural.

Pulmonary Endometriosis

The most accepted explanation of the etiology and pathophysiology of catamenial pneumothorax is pulmonary endometriosis in the presence or absence of diaphragmatic fenestrations. Lattes et al reported the first case of histologically proven endometriosis of the lung.[88] Since then well over 65 cases have been reported. It was proposed by Foster et al that endometriosis involving the pleura may be an extension of a surface phenomenon arising from the pelvic cavity.[89] Most of the patients in their series with purely pleural involvement had significant pelvic endometriosis. In contrast, patients with lung parenchymal endometriosis had pulmonary complaints without coexisting pelvic disease, suggesting that these lesions may arise from hematogenous spread of endometrial cells during menstruation. The mere presence of pulmonary endometriosis, however, still does not fully explain catamenial pneumothorax. Lillington et al. postulated that premenstrual enlargement of endometrial tissue would create a check-valve obstruction on a tributary bronchiole leading to localized hyperinflation and visceral pleural rupture.[78] Alternatively, immune and chemotactic proteins as well as prostaglandins secreted by the endometriotic implants could create local inflammation, leading to the rupture of pulmonary blebs and subsequent pneumothorax.[90] A third pathophysiologic explanation is the combination of pleural endometriosis and diaphragmatic perforations permitting the passage of air from the peritoneum to the pleura, as was documented via pleuroscopic examination and concomitant laparoscopy by Furman et al.[91]

The success of danazol and other hormonal ovulatory suppressants in the treatment of catamenial pneumothorax and hemoptysis further supports the relationship of pulmonary endometriosis to catamenial pneumothorax.[78,92] The prevalence and therefore the significance of pulmonary endometriosis in patients with catamenial pneumothorax remain unclear. Interestingly, pelvic endometriosis is found in only 22% to 37% of patients with catamenial pneumothorax, and pleural or diaphragmatic endometriosis in only 23% to 35% of patients with catamenial pneumothorax.[78,79,93]

Pulmonary endometriosis may also present in patients with catamenial pleural pain, hemoptysis, and hemothorax without concurrent pneumothorax.[94] In their review of the literature, Hibbard et al found pelvic endometriosis to be present in all patients with catamenial hemothorax, in half with catamenial pneumothorax, and in none with catamenial hemoptysis.[94]

In summary, relatively few cases of catamenial pneumothorax are described in the literature. It is quite possible that the true incidence of this condition is higher than we now suspect. Some women suspected of suffering with PMS and chest pain may be found to have a mild spontaneous pneumothorax during the menses that spontaneously resolves. This event would be missed unless a timely, thorough examination was performed.

Rheumatoid Arthritis

In the early 1960s it was reported that patients with rheumatoid arthritis (RA) may show either partial or complete remission of their disease while taking exogenous sex hormones.[95] Since that report, several investigators noted a protective effect of oral contraceptives on the development of RA. Wingrave reported data from the Royal College of General Practitioners' Oral Contraception Study suggesting the rate of development of RA in oral contraceptive users was one-half that of nonusers.[96] In addition, pregnancy was shown to be clinically beneficial in 75% of patients with RA, with postpartum exacerbation noted in 62%.[97,98] These data suggest that endogenous as well as exogenous gonadal sex steroids may play a significant role in the clinical course of RA.

The symptoms of RA characteristically wax and wane spontaneously. It was noted that a number of women complain of an exacerbation of symptoms just before or at the onset of menstruation, and such complaints are commonly attributed to an alteration of pain perception due to "premenstrual tension syndrome."[99] This phenomenon stimulated two independent investigators to further study the relation of menstrual cycle phase to the symptoms of RA. Latman evaluated 69 menstrual cycles in 14 patients with RA and noted that symptoms were significantly reduced during the postovulatory period when serum estradiol and progesterone concentrations were at their peak.[100] These clinical findings were corroborated by Goldstein et al.[101] Supporting this are data demonstrating statistically significant cyclical fluctuations of finger joint size, body weight, and grip strength in patients with RA.[99] Finger joint size was maximum within the first 6 days of menses while grip strength peaked in the periovulatory period with a nadir at the onset of menses.

The circatrigintan (30-day) rhythms of RA symptoms may be related to the hormonal effects on inflammation during the menstrual cycle. In 1972, Bodel et al described the suppressant actions of estradiol and progesterone on human lymphocytes in vitro.[102] Clinically, this correlates with the fact that RA symptoms are diminished in patients exposed to high serum concentrations of gonadal steroids due to pregnancy, oral contraceptives, and the luteal phase of the menstrual cycle.

Both cell mediated and humoral responses are influenced by estrogen and progesterone. Recently, estrogen receptors have been demonstrated specifically on suppressor/cytotoxic T lymphocytes (CD8) but not on helper/inducer T lymphocytes (CD4).[103] Estrogen receptors have also been demonstrated to be present on monocytes. Grossman et al demonstated that supplementation of estrogen to monocyte cultures produces antibody and complement membrane proteins.[104] In addition, using blastogenic T lymphocyte cultures, the same investigators clearly demonstrated a marked depression of mitogen-stimulated blastogenic transformation in the presence of estrogen. Similar results are seen with the addition of progesterone to the culture medium. In addition, progesterone is demonstrated to have an immunosuppressive effect in monkeys receiving hamster–rat and mouse–mouse skin grafts.[104] These in vitro data are complemented by in vivo data which demonstrate the immunomodulatory ability of estrogen to depress the phytohemagglutinin-induced mitogenesis of peripheral blood lymphocytes in patients with prostate cancer on estrogen and women taking oral contraceptives.[104] From these studies it is clear that estrogen and progesterone markedly suppress tissue rejection and mitogen reactivity of T lymphocytes. It is likely that this alteration of the immune system is at least partially responsible for the spontaneous circatrigintan rhythms of RA symptoms.

Asthma

The association of acute attacks of asthma with the menstrual cycle was first described in 1938 by Claude and Allemany Vall in a report of 36 asthmatic women who had exacerbations just before or during menses.[105] Several investigators have since noted similar findings.[106–108] The peak incidence of asthma attacks occurs 2 to 3 days prior to menses and during menses. This pattern, however, is not noted in all female asthmatics. Eliasson et al found by questioning 57 cycling women with asthma that only 33% had significant worsening of pulmonary symptoms during the premenstrual or menstrual period.[107] Premenstrual asthma is more prevalent in ovulatory than anovulatory cycles and has even been reported to respond to oophorectomy is some cases.[105] Aoyama et al could demonstrate no relation between allergies, infections, personality traits, or neurosis between asthmatic women with or without premenstrual exacerbations.[109]

It is possible that women with premenstrual exacerbations have a more severe form of asthma. Eliasson et al reported that 68% of asthmatic women with premenstrual asthma were previously hospitalized for asthma, whereas only 26% of noncatamenial asthmatics were hospitalized.[107] Pauli et al. examined this further by performing pulmonary function tests on 11 asthmatics and 28 normal controls during the follicular, midluteal, and late luteal phase for three consecutive menstrual cycles.[106] As expected, the normal group showed no significant cyclical changes in symptoms, peak flow rates, spirometric parameters, or airway reactivity. The asthmatic group also demonstrated no significant changes in their pulmonary function tests; however, their asthmatic symptoms, such as dyspnea, cough, wheeze, and chest tightness, deteriorated significantly from the follicular phase to the luteal phase.

The typical symptoms of the premenstrual syndrome are significantly more common in asthmatic women with premenstrual exacerbations than asthmatic women without menstrual variation.[110] The heightened awareness and anxiety concerning these asthmatic symptoms may explain the greater number of hospitalizations without significant changes in pulmonary function in patients with premenstrual asthma versus asthmatics without menstrual fluctuations. However, it is well known that asthma is affected by diurnal rhythms in circulating catecholamines, cyclic AMP, histamine, and cortisol, and it is certainly reasonable to postulate that circatrigintan rhythms of these same factors may affect asthmatic symptoms as well. In addition, the known immunomodulatory actions of gonadal sex steroids may also play a role in asthmatic exacerbations. When circulating levels of estradiol and progesterone fall premenstrually, their immunosuppressant actions also fall and asthmatic exacerbations appear at the time of menses.

There is no question that the symptoms of asthma worsen premenstually in a number of women but it is unclear whether this is actually due to worsening of bronchospasm or airway inflammation. Further investigation is necessary to better understand the pathophysiology of this phenomenon.

Diabetes Mellitus

Carbohydrate tolerance has been evaluated through the phases of the menstrual cycle using a variety of parameters: fasting glucose levels, oral glucose tolerance tests, intravenous glucose tolerance tests, insulin receptor status, and insulin sensitivity by the euglycemic-hyperinsulinemic clamp technique. Predicta-

bly, the results are conflicting, and usually the studies are inadequately controlled for possible confounding variables such as age, nutritional status, exercise, body weight, and the possible influence of the thermogenic effect of progesterone on blood flow and subcutaneous absorption of insulin. Nevertheless, there is a general impression that glucose tolerance is somewhat reduced during the luteal phase, and the better studies bear reviewing.

MacDonald and Crossley did oral glucose tolerance testing every 7 days in men and women and noted significantly greater variance in women, with the greatest deviation from the mean at midcycle. The slope of this variance against time was the same as for gastric emptying rate against time, from which the authors inferred that fluctuations in oral glucose tolerance could be related to changes in gastric emptying through the cycle.[111] Using intravenous glucose tolerance testing, two groups found no differences between the first and second halves of the cycle in women on and off exogenous estrogens.[112,113]

Modifications of insulin receptor binding during the menstrual cycle have been the subject of several studies, some of which seem to suggest decreased binding to erythrocytes and monocytes in the luteal phase of normal women with the changes generally being due to alteration in receptor concentration rather than affinity.[113-116] However, this is not undisputed,[116] and in any case the clinical significance of small changes in tissue binding in vitro is probably negligible. In vivo studies of insulin-mediated glucose utilization using the sensitive euglycemic-hyperinsulinemic clamp technique have failed to demonstrate fluctuations in insulin sensitivity during the menstrual cycle.[117-119]

All the reports mentioned above deal with nondiabetic women. The few investigations of diabetic women are often no better than anecdotal impressions that metabolic control is erratic during the late luteal phase. There are scattered but striking reports of acute deterioration of diabetic control during the menses, such as that of the young woman with repeated episodes of diabetic ketoacidosis (DKA) during menstruation.[120] In a large, retrospective study, Cramer noted that three quarters of hospital admissions for DKA in the 14- to 42-year old age group were female, and half of these were menstruating or just premenstrual at the time of admission. Data regarding other precipitating factors are unclear.[121]

Walsh and O'Sullivan performed serial oral glucose tolerance tests in 22 diabetic women and noted that, although glucose tolerance varied in all the patients, it significantly worsened during the menses only in women over 35 years.[122] Scott et al used the hyperinsulinemic clamp to examine insulin sensitivity and forearm venous plethysmography to look for blood flow alterations that might change subcutaneous insulin absorption in nine Type 1 diabetics during the follicular and luteal phases. They noted no significant differences in glucose utilization rates or forearm blood flow between the two phases. Of interest, however, is that basal growth hormone levels were significantly higher during the luteal phase.[123] Growth hormone levels are known to be elevated at the time of ovulation in nondiabetic women, and growth hormone responsiveness to arginine infusion is elevated in normal women during the luteal phase and in normal men pretreated with diethylstilbestrol.[124,125] It is possible that increased pulsatile growth hormone secretion could cause decreased glucose tolerance during the luteal phase in a manner that might not be detected by a short period of hyperinsulinemic clamping because of the delayed effects of growth hormone on glucose metabolism. There is no experimental support for this hypothesis at present.

Overall, the nature of catamenial fluctuations in energy metabolism and their clinical significance for diabetic management remains inconclusive and awaits further detailed study.

Porphyria

The porphyrias are a group of rare inheritable diseases caused by several enzymatic defects along the biosynthetic pathway of heme. The manifestations are due to the accumulation of toxic porphyric precursors proximal to the enzymatic block. Biochemically the enzyme defects appear to be expressed in many tissues; this has facilitated the elucidation of these disorders, permitting the use of circulating monocytes rather than liver or neural tissues for study. Depending on the site of the defect and the major tissues affected, the clinical features include neuropsychiatric manifestations, abdominal pain due to autonomic neuropathy, and photodermatitis. The presentation can be acute and episodic, as in acute intermittent porphyria, or chronic and remittent, as in porphyria cutanea tarda.[126]

Acute intermittent porphyria (AIP) is caused by a block at the level of porphobilinogen desaminase (also called urosporphyrinogen I (Uro I) synthase), the third enzyme in heme biosynthesis. The prevalence of the abnormal gene for this autosomal dominant disease is estimated to be 0.0005% to 0.001% of the United States population, but far fewer than this number are clinically affected by the defect. This suggests that other endogenous or exogenous factors are important in pathogenesis, especially in the precipitation of acute attacks. Many of these factors (such as alcohol, starvation, and lipid-soluble drugs metabolized by the cytochrome P-450 system) probably provoke attacks by directly or indirectly inducing the rate-limiting enzyme in heme synthesis, delta-amino levulinic acid (ALA) synthesis. The increase in the rate of heme synthesis unmasks the enzymatic defect and the buildup of precursors provokes an acute attack.[126] Sex hormones are suspected of being endogenous provocateurs since AIP is most common in postpubertal females, and since many women experience exacerbations during menstruation.[126,127] McColl et al performed a careful study of alterations in heme biosynthesis during the menstrual cycle in normal and AIP-afflicted patients.[128] Fluctuating activity of leukocyte ALA synthase was noted in both groups, but fluctuation was most marked in the patients with the greatest increase in enzyme activity at the time of menses. This appeared to correspond to an increased frequency of acute attacks in the week prior to menstruation, but there was no statistically significant correlation between sex steroid levels and ALA synthase activity. Of note, the defective enzyme in AIP, Uro I synthase, did not exhibit fluctuation, suggesting that the catamenial factor involved exerts its effect by induction of the earlier, rate-limiting enzyme with consequent build-up of toxic precursors.[126]

Estrogens, androgens, and oral contraceptive combinations are used to interrupt ovulation and eliminate sex hormone surges in AIP.[126-131] These attempts meet with some success in suppressing catamenial attacks in some patients but exacerbate AIP in others. Inconsistency in the results is probably due to the fact that 5 beta-hydroxy metabolites of endogenous and exogenous sex steroids can themselves precipitate attacks by inducing ALA-synthase. In fact, AIP is associated with an additional, partial defect in the enzyme 5-alpha-hydroxylase, so that porphyrinogenic 5-beta-hydroxy metabolites are produced in excess of 5-alpha-hydroxy metabolites in some patients. In general, estrogens and progestins are contraindicated in this disease. When danazol, used because it would suppress gonadotropin secretion without exposure to estrogen or progesterone, was tried on two women with catamenial AIP, attacks were exacerbated. This was possibly because danazol, which has a double bond in the 4–5 position, can be reduced to either the 5-alpha or the 5-beta configurations by the stereo-specific 5-reductase enzymes. With a 5-alpha-reductase deficiency, 5-beta-hydroxy metabolites might be produced in excess, resulting in induction of ALA-synthase and precipitation of acute attacks.[132,133] Gonadotropin-releasing hormone analogues have been tried with the same rationale as the danazol trial, but to better effect. Two recent reports using buserelin intranasally and the D-His analogue intranasally or subcutaneously noted modest to significant reduction in premenstrual attacks of AIP.[134,135]

Hemostatic Disorders

Disorders of hemostasis are rarely associated with cyclical fluctuation in relation to menses. These are usually platelet disorders, generally with low platelet counts during the menses with normal to high counts at midcycle.[136,137] Sex steroids are associated with thrombocytopenia.[138] Scattered reports note the presence of platelet-associated IgG antibodies in these conditions, but it is unclear how the regular fluctuations could be explained on the basis of an immune thrombocytopenia.[139,140] One well-studied condition, which is probably a single manifestation of a cyclical immune phenomenon, is termed menstrual cyclic thrombocytopenia. Tomer et al. studied three patients who presented with menorrhagia and other bleeding phenomena because of a regular drop of platelet counts to 5000 to $20,000/mm^3$ at the onset of menses, with normalization of platelet counts by midcycle. It was found that the problem was excessive platelet consumption rather than underproduction, and the patients had elevated levels of antibodies to platelet glycoprotein Ib at all times of the menstrual cycle.[141] The cyclical nature of the disease might be explained by a catamenial increase in the expression of monocyte Fc gamma receptors. These receptors mediate clearance of antibody-coated platelets by macrophages, and their expression is known to be enhanced by estrogens.[142,143]

Thrombotic thrombocytopenic purpura (TTP), a potentially devastating condition associated with platelet consumption and intravascular coagulation, is known to be hormonally influenced, with episodes coinciding with pregnancy and oral contraceptive use.[143,144] Although usually acute and fulminating, a chronic, recurrent form of TTP exists,[144] and the patients require regular treatment with fresh frozen plasma infusions. In one well-documented case of a patient who manifested TTP both with pregnancy and on using an oral contraceptive, declines in platelet count and haptoglobin levels were noted in the luteal phase of repeated normal menstrual cycles. Delay or absence of ovulation caused delay or absence of the platelet and haptoglobin fluctuations.[145] The most common theory of TTP pathogenesis involves the aggregation of endothelially derived abnormal von Willebrand factor (VWF) multimers which trigger a cascade resulting in platelet consumption and thrombosis.[146] A role for sex steroids in the cyclic modulation of this phenomenon is an interesting possibility, supported by a study noting elevated production of VWF from cultured endothelial cells in response to large doses of estrogens[147] and by the fact that VWF levels are elevated in late pregnancy in both normal women and those with von Willebrand's disease.

Appendicitis

It is postulated that gonadal sex steroids can influence an established inflammatory process in the appendix, thereby influencing the timing of symptoms of acute appendicitis. Short first noted that the advent of the monthly period often coincided with an acute attack.[148] Arnbjornsson studied this further in a retrospective review of 524 women between the ages of 15 and 45 years who underwent surgery for acute appendicitis.[149] He found that twice as many surgeries occurred in the luteal and menstrual phases as in the follicular phase. This may not seem surprising in view of the fact that women often have premenstrual and menstrual pain and that surgery would be more likely to occur during this period to rule out acute abdominal disease. Interestingly, Arnbjornsson noted by histological examination that the greatest proportion of normal as well as gangrenous or perforated appendices were removed during the menstrual and follicular phase, while a phlegmonous appendix was the most likely finding in the luteal phase.[149] The significantly higher proportion of gangrenous and perforated appendices removed in the menstrual and follicular phase might be explained by the existence of recurrent monthly pain that can be confused with pain associated with acute appendicitis and therefore cause delay in the patient seeking medical care. Very few normal appendices were removed during the luteal phase. These data suggest that female sex hormones may have some influence on the inflammatory process in the appendix.

This concept of sex steroid influence on the timing of acute appendicitis is supported by additional data gathered from patients on monophasic oral contraceptives.[150] In this patient population no cyclical fluctuation was noted in the presentation of acute appendicitis. There was no difference noted in the incidence of acute appendicitis in patients who were or were not using oral contraceptives. Given the current popularity of multiphasic oral contraceptives, it will be interesting to note if the presentation of acute appendicitis varies in different phases of the cycle. Certainly, further study on the effect of sex steroids on the biologic nature of acute appendicitis is indicated.

Cholelithiasis

It is generally accepted that women develop gall-stones more frequently than men. In addition, data suggest that oral contraceptives encourage the oversaturation of bile with cholesterol and that gallstones seem to be more common in women taking estrogen for relief of postmenopausal symptoms.[151–153] Since cholelithiasis depends on a disturbance of the solubility relationships between biliary lipids, cholesterol, bile acids, and phospholipids (expressed as the cholesterol saturation index) the question arises as to what effect other steroidal moieties such as the endogenous sex steroids have on the formation of gallstones.[154]

Low-Beer et al evaluated the cholesterol saturation index (CSI) in 11 healthy females with regular cycles by collecting serum and duodenal bile during the early follicular, ovulatory, and midluteal phase of the menstrual cycle.[155] In 9 of the 11 women, the CSI was higher in the midluteal phase than in the early follicular or ovulatory phases and no difference in the CSI was seen between the latter two phases. An additional finding was the significant fall in serum cholesterol and triglycerides in the midluteal phase, with very little change from the early follicular to the ovulatory phases. These authors concluded that the tendency for cholesterol-rich gallstones to form fluctuates with the menstrual cycle. They postulated that this phenomenon is probably due to a direct effect of sex steroids on the liver and on the gallbladder's emptying time, which has been shown to be slower in the luteal phase.[156] However, Whiting et al and Bennion et al, who also examined the CSI throughout the menstrual cycle in normal women, found no significant change in the mean CSI at each phase of the menstrual cycle.[153,157]

There has been no demonstration of cyclical variation in the incidence of acute cholelithiasis or gallbladder pain. In addition, it has not been suggested that anovulatory women have a different rate of gallstone formation than women with regular cycles. The fact is that the highest incidence of gallbladder disease occurs in postmenopausal women. Therefore, the clinical significance of bile content variations that may occur during the normal menstrual cycle remains undetermined.

Hepatic Disease

Two patients were described with recurrent premenstrual rise in unconjugated bilirubin without evidence of hemolysis or chronic liver disease.[158] This entity possibly represents a subset of Gilbert's disease, although the luteal phase periodicity suggests a kinship to transient nonhemolytic unconjugated jaundice associated with breast-feeding, which is thought to be due to 3-α-20-β-pregnanediol in breast milk.[159] The effect of progesterone on heme catabolism and bilirubin turnover is unclear, so a role of progesterone or its metabolites in the etiology of this condition is still speculative.

Genital Herpes

Recurrent herpes labialis often follows various physiologic states such as fever, sunburn, and trauma as well as psychological states such as emotional stress or discomfort.[160] In addition, women frequently report an association between the menstrual cycle and the onset of herpetic outbreaks. This latter association was investigated by several authors with conflicting results. Segal et al noted a predilection of outbreaks in the premenstrual and menstrual phases of the cycle.[161] However, a 3-year prospective study of 149 women carried out by this same group demonstrated recurrent herpetic episodes as being related only to previous experience with recurrent herpes, upper respiratory infections, socioeconomic status, and mood traits. The timing of recurrent herpes episodes was not related to the phase of the menstrual cycle.[160]

These findings are supported by laboratory data examining menstrual cycle variations on natural killer cytotoxicity (NKC) and antibody-dependent cellular cytotoxicity (ADCC) to cells infected with the herpes simplex virus. Both of these viral defense systems play a particularly important role in regard to the herpes simplex virus and both can be modulated by circulating prostaglandins.[162,163] NKC and ADCC activity was not found to be significantly different between any phase of the menstrual cycle among 13 normal women.[164] This study supports the clinical data suggesting no linkage between the onset of recurrent herpetic labialis and the phase of the menstrual cycle.

Recurrent Urticaria and Anaphylaxis

Recurrent urticaria and anaphylaxis is a condition characterized by recurring attacks of some or all of the following without evidence of an external inciting cause: urticaria, angioedema, upper and lower airway obstruction, vomiting, diarrhea, abdominal bloating, syncope, hypotension, and flushing.[165] This syndrome occurs equally in men and women. A subset of women, however, have exacerbations as a result of endogenous progesterone sensitivity.

There are several case reports of patients who present with recurrent urticaria in the premenstrual and menstrual phase of the cycle.[166-168] Farah and Shbaklu reported two patients with recurrent mid- and premenstrual urticaria that was inhibited with ovulation suppression and exacerbated with exogenous progesterone administration. In addition, these patients demonstrated a positive skin test with progesterone and immunofluorescence of antibodies reactive to the luteinized cells of the corpus luteum.[169] Meggs et al reported one patient with weekly life-threatening anaphylactic episodes that responded to bilateral oophrectomy,[170] and Slater et al reported two women with this syndrome who responded to gonadotropin-releasing hormone agonist therapy.[171] These studies suggest that patients may experience immediate hypersensitivity responses to endogenous progesterone or other hormones associated with the menstrual cycle. Slater and Kaliner hypothesized that cyclic urticaria and anaphylaxis are not due to a hypersensitivity response to progesterone but rather to progesterone's alteration of mast cell function and histamine release. However, they could not demonstrate any effect of either estrogen or progesterone on basophil histamine release.[165]

A variation of recurrent urticaria and angioedema exists which is associated with eosinophilia and improves with progesterone supplementation. Cooper and Patterson were the first to report a patient who developed premenstrual fatigue, edema, hypereosinophilia, and elevated circulating IgM.[172] Subsequently, Mittman et al reported a woman with a 4-year history of monthly urticarial episodes associated with hypereosinophilia which began at the end of menses and lasted to midcycle.[173] When this patient's concentration of serum progesterone naturally rose in the luteal phase, the hives were quiescent, and treatment with oral medroxyprogesterone resulted in remission of the urticarial episodes and a decrease in the eosinophil count. It is apparent that the immunomodulatory effects of gonadal sex steroids play a major role in the etiology of recurrent urticaria and anaphylaxis. However, it is not clear whether this phenomenon occurs as a direct result of invoking a hypersensitivity response or as an indirect result of sex steroid binding to immunoactive cells.

Glaucoma

A few studies suggest that intraocular pressure and outflow of aqueous humor vary through the menstrual cycle in normal women. Without hormonal measurements, peaks of pressure were noted during the mid-follicular period and less uniformly during the luteal phase.[174,175] Feldman et al noted no significant correlation between sex hormone levels and ocular pressure or aqueous flow parameters throughout a menstrual cycle, although there was a tendency for pressure to be lowest when estrogen was highest just before midcycle.[176]

A small study of glaucomatous women showed a premenstrual rise in intraocular pressure, but hormone levels were not measured.[177] Although inconclusive, the association is potentially significant since administration of progesterone (and possibly estrogen as well) was shown to decrease intraocular pressure, both acutely[174,178] and chronically.[179]

Exotica

Some opera singers are apparently troubled by hoarseness of voice premenstrually—even to the extent that their contracts with opera houses explicitly exempt them from having to perform during that portion of their menstrual cycle.[180] While women with such highly trained voices have not been systematically investigated, a careful acoustical analysis of untrained women showed no difference in voice quality between midcycle and premenstrual periods.[181]

SUMMARY

A study of the catamenial syndrome begins with a fascinating potpourri of clinical observations but ends with many unanswered questions. Why is there a luteal phase predilection for so many disparate symptoms? Are the noted effects caused by sex steroid fluctuations or are they altered pari passu with hormonal changes by higher signals? What are the causes of the less common but well-documented cyclic exacerbations of similar disorders in men? These questions extend the field beyond clinical interest to areas of fundamental cellular and molecular importance. Basic research advances are needed to improve our understanding of the interactions of steroid hormones with diverse signaling pathways (as in the central nervous and immune systems) and to provide a rational basis for possible hormonal treatment of these disorders.

REFERENCES

1. Smith S, Schiff I. The premenstrual syndrome—diagnosis and management. *Fertil Steril.* 1989;52:527.

2. Jeliffe SE. Aphasia, hemiparesis, and hemianesthesia in migraine. *NY State J Med.* 1906;83:33

3. Gowers WR. *Epilepsy and Other Chronic Convulsive Diseases. Their Causes, Symptoms and Treatment.* New York, NY: William Wood; 1885.

4. Bandler B, Kaufman IC, Dykens JW, et al. Seizures and the menstrual cycle. *Am J Psych.* 1957;113:704.

5. Laidlaw J. Catamenial epilepsy. *Lancet.* 1956;271:1235.

6. Logothetis J, Harner R, Morrell F, et al. The role of estrogens in catamenial exacerbations of epilepsy. *Neurology (Minneap).* 1959;9:352.

7. Sanchez-Longo LP, Gonzalez Saldana LE. Hormones and their influence in epilepsy. *Acta Neurol Lat Am.* 1966;12:29.

8. Rosciszewska D. In: Hopkins A, ed. *Epilepsy.* London, UK: Chapman and Hall; 1987:374.

9. Backstrom T. Epileptic seiures in women related to plasma estrogen and progesterone during the menstrual cycle. *Acta Neurol Scand.* 1976;54:321.

10. Helmchen H, Kunkel H, Selbach H. Periodic influences on the individual frequency of epileptic seizures. *Arch Psychiatr Nervenkr.* 1964;206:293.

11. Diamantopoulos N, Crumrine PK. The effect of puberty on the course of epilepsy. *Arch Neurol.* 1986;43:873.

12. Lennox WG, Lennox MA. *Epilepsy and Related Disorders,* vol. 2. Boston, MA: Little, Brown; 1960:645.

13. Loiseau P, Legroux M, Henry P. Epilepsies et grossesses. *Bordeaux Med.* 1974;7:1157.

14. Rosciszewska D, Grudzinska B. Influence of pregnancy on the course of epilepsy. *Neurol Neurochir Pol.* 1970;4:71.

15. Huhmar E, Jarvinen PA. Relation of epileptic symptoms to pregnancy, delivery and puerperium. *Ann Chir Gynaecol.* 1961;50:49.

16. Ramsay RE. Effect of hormones on seizure activity during pregnancy. *J Clin Neurophysiol.* 1987;4:23.

17. Gastaut H, Tarsinari C. Triggering mechanism in epilepsy. *Epilepsia.* 1966;7:86.

18. Rosciszewska D, Buntner B, Guz I, et al. *J Neurol Neurosurg Psychiatr.* 1986;49:47.

19. Narbone MC, Ruello C, Oliva A, et al. Hormonal dysregulation and catamenial epilepsy. *Funct Neurol.* 1990;5:49.

20. Murri L, Bonuccelli U, Melis GB. Neuroendocrine evaluation in catamenial epilepsy. *Funct Neurol.* 1986;1:399.

21. Wooley DE, Timiras PS. Estrous and circadian periodicity and electroshock convulsions in rats. *Am J Physiol.* 1962;202:379.

22. Wooley DE, Timiras PS. The gonad-brain relationship: effects of female sex hormones on electroshock convulsions in the rat. *Endocrinology.* 1962;70:169.

23. Terasawa E, Timiras PS. Electrical activity during the estrous cycle of the rat: cyclic changes in limbic structures. *Endocrinology.* 1968;83:207.

24. Logothetis J, Harner R. Electrocortical activation by estrogens. *Arch Neurol.* 1960;3:290.

25. Buterbaugh GG. Estradiol replacement facilitates the acquisition of seizures kindled from the anterior neocortex in female rats. *Epilepsy Res.* 1989;4:207.

26. Costa PJ, Bonnycastle DD. The effect of DCA, compound E, testosterone, progesterone and ACTH in modifying "agene-induced" convulsions in dogs. *Arch Int Pharmacodyn Ther.* 1952;91:330.

27. Craig CR. Anticonvulsant activity of steroids: separation of anticonvulsant from hormonal effects. *J Pharmacol Exp Ther.* 1966;153:337.

28. Nicoletti F, Speciale C, Sortino MA, et al. Comparative effects of estradiol benzoate, the antiestrogen clomiphene citrate, and the progestin medroxyprogesterone acetate on kainic acid-induced seizures in male and female rates. *Epilepsia.* 1985;26:252.

29. Leary PM, Batho K. Changes in the electroencephalogram related to the menstrual cycle. *S Afr Med J.* 1979;55:666.

30. Becker D, Creutzfeld OD, Schwibbe M, et al. Changes in physiological, EEG and psychological parameters in women during the spontaneous menstrual cycle and following oral contraceptives. *Psychoneuroendocrinology.* 1982;7:75.

31. Backstrom T, Carstensen H, Sodergard R. Concentration of estradiol, testosterone and progesterone in cerebrospinal fluid compared to plasma unbound and total concentrations. *J Steroid Biochem.* 1976;7:469.

32. Backstrom T, Zetterlund B, Blom S, et al. Effects of intravenous progesterone infusions on the epileptic discharge frequency in women with partial epilepsy. *Acta Neurol Scand.* 1984;69:240.

33. Nabeem J, Oomura Y, Minami T, et al. Mechanism of the rapid effect of 17-beta estradiol on medial amygdala neurons. *Science.* 1986;233:226.

34. Gee KW. Steroid modulation of the GABA/benzodiazepine receptor-linked chloride ionophore. *Mol Neurobiol.* 1988;2:291.

35. Shavit G, Lerman P, Korczyn AD, et al. Phenytoin pharmacokinetics in catamenial epilepsy. *Neurology.* 1984;34:959.

36. Back DJ, Bates M, Bowden A, et al. The interaction of anticonvulsants with oral contraceptive steroid therapy. *Contraception.* 1980;22:495.

37. Mattson RH, Cramer JA. Epilepsy, sex hormones and antiepileptic drugs. *Epilepsia.* 1985;26(suppl 1):S4-S51.

38. Backstrom T, Jorpes P. Serum phenytoin, phenobarbital, carbamazepine, albumin and plasma estradiol, progesterone concentrations during the menstrual cycle in women with epilepsy. *Acta Neurol Scand.* 1979;59:63.

39. Kumar N, Behari M, Ahuja GK, et al. Phenytoin levels in catamenial epilepsy. *Epilepsia.* 1988;29:155.

40. Herkes GK, Eadie MJ. Possible roles for frequent salivary antiepileptic drug monitoring in the management of epilepsy. *Epilepsy Res.* 1990;6:146.

41. Lennox WG, Cobb S. Epilepsy. *Medicine.* 1928;7:105.

42. Groff DN. Suggestion for control of epilepsy (letter). *NY State J Med.* 1962;62:3017.

43. Zimmerman AW, Holden KR, Reiter EO, et al. Medroxyprogesterone acetate in the pretreatment of seizures associated with menstruation. *J Pediatr.* 1973;83:959.

44. Hall SM. Treatment of menstrual epilepsy with a progesterone-only oral contraceptive. *Epilepsia.* 1977;18:235.

45. Mattson RH, Klein PE, Caldwell BV, et al. Medroxyprogesterone treatment of women with uncontrolled seizures. *Epilepsia.* 1982;23:436.

46. Mattson RH, Cramer JA, Caldwell BV, et all. Treatment of seizures with medroxyprogesterone acetate: preliminary report. *Neurology.* 1984;34:1255.

47. Herzog AG. Intermittent progesterone therapy and frequency of complex partial seizures in women with menstrual disorders. *Neurology.* 1986;36:1607.

48. Dana-Haeri J, Richens A. Effect of norethisterone on seizures associated with menstruation. *Epilepsia.* 1983;24:377.

49. Feely M, Gibson J. Intermittent clobazam for catamenial epilepsy: tolerance avoided. *J Neurol Neurosurg, Psychiatr.* 1984; 47:1279.

50. Ryan RJ, Swanson DW, Faiman C, et al. Effects of convulsive electroshock on serum concentrations of follicle stimulating hormone, luteinizing hormone, thyroid stimulating hormone and growth hormone in man. *J Clin Endocrinol Metab.* 1970;30:51.

51. Trimble MR. Serum prolactin in epilepsy and hysteria. *Br Med J.* 1978;2:1682.

52. Newmark ME, Penry JK. Catamenial epilepsy: a review. *Epilepsia.* 1980;21:281.

53. Herzog AG, Seibel MM, Schomer DL, et al. Reproductive endocrine disorders in women with partial seizures of temporal lobe origin. *Arch Neurol.* 1986;43:341.

54. Lundberg PO. Prophylactic treatment of migraine with flumedroxone. *Acta Neurol Scand.* 1969;45:309.

55. Epstein MT, Hockaday JM, Hockaday TDR. Migraine and reproductive hormones throughout the menstrual cycle. *Lancet.* 1975;i:534.

56. Horth CE, Wainscott G, Neylar C, et al. Progesterone, estradiol and aldosterone levels in plasma during the menstrual cycle of women suffering from migraine. *J Endocrinol.* 1975;65:24.

57. Lance JW, Anthony M. Some clinical aspects of migraine. *Arch Neurol.* 1966;15:356.

58. Murialdo G, Martignoni E, DeMaria A, et al. Changes in the dopaminergic control of prolactin secretion and in ovarian steroids in migraine. *Cephalalgia.* 1985;6:43.

59. Whitty CWM, Hockaday JM, Whitty MM. The effect of oral contraceptives on migraine. *Lancet.* 1966;i:856.

60. Somerville BW. The role of estradiol withdrawal in the etiology of menstrual migraine. *Neurology* (Minneap). 1972;22:355.

61. Somerville BW. Estrogen-withdrawal migraine. *Neurology* (Minneap). 1975;25:239.

62. Volavka J, Bauman J, Pevnick J, et al. Short-term hormonal effects of naloxone in man. *Psychoneuroendocrinology.* 1980;5:225.

63. Stubbs WA, Jones A, Edwards CRW, et al. Hormonal and metabolic responses to an enkephalin analogue in normal man. *Lancet.* 1978;ii:1225.

64. Ferin M. Endogenous opioid peptides and the menstrual cycle. *Trends Neurosci.* 1984;3:194.

65. Moult PJA, Cunnah D, Besser GM. Different opioid mechanisms are involved in the modulation of ACTH and gonadotropin release in man. *Neuroendocrinology.* 1986;42:357.

66. Facchinetti F, Martignoni E, Fioroni L, et al. Opioid control of the hypothalamic-pituitary-adrenal axis cyclically fails in menstrual migraine. *Cepahalalgia.* 1990;10:51.

67. Nappi G, Martignoni E, Bono G, et al. THDA system function in migraine. In: Clifford Rose F, Zilkha KJ, eds. *Progress in Migraine Research.* London: Pitman; 1981:110.

68. Rand CW, Andler M. Tumors of the brain complicating pregnancy. *Arch Neurol Psychiatry.* 1950;63:1.

69. Schoenberg BS, Christine BW, Whisnant JP. Nervous system neoplasms and primary malignancies of other sites. *Neurology.* 1975;25:705.

70. Cahill DW, Bashirelahi N, Solomon LW, et al. Estrogen and progesterone receptors in meningiomas. *J Neurosurg.* 1984;60:985.

71. Schwartz MR, Randolph RL, Cech DA, et al. Steroid hormone binding macromolecules in meningiomas. *Cancer.* 1984;53:922.

72. Billiard M, Guilleminault C, Dement WC. A menstrual-linked periodic hypersomnia. Kleine-Levin syndrome or new clinical entity? *Neurology.* 1975;25:436.

73. Sachs C, Persson HE, Hagenfeldt K. Menstruation-related periodic hypersomnia: a case study with successful treatement. *Neurology* (NY). 1982;32:1376.

74. Goetting M. Menstrual exacerbation of action myoclonus and successful treatment with acetazolamide (letter). *Neurology.* 1985;40:1304.

75. Massey EW. menstrual meralgia (letter). *Arch Neurol.* 1978;35:549.

76. Martin RA, Howard FM, Salamone CR, et al. Spinal cord vascular malformations with symptoms during menstruation. *J Neurosurg.* 1977;47:626.

77. Maurer ER, Schaal JA, Mendez FL. Chronic recurrence of spontaneous pneumothorax due to endometriosis of the diaphragm. *JAMA.* 1958;168:2013.

78. Lillington GA, Mitchell SP, Wood GA. Catamenial pneumothorax. *JAMA.* 1972;219:1328.

79. Barrocas A. Catamenial pneumothorax: case report and a review of the literature. *Am Surg.* 1979;45:340.

80. Watt AG. Spontaneous pneumothorax: a retrospective review of 210 consecutive admissions to Royal Perth Hospital. *Med J Aust.* 1978;1:186.

81. Schoenfeld A, Ziv E, Zeelel Y, et al. Catamenial pneumothorax—a literature review and report of an unusual case. *Ob Gyn Surv.* 1986;41:20.

82. Crutcher RR, Waltuch TL, Blue ME. Recurring spontaneous pneumothorax associated with menstruation. *J Thorac Cardiovasc Surg.* 1967;54:599.

83. Muller N, Nelms B. Postcoital catamenial pneumothorax. Report of a case not associated with endometriosis and successfully treated with tubal ligation. *Am Rev Respir Dis.* 1986;134:803.

84. Lozman H, Newman AJ. Spontaneous pneumoperitoneum occurring during postpartum exercises in the knee-chest position. *Am J Obstet Gynecol.* 1956;72:903.

85. Mayo P. Recurrent spontaneous pneumothorax concomitant with menstruation. *J Thorac Cardiovasc Surg.* 1963;46:415.

86. Rossi NP, Goplerad CP. Recurrent catamenial pneumothorax. *Arch Surg.* 1974;109:173.

87. Vernon MW, Beard JS, Graves K, et al. Classification of endometriotic implants by morphologic appearance and capacity to synthesize prostaglandin F *Fertil Steril.* 1986;46:801.

88. Lattes R, Shepard F, Tovell H, et al. A clinical and pathologic study of endometriosis of the lung. *Surg Genec Obstet.* 1956;103:552.

89. Foster DC, Stern JL, Buscema J, et al. Pleural and parenchymal pulmonary endometriosis. *Obstet Gynecol.* 1981;58:552.

90. Isaacson KB, Coutifaris C, Garcia CR, et al. Production and secretion of complement component 3 by endometriotic tissue. *J Clin Endocrinol Metab.* 1989;69:1003.

91. Furman WR, Wang KP, Summer WR, et al. Catamenial pneumothorax: evaluation by fiberoptic pleuroscopy. *Am Rev Resp Dis.* 1980;121:137.

92. Johnson WM, Tyndal CM. Pulmonary endometriosis: treatment with danazol. *Obstet Gynecol.* 1987;69:507.

93. Yeh T. Endometriosis within the thorax: metaplasia, implantation or metastasis? *J Thorac Cardiovasc Surg.* 1967;53:201.

94. Hibbard LT, Schumann WR, Goldstein GE. Thoracic endometriosis: a review and report of two cases. *Am J Obstet Gynecol.* 1981;140:227.

95. Blais JA, Demers R. The use of norethynodrel (Enovid) in the treatment of rheumatoid arthritis. *Arthritis Rheum.* 1962;5:284.

96. Wingrave SJ, Kay CR. Reduction in incidence of rheumatoid arthritis associated with oral contraceptives. *Lancet.* 1978;8064:569.

97. Oka M, Vaino U. Effect of pregnancy on the prognosis and serology of rheumatoid arthritis. *Acta Rheum Scand.* 1966;12:47.

98. Ostensen M, Aune B, Husby G. Effect of pregnancy and hormonal changes on the activity of rheumatoid arthritis. *Scand J Rheumatol.* 1983;12:69.

99. Rudge SR, Kawanko IC, Drury PL. Menstrual cyclicity of finger joint size and grip strength in patients with rheumatoid arthritis. *Ann Rheum Dis.* 1983;42:425.

100. Latman NS. Relation of menstrual cycle phase to symptoms of rheumatoid arthritis. *Am J Med.* 1983;74:957.

101. Goldstein R, Duff S, Karsh J. Functional assessment and symptoms of rheumatoid arthritis in relation to menstrual cycle phase (letter). *J Rheumatol.* 1987;14:395.

102. Bodel P, Dillard MG Jr, Kaplan SS, et al. Anti-inflammatory effects of estradiol on human blood leukocytes. *J Lab Clin Med.* 1972;80:373.

103. Simpson WH. Oestrogen and human T-lymphocytes: presence of specific receptors in the T-suppressor/cytotoxic subset. *Scand J Immunol.* 1988;28:345.

104. Grossman CJ. Regulation of the immune system by sex steroids. *Endocrin Rev.* 1984;5:435.

105. Claude F, Allemany Vall R. Asthme et menstruation. *Presse Med.* 1938;38:755.

106. Pauli BD, Reid RL, Munt PW, et al. Influence of the menstrual cycle on airway function in asthmatic and normal subjects. *Am Rev Resp Dis.* 1989;140:358.

107. Eliasson O, Scherzer HH, DeGraff AC. Morbidity in asthma in relation to the menstrual cycle. *J Allergy Clin Immunol.* 1986;77:87.

108. Wulfsohn NL, Politzer WM. Bronchial asthma during menses and pregnancy. *S Afr Med J.* 1964;38:173.

109. Aoyama Y, Toyoizumi K, Fueki R, et al. Relation between bronchial asthma and the menstrual cycle. *Jap J Allerg.* 1965;4:583.

110. Rees L. An aetiological study of premenstrual asthma. *J Psychosom Res.* 1963;7:191.

111. MacDonald I, Crossley JN. Glucose tolerance during the menstrual cycle. *Diabetes.* 1970;19:450.

112. Goldman JA, Eckerling B. Glucose metabolism during the menstrual cycle. *Obstet Gynecol.* 1970;35:207.

113. Spellacy WN, Carlson KL, Schade SL. Menstrual cycle carbohydrate metabolism. *Am J Obstet Gynecol.* 1967;99:382.

114. DePirro R, Fusco A, Bertoli A, et al. Insulin receptors during the menstrual cycle in normal women. *J Clin Endocrinol Metab.* 1978;47:1387.

115. Bertoli A, DePirro R, Fusco A, et al. Differences in insulin receptors between men and menstruating women and influence of sex hormones on insulin binding during the menstrual cycle. *J Clin Endocrinol Metab.* 1980;50:246.

116. Moore P, Kolterman O, Weyant T, et al. Insulin binding in human pregnancy: comparisons to the postpartum, luteal and follicular states. *J Clin Endocrinol Metab.* 1981;52:937.

117. Toyoda N. Insulin receptors on erythrocytes in normal and obese pregnant women: comparisons to those in nonpregnant women during the follicular and luteal phases. *Am J Obstet Gynecol.* 1982;144:679.

118. Toth EL, Suthijumroom A, Crockford PM, et al. Insulin action does not change during the menstrual cycle in normal women. *J Clin Endocrinol Metab.* 1987;64:74.

119. Yki-Jarvinen H. Insulin sensitivity during the menstrual cycle. *J Clin Endocrinol Metab.* 1984;59:350.

120. Harrop GA, Mosenthal HO. The influence of menstruation on acidosis in diabetes mellitus; report of a case. *Bull Johns Hopkins Hosp.* 1918;29:161.

121. Cramer HI. The influence of menstruation on carbohydrate tolerance in diabetes mellitus. *Can Med Assoc J.* 1942;47:51.

122. Walsh CH, O'Sullivan DJ. Carbohydrate tolerance during the menstrual cycle in diabetics. *Lancet.* 1973;i:413.

123. Scott AR, Macdonald IA, Bowman CA, et al. Effect of phase of menstrual cycle on insulin sensitivity, peripheral blood flow and cardiovascular responses to hyperinsulinemia in young women with Type 1 diabetes. *Diabetic Medicine.* 1990;7:57.

124. Merimee TJ, Fineberg SE. Studies of the sex-based variation of human growth hormone secretion. *J Clin Endocrinol.* 1971;33:896.

125. Merimee RTJ, Burgess JA, Rabinowitz D. Sex-determined variation in serum insulin and growth responses to amino acid stimulation. *J Clin Endocrinol.* 1966;26:791.

126. Bloomer JR, Bonkovsky HL. The porphyrias. *Disease-A-Month.* 1989;1:54.

127. Zimmerman TS, McMillin JM, Watson CJ. Onset of manifestations of hepatic porphyria in relation to the influence of female sex hormones. *Arch Intern Med.* 1966;118:229.

128. McColl KEL, Wallace AM, Moore MR, et al. Alterations in heme biosynthesis during the human menstrual cycle: studies in normal subjects and patients with latent and active acute intermittent porphyria. *Clin Sci.* 1982;62:183.

129. Levit EJ, Nodine JH, Perloff WH. Progesterone-induced porphyria. *Am J Med.* 1957;22:831.

130. Perlroth MG, Marner HS, Tschudy DP. Oral contraceptive agents and the management of acute intermittent porphyria. *JAMA.* 1965;194:1037.

131. Wetterberg L. Oral contraceptives and acute intermittent porphyria. *Lancet.* 1964;ii:1178.

132. Bradlow HL, Gillete PN, Gallagher TF, et al. Studies in porphyria II. Evidence for a deficiency of steroid delta 4-5 alpha-reductase activity in acute intermittent porphyria. *J Exp Med.* 1973;138:754.

133. Lamon JL, Frykholm BC, Herrera W, et al. Danazol administration to females with menses-associated exacerbations of acute intermittent porphyria. *J Clin Endocrinol Metab.* 1979;48:123.

134. Herrick AL, McColl KEL, Wallace AM, et al. LHRH analogue treatment for the prevention of premenstrual attacks of acute porphyria. *Quarterly J Med.* 1990;75:355.

135. Anderson KE, Spitz IM, Bardin W, et al. A gonadotropin-releasing hormone analogue prevents cyclical attacks of porphyria. *Arch Intern Med.* 1990;150:1469.

136. Cohen T, Cooney DP. Cyclic thrombocytopenia. Case report and review of literature. *Scand J Hematol.* 1974;12:9.

137. Wahlberg P, Nyman D, Ecklund P, et al. Cyclical thrombocytopenia with remission during lynestrenol treatment in a woman. *Ann Clin Res.* 1977;9:356.

138. Cooper BA, Bigelow FS. Thrombocytopenia associated with the administration of diethystilbestrol in man. *Ann Int Med.* 1960;52:907.

139. Cines DB, Schreiber AD. Immune thrombocytopenia: use of Coombs antiglobulin test to detect IgG and C3 on platelets. *N Engl J Med.* 1979;300:106.

140. Cines DB, Wilson SB, Tomaski A, et al. Platelet antibodies of the IgM class in immune thrombocytopenia. *J Clin Invest.* 1985;75:1183.

141. Tomer A, Schreiber AD, McMillan R, et al. Menstrual cyclic thrombocytopenia. *Br J Haematol.* 1989;71:519.

142. Schreiber AD, Chien P, Tomaski A, et al. Effect of danazol in immune thrombocytopenic purpura. *N Engl J Med.* 1987;316:503.

143. Friedman D, Nettl F, Schreiber AD. Effect of estradiol and steroid analogues on the clearance of immunoglobulin G-coated erythrocytes. *J Clin Invest.* 1985;75:162.

144. Byrnes JJ, Khurana M. Treatment of thrombotic thrombocytopenic purpura with plasma. *N Engl J Med.* 1977;297:1386.

145. Cuttner J. Thrombotic thrombocytopenic purpura: a ten-year experience. *Blood.* 1980;56:302.

146. Moake J, Rudy CK, Troll JH, et al. Unusually large plasma factor VIII: von Willebrand factor multimers in chronic relapsing thrombotic thrombocytopenic purpura. *N Engl J Med.* 1982;307:1432.

147. Holdrinet RSG, de Pauw BE, Haanan C. Hormonal dependent thrombotic thrombocytopenic purpura (TTP). *Scand J Hematol.* 1983;30:250.

148. Short AR. The causation of appendicitis. *Br. J. Surg.* 1920;8:171.

149. Arnbjornsson E. Acute appendicitis risk in various phases of the menstual cycle. *Acta Chir Scand.* 1983;149:603.

150. Arnbjornsson E. The influence of oral contraceptives on the frequency of acute appendicitis in different phases of the menstrual cycle. *Surg Gynecol Obstet.* 1984;158:464.

151. Pertsemelidis D, Panveliwalla D, Ahrens EH. Effects of clofibrate and an estrogen-progestin combination on fasting biliary lipids and cholic acid kinetics in man. *Gastroenterology.* 1974;66:565.

152. Boston Collaborative Drug Surveillance Program. *N Engl J Med.* 1974;290:15.

153. Bennion LJ, Ginsberg RL, Garnick MB, et al. Effects of the normal menstrual cycle on human gallbladder bile. (letter) *N Engl J Med.* 1976;292:189.

154. Admirand WH, Small DM. The physico-chemical basis of cholesterol gallstone formation in man. *J Clin Invest.* 1968;47:1043.

155. Low-Beer TS, Wicks AC, Heaton KW, et al. Fluctuations of serum and bile lipid concentrations during the menstrual cycle. *Fr Med J.* 1977;1:1568.

156. Nilsson S, Stattin S. Gallbladder emptying during the normal menstrual cycle. A cholecystographic study. *Acta Chirurgica Scandinavia.* 1967;133:638.

157. Whiting MJ, Down RH, Watts JM. Precision and accuracy in the measurement of the cholesterol saturation index of duodenal bile. Lack of variation due to the menstrual cycle. *Gastroenterology.* 1981;80:533.

158. Yamaguchi K, Okuda K, Yonemitsu H, et al. Cyclic premen-

strual unconjugated hyperbilirubinemia. *Ann Int Med.* 1975;83: 524.

159. Arias IM, Wolfson S, Lucey, et al. Transient familial neonatal hyperbilirubinemia. *J Clin Invest.* 1965;44:1142.

160. Friedman E, Katcher AH, Brightman VJ. Incidence of recurrent herpes labialis and upper respiratory infection: a prospective study of the influence of biologic, social and psychologic predictors. *Oral Surg Oral Med Oral Pathol.* 1977;43:873.

161. Segal AL, Katcher AH, Brightman VJ, et al. Recurrent herpes labialis, recurrent apthous ulcers and the menstrual cycle. *J Dent Res.* 1974;53:797.

162. Kohl S, Loo LS, Greenberg SB. Protection of newborn mice from herpes simplex virus by human interferon, antibody and leukocytes. *J Immunol.* 1982;128:1107.

163. Bankhurst AD. The modulation of human natural killer cell activity by prostaglandins. *J Clin Lab Immunol.* 1982;7:85.

164. Gonik B, Loo L, Bigelow R, et al. Influence of menstrual cycle variations on natural killer cytotoxicity and antibody-dependent cellular cytotoxicity to cells infected with herpes simplex virus. *J Reprod Med.* 1985;30:493.

165. Slater JE, Kaliner M. Effects of sex hormones on basophil histamine release in recurrent idiopathic anaphylaxis. *J Allergy Clin Immunol.* 1987;80:285.

166. Guy WH, Jacob FN, Guy WB. Sex hormone sensitization (corpus luteum). *Arch Dermatol.* 1951;63;377.

167. Zondek B, Bromberg YM. Endocrine allergy I. Allergic sensitivity to endogenous hormones. *J Allergy.* 1945;16:1.

168. Phillips EW. Clinical evidence of sensitivity to gonadotropins in allergic women. *Ann Intern Med.* 1949;30:364.

169. Farah FS, Shbaklu Z. Autoimmune progesterone urticaria. *J Allergy Clin Immunol.* 1971;48:257.

170. Meggs WJ, Pescovits OH, Metcalfe D, et al. Progesterone sensitivity as a cause of recurrent anaphylaxis. *N Engl J Med.* 1984; 311:1236.

171. Slater JE, Raphael G, Cutler GB, et al. Recurrent anaphylaxis in menstruating women: treatment with a luteinizing hormone-releasing hormone agonist—a preliminary report. *Obstet Gynecol.* 1987;70:542.

172. Cooper BJ, Patterson R. Elevated IgM levels, edema, and fatigue syndrome. *Arch Intern Med.* 1976;136:1366.

173. Mittman RJ, Bernstein DI, Steinberg DR, et al. Progesterone-responsive urticaria and eosinophilia. *J Allergy Clin Immunol.* 1989;84:304.

174. Paterson GD, Miller SJH. Hormonal influence in simple glaucoma. *Br J Ophthalmol.* 1963;47:129.

175. Becker B, Friedenwald JS. Clinical aqueous outflow. *Arch Ophthalmol.* 1953;50:557.

176. Feldman F, Bain J, Matuk AR. Daily assessment of ocular and hormonal variables throughout the menstrual cycle. *Arch Ophthalmol.* 1978;96:1835.

177. Dalton K. Influence of menstruation on glaucoma. *Br J Ophthalmol.* 1967;51:692.

178. Avasthi P, Luthra MD. Effect of sex hormones on intraocular pressure. *Int Surg.* 1967;48:350.

179. Freister G, Mannor S. Intraocular pressure and outflow facility: effect of estrogen and combined estrogen-progestin treatment in normal human eyes. *Arch Ophthalmol.* 1970;83:311.

180. Luchsinger R, Arnold G. *Voice-Speech-Language.* Belmont, Calif: Wadsworth Publishing Co; 1965:157.

181. Silverman E-M, Zimmer CH. Effect of menstrual cycle on voice quality. *Arch Otolaryngol.* 1978;104:7.

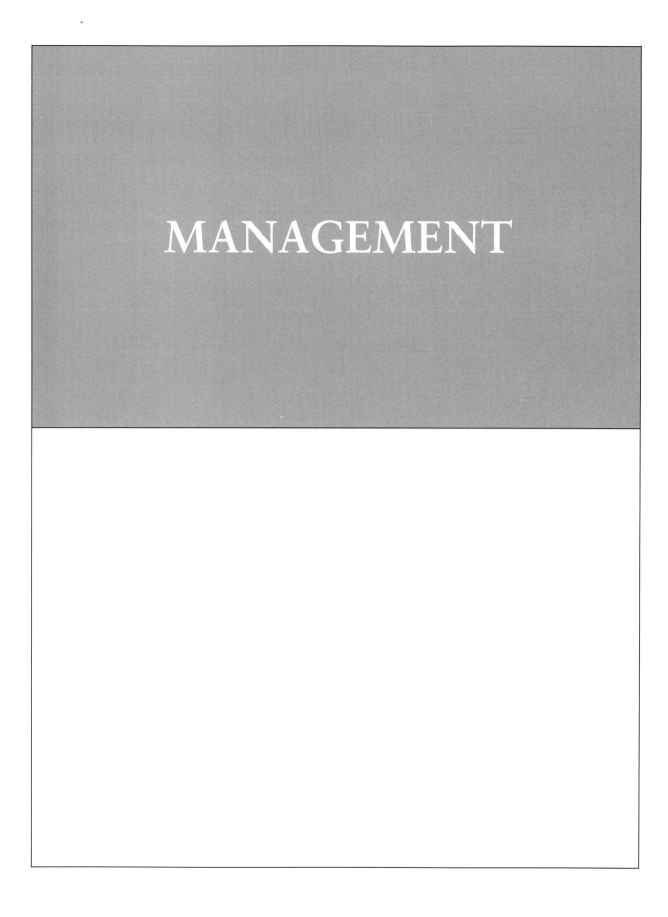

MANAGEMENT

CHAPTER 9

Nutritional Intervention in Premenstrual Syndrome

Judith J. Wurtman

Nutrition clearly plays a role in premenstrual syndrome (PMS), and nutritional modification can frequently help to reduce distressing symptoms. This chapter reviews menstrual cycle-related changes in nutrition, the relationship of nutrient intake to the pathophysiology of PMS, and the use of dietary modification as a treatment for PMS.

OVERVIEW

An increase in appetite, especially for carbohydrate-rich foods, has long been known as one of the many characteristic behavioral changes of premenstrual syndrome. A 1988 calendar describing in cartoon form the various behavioral and somatic changes in the premenstrual woman showed a rather thin young woman attempting to devour the state of Pennsylvania in order to consume the city of Hershey, a presumed source for the chocolate she was craving. Because these changes in appetite are so closely associated with a deterioration in mood, many have assumed that eliminating the craved foods from the diet of the premenstrual woman would produce an improvement in mood.[1-3] Thus medical and popular literature is replete with diets for PMS that admonish the premenstrual woman to eliminate foods rich in refined flour, sugar, and chocolate to control and decrease her PMS symptoms.

The prevalence of reported changes in appetite during the late luteal phase may also account, in part, for the scrutiny given to the adequacy of nutrient intake of premenstrual women. The theory that the appetitive and affective changes of PMS may be caused by inadequate nutrient intake or enhanced requirements for specific nutrients was based on the association between vitamin B_6 and the biosynthesis of two neurotransmitters, dopamine and serotonin. Because these two neurotransmitters are known to affect a variety of mood states, it seemed reasonable to infer that alterations in their synthesis or activity may be responsible for the dysphoria of PMS. The relief of premenstrual symptoms by vitamin B_6 supplementation became a commonly advised therapy despite the absence of agreement on its effectiveness. The concomitant use of large doses of other vitamins and minerals has also been recommended, presumably based on the assumption that the food cravings of many premenstrual women result from inadequate nutrient intake or an increased need for specific vitamins and minerals.

Recent studies on the appetitive changes in the menstrual cycle focus on the relationship between dietary intake and neurotransmitter synthesis. It now appears that the late luteal increase in carbohydrate appetite may reflect an attempt by the premenstrual woman to use food as a form of self-medication.[4] The consumption of carbohydrate-rich, protein-poor foods results in an increased synthesis in brain serotonin and measurable improvements in several of the behavioral characteristics of PMS. Evidence for menstrual cycle changes in brain serotonin has been accumulating for several years based largely on changes in peripheral levels of this neurotransmitter. The recent availability of pharmacologic agents that increase central serotoninergic activity has now made it possible to examine more directly the relationship between serotonin and changes in premenstrual appetite and affect. In a study described here, such treatment improved the mood of women with PMS and returned their food intake to levels demonstrated in the follicular phase of the cycle.[5] Confirmation of the involvement of brain serotonin in the behavioral changes of PMS awaits the results of other studies using drugs that have similar effects on the neurotransmitter. However, until such therapeutic agents become available, it may be possible to improve, to some extent, the dysphoria of PMS by using carbohydrate intake itself to increase the availability of brain serotonin. Rather than restricting the consumption of this craved macronutrient, it now appears beneficial to increase its intake. The resulting enhancement of serotonin synthesis and activity should, to some extent, relieve the negative affect and satisfy the carbohydrate hunger of the premenstrual women. The side effects of such treatments (weight gain, water retention) can be minimized by recommending carbohydrate foods low in fat and salt.

MENSTRUAL CYCLE CHANGES IN FOOD INTAKE

Premenstrual Changes in Nutrient Intake

The concept that changes in food intake occur premenstrually was originally based on subjective descriptions of premenstrual increases in appetite. Women described themselves in self-reports as increasing their desire for and consumption of sweet carbohydrates, and occasionally salty, starchy foods as well (chocolate, cookies, pastries, crackers, potato chips). Usually these changes in appetite were associated with the affective characteristics of PMS; for example, in a study of 300 nurses, Smith and Sauder found a significant association between the craving for sweets and premenstrual tension.[6] The association between premenstrual dysphoria and increased appetite was strengthened in a study by Both-Orthman et al in which premenstrual increases in appetite were found only among women

with premenstrual mood changes. Subjects with no evidence of menstrually related mood disorder showed no changes in their appetite throughout the menstrual cycle.[7]

Information on actual caloric and nutrient intake throughout the menstrual cycle comes largely from self-monitoring. Typically, women are asked to keep track of their food intake on an outpatient basis. This is accomplished with a diary in which women write down everything they eat each day, or by having women report to a trained interviewer everything they consumed on the previous day. Often, but not always, the subjects are asked to monitor their daily mood changes as well. Some of these studies supported self-reports of an increased appetite for carbohydrate-rich foods during the late luteal phase of the cycle. Women increased their carbohydrate intake by approximately 53% above preovulatory levels in a study of eight women who reported their food intake to a trained interviewer over two menstrual cycles.[8] No information concerning the presence of premenstrual syndrome was obtained in this study. Three-day food intake records were used to compare food intake during the follicular and luteal phases of the cycle in a study of pyridoxine and magnesium status of women with PMS.[9] Although average magnesium intakes were higher among controls in the premenstrual phase than test subjects, no significant differences in plasma magnesium levels were found. Pyridoxine intakes did not differ between the groups during either phase of the food intake measurement, and both groups had an adequate pyridoxine status. There were differences, however, in calorie and nutrient intakes between the pre- and postmenstrual phases. The control subjects increased their carbohydrate intakes during the postmenstrual phase and consumed proportionately more calories, protein, fat, and vitamin B$_6$ premenstrually. The increases reported by the test subjects were of the same nature but to a lesser degree. These findings contrast with self-reports of premenstrual carbohydrate craving and the increase in carbohydrate intake described in the survey of Dalvit-McPhillips.[8] An absence of premenstrual craving for or consumption of sweets was also reported in a study of 11 women living in a hostel. However, no measurement of menstrual mood changes were made nor were the women allowed free food choice; they were restricted to the fixed menu of the hostel dining room. Whether access to sweet carbohydrates would have altered premenstrual food patterns cannot be determined in this study.[10] In a similar type study, Tomelleri et al obtained weekly reports of food cravings of 83 college women who obtained their food in a college dining room.[11]

Women reported greater preference for chocolate during the week of menstrual flow; otherwise, no change in food cravings were noted. However, here too, no measure of menstrual cycle mood changes was made.

Premenstrual Changes in Caloric Intake

Energy and macronutrient intakes were examined in a study of 14 women who took part in a 1-year dietary intake study.[12] The women, whose ages ranged from 20 to 47 years, were instructed to keep food intake diaries over this period; a restrospective analysis was made of their food intake during the pre- and postmenstrual phases of their cycle. The number of cycles used for the analysis ranged from 1 to 4, and no information concerning the presence of premenstrual symptoms was given.

A significant but functionally small increment in energy intake was noted during the premenstrual food intake measurement period. The subjects consumed approximately 90 calories more per day (the equivalent of a large apple). No significant increase in macronutrient intake was detected, although a small rise in fat consumption probably accounted for the increase in calories.[12]

One problem with most of these studies is that the information on food intake is provided by the subjects with little or no objective confirmation. Therefore, underreporting of food intake or food cravings because of forgetfulness or desire to present a nutritionally sound diet to the investigator can result in an erroneous estimate of menstrual cycle food changes. More recent studies attempted to correct this error by monitoring directly the amount and types of food consumed rather than relying on record keeping by the subjects. Lissner et al[13] measured food choices of more than 60 nonsmoking females between the ages of 22 and 41 who consumed their meals in a research unit at Cornell University. The subjects were able to select the types and portions of food they wanted to eat and were instructed to eat to satiety. Both meal and snack items were provided. Their average energy intake was about 87 kcal higher during the 10 days before menstruation than 10 days after its onset; Tarasuk and Beaton had similar findings.[12] Again, no information was provided as to the premenstrual symptoms of the subjects.[13] A significant increase in luteal phase calorie intake and a trend to greater sucrose intake was reported in a study by Gong et al.[14] Nine women, aged 24 to 43, ate a self-selected diet served in a dormitory throughout one menstrual cycle. After foods and beverages were selected, the foods were weighed and recorded; plate waste was measured at the end of the meal. As in the previous study, no measurement of premenstrual symptoms was made.

The either/or nature of these studies, ie, *either* the study uses subjective evaluation to measure changes in mood and cravings, *or* food intake is measured directly, but premenstrual changes in mood are not), prevents adequate confirmation of a link between increased carbohydrate intake and the dysphoria of PMS. Moreover, few of the studies in which food intake was monitored directly distinguished between the food choices of subjects with premenstrual syndrome and those who were symptom free.

Relationship between Carbohydrate Intake and Mood

To examine the occurrence and coincidence of depressed mood and excessive carbohydrate intake, we admitted to the Massachusetts Institute of Technology clinical research center 19 patients who claimed to suffer from severe PMS, and 9 control subjects, during the early follicular and late luteal phases of their menstrual cycles.[5] Mood was assessed with the Hamilton depression scale and an addendum that evaluated fatigue, sociability, appetite, and carbohydrate craving. Calorie and nutrient intakes were measured directly over 48 hours by providing subjects with a variety of isocaloric carbohydrate-rich and protein-rich meal and snack foods. Both calorie and carbohydrate intakes increased significantly among the test subjects during the luteal phase; calorie intake increased by about 500 kcal and carbohydrate intake increased by 24% from meals and 43% from snacks. The control subjects did not alter their intake of calories or any macronutrient. We also found a significant increase in the ratings of depression concurrent with the excessive intake of carbohydrate-rich foods. These results support the earlier studies of self-reported mood and food intake changes; that is, only those subjects who experienced the symptoms of PMS altered their food choices. The presence of significant changes in carbohydrate intake among the subjects with PMS and the absence of such changes among the control subjects also helps explain the contradictory findings among the previous studies on food intake. Few of those studies evaluated the presence and severity of premenstrual syndrome among the subjects. Thus whether menstrual cycle changes in food intake patterns were found might have depended simply on the proportion of subjects in the study population who suffered from PMS.

The premenstrual increase in calorie intake noted in several of the studies cited corresponds in part to the postovulatory increase in energy expenditure described by Webb.[15] He used direct calorimetry to monitor energy expenditure throughout the menstrual cycle in 11 women with normal menstrual cycles. Measurements carried out for 2 days each week across the entire menstrual cycle revealed an increase in postovulatory energy expenditure ranging from 8% to 16%. Of interest is the response of 1 subject who showed no increase in postovulatory energy expenditure when on oral contraceptives, but demonstrated a 14% increase when she was not on the medication. Since menus were fixed to correspond to energy expenditure, no measurements were made of changes in food choice, nor was there any evaluation of premenstrual symptoms.

THE USE OF NUTRIENTS AS TREATMENT FOR MENSTRUAL CYCLE CHANGES

Pyridoxine Phosphate (Vitamin B₆)

The use of nutritional supplementation to relieve the symptoms of PMS was first proposed by the Biskinds in the 1940s.[16] They suggested that a deficiency in the vitamin B complex might be indirectly responsible for the premenstrual changes in mood and physical complaints. Subsequently vitamin B₆ was targeted as the critical nutrient in the somatic and behavioral complaints of PMS based on its function as a coenzyme (pyridoxal phosphate) in the biosynthesis of dopamine and serotonin. It was thought that an estrogen-induced deficiency in the coenzyme might influence the synthesis of serotonin from tryptophan. Although pyridoxal phosphate levels are similar in women with PMS and those who are symptom free,[9,17] numerous studies have been done to establish a role for this vitamin in the relief of menstrual cycle mood changes. The earlier studies used megadoses of the vitamin; for example, in a double-blind crossover study, Abraham and Hargove administered 500 mg of vitamin B₆ daily for three consecutive menstrual cycles. They reported that 21 of 25 subjects showed significant symptomatic improvement.[18,19] Improvement with lower doses of vitamin B₆ has also been reported. Williams et al treated 617 women with either 100 or 200 mg of vitamin B₆ or placebo daily for three menstrual cycles. The group treated with the vitamin showed a significant improvement in their symptoms[20] as did the placebo group. Improvement among 64% of subjects was also found in a study using 100 mg of vitamin B₆ or placebo in a single-blind study.[21] Considerably smaller amounts of pyridoxine were also found to be effective in relieving the emotional symptoms of PMS. Doll et al. carried out a double-blind study over 3 months using 50 mg of vitamin B₆.[22] The 32 subjects reported a significant improvement in mood.

Other studies failed to find positive effects. Stokes and Mendels found no significant improvement in 13 women treated with 50 mg of vitamin B₆,[23] and placebo was as effective as the vitamin therapy in two studies using 150 to 250 mg of pyridoxine.[24,25]

These contradictory findings indicate that the effectiveness of vitamin B₆ as therapy for the behavioral complaints of PMS is uncertain. Moreover, because excessive ingestion of pyridoxine is associated with peripheral neuropathy that is relieved when therapy is stopped, administration of doses greater than 200 mg are not recommended.[26] It should be noted that the recommended daily dietary allowance for vitamin B₆ is 2 mg.

Calcium

The effectiveness of supplementation of other nutrients as a therapy for PMS has not been as widely studied. The administration of 1 g of calcium carbonate (an amount close to the daily recommended intake of calcium) was associated with an improvement in mood, water retention, and pain[27] premenstrually and pain during the menstrual cycle. Obviously, more studies must be performed to confirm this finding and to elucidate the underlying mechanisms. Since calcium requirements are often neglected or difficult to meet unless substantial amounts of dairy products are consumed, supplementation with calcium may be recommended.

Magnesium

Magnesium deficiency is considered etiologic in the symptoms of PMS. Abraham suggested that a particular cluster of premenstrual symptoms reflected intracellular magnesium deficiency[28] and recommended supplementation with this mineral. In a more recent study comparing magnesium consumption of symptomatic and control subjects, Gallant et al[9] did not find any difference in plasma magnesium levels between the two groups. The control group consumed more magnesium in their diet; however, this may be related to the greater caloric intake of this group.

An association between specific symptomatic complaints of PMS and decreased monocyte magnesium levels was reported by an Italian study.[29] Eighteen subjects and 11 controls were evaluated prospectively for menstrual cycle symptoms for two consecutive menstrual cycles. The severity of PMS symptoms ranged from mild to severe, according to daily assessments made with the menstrual distress questionnaire. Although no significant variations in plasma and red blood cell magnesium levels throughout the menstrual cycle were detected between controls and patients, monocyte magnesium levels were significantly increased premenstrually among controls but not among the patients. The possible relationship between premenstrual magnesium concentrations and the presence of individual symptoms was examined. Red blood cell magnesium levels were decreased premenstrually among the 4 patients suffering pain, and 1 patient suffering behavioral changes. Polymorphonucleated blood cells showed a decreased magnesium concentration premenstrually among 2 patients suffering from inability to concentrate and 1 patient with behavioral changes. There was no correlation between magnesium levels and the overall severity of PMS.

The authors suggest that a magnesium deficit might be involved indirectly with the symptoms of PMS by interfering with neurotransmitter activity, renal water handling, and hormone metabolism. However, there is no evidence from these results that the magnesium levels of the patients represented a deficit merely because the levels failed to rise premenstrually compared to controls. Moreover, the very few patients who showed an association between magnesium concentrations and behavioral changes (3 of 18) suggest that a deficit in the level of this trace element may not be a major contributor to the etiology of premenstrual behavioral changes.[29]

Vitamin E

The involvement of yet another nutrient in the symptoms of PMS was evaluated in a study at the University of Texas. Chuong et al measured blood levels of vitamin E in asymptomatic women and women with premenstrual syndrome at 2- to 3-day intervals through three menstrual cycles. Pre- and postmenstrual vitamin E did not change significantly within the control and premenstrual groups, nor were there any differences between the two groups in either the luteal or follicular phase values. Thus, their results fail to support any relationship between vitamin E deficiency and premenstrual syndrome.[30]

NUTRIENT INTAKE, BRAIN SEROTONIN, AND PMS

Carbohydrate Craving

The association of a premenstrual increase in carbohydrate consumption concurrent with significantly depressed mood suggests a possible involvement of brain serotonin in this cyclical disorder of mood and food intake. A similar association of affective and appetitive symptoms is observed in patients with seasonal affective disorder[31] and in many carbohydrate-craving obese people.[32] In both of these disorders, as in PMS, patients typically complain of mood disturbances, diminished interest in previously enjoyed activities, decreased energy and increased fatigue, reduced productivity, social withdrawal, and an increased appetite for carbohydrate-rich foods leading to weight gain. Moreover, like PMS, these disorders also recur cyclically. Seasonal affective disorder is experienced each fall as the days grow shorter, and the syndrome disappears spontaneously each spring as the days grow longer. Obese people with carbohydrate craving experience the need to consume carbohydrate-rich foods at times of day or evening specific for each individual; this appetite for carbohydrate is often accompanied by a slight but real deterioration in mood.[32]

Serotonin and Carbohydrate Craving

The possible involvement of serotonin in the disturbed food intake and mood of patients with seasonal affective disorder and carbohydrate-craving obesity was supported by studies using dex-fenfluramine, a drug that selectively enhances serotonin-mediated neurotransmission. In a series of studies in which obese carbohydrate-craving patients were treated with dex-fenfluramine, the drug selectively diminished carbohydrate intake without significantly decreasing protein consumption.[32] Similarly, administration of dex-fenfluramine to subjects suffering from seasonal affective disorder also decreased their excessive carbohydrate craving and normalized their mood.[33] These responses to dex-fenfluramine are consistent with the known role of serotoninergic neurons in the control of mood and the more recently described role of serotoninergic neurons in the control of appetite.[34] The release of the transmitter from these neurons is affected by food consumption and, in turn, may influence subsequent food choice. Consumption of carbohydrate-rich, protein-poor foods can enhance serotonin synthesis via insulin-mediated changes in the plasma amino acid patterns, which facilitates the uptake of circulating tryptophan, serotonin's precursor, into the brain.[35] Moreover, the consumption of carbohydrate-rich meals by patients with seasonal affective disorder and individuals suffering from carbohydrate-craving obesity produced significant improvements in self-reported depression, fatigue, and anger, presumably by the dietary-induced increase in serotonin activity.[36]

The significant premenstrual increase in caloric intake from carbohydrate-rich foods in association with abnormal depression scores reported by direct measurements[4] and self-reports[6,7] suggests an involvement of brain serotonin in this condition as well. The involvement of peripheral serotonin in the affective component of PMS has already been proposed, based on observations that platelet serotonin is decreased in patients with PMS compared to controls[37,38] and on measurements of plasma[39] and whole blood[40] serotonin levels. Circulating serotonin is not thought to cross the blood–brain barrier; hence, these findings may not reflect mechanisms regulating the production and release of serotonin from brain neurons. Hrboticky et al[41] suggest that tryptophan uptake into the brain may be decreased premenstrually, leading to decreased synthesis of brain serotonin. They found an increased catabolism of tryptophan through the kynurenine metabolic pathway when the amino acid was administered during the luteal phase of the menstrual cycle. This change from the levels seen during the follicular phase was not due to inadequate vitamin B_6 levels, because subjects were supplemented with pyridoxine.

We found that subjects with severe premenstrual depression demonstrated significant improvements in mood after consuming a carbohydrate-rich, protein-poor test meal.[4] These changes were observed only during the late luteal stage of the cycle and were not found among symptom-free controls. As the intake of dietary carbohydrate was sufficient to accelerate brain serotonin synthesis,[35] these observations also suggest the possible involvement of serotonin in the premenstrual mood disorder.

Serotonin and PMS

To examine further the role of serotonin in the appetitive and affective components of PMS, we administered dex-fenfluramine to 17 women with PMS.[5] Subjects received the drug (the dextro-isomer of dl-fenfluramine, 15 mg twice daily) or placebo in random order during the luteal phases of six menstrual cycles (ie, for three control and three treatment cycles).

The drug fully suppressed the premenstrual rise in kilocalorie, carbohydrate, and fat intake; placebo had no effect. Behavioral changes, which were measured on the Hamilton rating scale for depression and its addendum (a scale that evaluates symptoms of fatigue, social withdrawal, and changes in appetite and carbohydrate craving), showed a significant improvement on the drug.

Additional evidence for the role of central serotonin in the mood disturbances and to some extent appetitive changes of PMS comes from a recent study using fluoxetine.[42] Women who met criteria for severe PMS were randomly assigned to treatment with fluoxetine (20 mg) or placebo for two menstrual cycles. Five of the nine drug-treated subjects no longer met criteria for severe PMS and three experienced milder symptoms than prior to treatment. One did not respond. No mention was made in the report of changes in carbohydrate appetite as an effect of the treatment. However, the authors reported that one of the fluoxetine-treated subjects experienced a decrease in appetite as a side effect. Since the drug was administered continuously throughout two menstrual cycles, measurements of intracycle changes in appetite were not possible.[42] Moreover, the effect of administering the drug only when women are experiencing the symptoms of PMS was not tested. Hence, no information is available as to how quickly symptomatic relief would be experienced with intermittent drug administration.

The improvement in the affective and appetitive symptoms of PMS with dietary and drug treatments that increase brain serotonin availability supports the possible involvement of serotonin-releasing raphe neurons. It is likely that such findings will generate pharmacologic therapies based on drugs that, like dex-fenfluramine and fluoxetine, increase serotoninergic transmission or block its reuptake. However, it is important not to overlook the utility of carbohydrate consumption itself in producing some symptomatic relief. Simple and complex carbohydrates have similar effects on brain serotonin[35]; when consumed with little or no protein, both types of carbohydrate will cause an increase in brain tryptophan uptake and subsequently, brain serotonin synthesis and release. The claims of increased carbohydrate craving and consumption by women who suffer from severe PMS, and our findings that eating carbohydrates decreases PMS symptoms, suggest that carbohydrate may act as a type of edible tranquilizer. Clearly there is no reason to support the notion that avoiding carbohydrate-rich foods will improve the affective symptoms of PMS, and much reason to recommend consumption of a carbohydrate-rich diet during the premenstrual week. Since the effects of carbohydrate intake on brain serotonin are relatively short-lived (the peak effect is found between 60 and 90 minutes after carbohydrate intake), it will be necessary to recommend eating carbohydrate-rich meals or snacks at frequent intervals to sustain an improvement in mood. Such a food plan is presented in the appendix of this chapter. However, since increased carbohydrate consumption is compatible with the food choices preferred by women with PMS, these recommendations should be well accepted.

SUMMARY

Deficiency of nutrients, such as pyridoxine, calcium, magnesium, and vitamin E, is theorized to contribute to PMS, but the available evidence suggests a minor role for these nutrients. In contrast, data consistently suggest that central nervous system serotonin deficiency is involved in the carbohydrate cravings and mood disturbances of PMS. Carbohydrate consumption transiently increases brain serotonin levels and temporarily reduces mood symptoms. Consequently, high-carbohydrate, but low-salt and low-fat diets are recommended for PMS patients. Similarly, medications that increase central nervous system serotonin levels are useful treatments for the emotional symptoms of PMS.

REFERENCES

1. Abraham G. Premenstrual tension. *Curr Prob Obstet Gyn* 1981; 3:1.
2. Davalon M, Bachman J. Premenstrual syndrome. A practical approach to management. *Postgrad Med.* 1989;86:51.
3. Coupey S, Ahlstrom P. Common menstrual disorders. *Pediatr Clin North Am.* 1989;36:551.
4. Wurtman J, Brzezinski A, Wurtman R, et al. Effect of nutrient intake on premenstrual depression. *Am J Obstet Gynecol.* 1989; 161:1228.
5. Brzezinski A, Wurtman J, Wurtman R, et al. D-Fenfluramine suppresses the increased calorie and carbohydrate intakes and improves the mood of women with premenstrual depression. *Obstet Gynecol.* 1990;76:296.
6. Smith S, Sauder C. Food cravings, depression and premenstrual problems. *Psychosom Med.* 1969;36:281.
7. Both-Orthman B, Rubinow D, Hoban C, et al. Menstrual cycle phase-Related Changes in appetite in patients with premenstrual syndrome and in control subjects. *Am J Psych.* 1988;145:628.
8. Dalvit-McPhillips S. The effect of the human menstrual cycle on nutrient intake. *Phys Beh.* 1983;31:209.
9. Gallant M, Bowering J, Short S, et al. Pyridoxine and magnesium status of women with premenstrual syndrome. *Nutr Res.* 1987;7: 243.
10. Manocha S, Coudhuri G, Taylor B. A study of dietary intake in

11. Tomelleri R, Gruewald K. Menstrual cycle and food cravings in young college women. *J Am Diet Assoc.* 1987;87:311.
12. Tarasuk V, Beaton G. Menstrual-cycle patterns in energy and macronutrient intake. *Am J Clin Nutr.* 1991;442.
13. Lissner L, Stevens J, Levitsky D, et al. Variation in energy intake during the menstrual cycle. *Am J Clin Nutr.* 1988;48:956.
14. Gong E, Garrel D, Calloway D. Menstrual cycle and voluntary food intake. *Am J Clin Nutr.* 1989;49:252.
15. Webb P. Twenty-four hour energy expenditure cycle. *Am J Clin Nutr.* 1989;49:252.
16. Biskind M, Biskind G, Biskind L. Nutritional deficiencies in the etiology of menorrhagia, metrorrhagia, cystic mastitis, and premenstrual tension. *Surg Gynecol Obstet.* 1944;78:49.
17. Ritchie C, Singkamani R. Plasma pyridoxal 5'-phosphate in women with the premenstrual syndrome. *Hum Nut: Clin Nutr.* 1986;40C:75.
18. Abraham G, Hargove J. Effect of vitamin B-6 on premenstrual syndromes: a double-blind crossover study. *Infertility.* 1980;3: 155.
19. Goei G, Abraham G. Effect of a nutritional supplement, optivite, on symptoms of premenstrual tension. *J Repro Med.* 1983;28:527.
20. Williams M, Harris R, Dean R. Controlled trial of pyridoxine in the premenstrual syndrome. *J Int Med Res.* 1985;13:174.
21. Day J. Clinical trials in the premenstrual syndrome. *Curr Med Res Opin.* 1979;6:40.
22. Doll H, Brown S, Thurston A, et al. Pyridoxine and the premenstrual syndrome: a randomized crossover trial. *J R Coll Gen Pract.* 1989;39:364.
23. Stokes J, Mendels J. Pyridoxine and premenstrual tension. *Lancet.* 1972;ii:77.
24. Taylor M, Krutan M, Freeman E. Vitamin B-6 status of women with premenstrual syndrome. *Fed Proc.* 1985;44:776.
25. Kendall K, Schnurr P. The effects of vitamin B-6 supplementation on premenstrual symptoms. *Obstet Gynecol.* 1987;70:145.
26. Schaumburg H, Kaplan J, Widebank A. Sensory neuropathy from pyridoxine abuse. *N Engl J Med.* 1983;138:405.
27. Thys-Jacobs S, Ceccarelli S, Bierman A, et al. Calcium supplementation in premenstrual syndrome: a randomized cross-over trial *J Gen Intern Med.* 1989;4:183.
28. Abraham G, Magnesium deficiency in premenstrual tension. *Magnesium Bull.* 1982;4:68.
29. Facchinetti F, Borella P, Fioroni L, et al. Reduction of monocyte magnesium in patients affected by premenstrual syndrome. *J Psychosom Obstet Gynaecol.* 1990;11:221.
30. Chuong C, Dawson E, Smith E. Vitamin E levels in premenstrual syndrome. *Am J Obstet Gynecol.* 1990;163:1591.
31. Rosenthal N, Genhart M, Cabellero B. Psychobiological effects of carbohydrate- and protein-rich meals in patients with seasonal affective disorder and normal controls. *Biol Psych.* 1989;25:1029.
32. Wurtman J, Wurtman R, Tsay R, et al. D-fenfluramine selectively suppresses carbohydrate snacking in obese subjects. *Int J Eating Disor.* 1985;50:343.
33. O'Rourke D, Wurtman J, Wurtman R, et al. Responses of patients with seasonal affective disorder to d-fenfluramine. *J Clin Psych.* 1989;50:343.
34. Silverston R, Smith G, Richards R. A comparative evaluation of dexfenfluramine and d-fenfluramine on hunger, food intake, psychomotor function and side effects in normal human subjects. In: Bender AE, Brooks LJ, eds. *Body Weight Control: The Physiology, Clinical Treatment, and Prevention of Obesity.* London: Churchill Livingstone; 1987:240.
35. Fernstrom J, Wurtman R. Brain serotonin content: physiological dependence on plasma tryptophan levels. *Science.* 1971;173:149.
36. Lieberman H, Wurtman J, Chew B. Changes in mood after carbohydrate consumption may influence snack choices of obese individuals. *Am J Clin Nutr.* 1986;45:772.
37. Taylor D, Matthew R, Ho B, et al. Serotonin levels and platelet

uptake during premenstrual tension. *Neuropsychobiol.* 1984;12: 16.

38. Ashby C, Carr L, Cook C, et al. Alteration of platelet serotonergic mechanisms and monoamine oxidase activity in premenstrual syndrome. *Biol Psych.* 1988;24:225.

39. Rapkin A, Edelmuth E, Chang L, et al. Whole-blood serotonin in premenstrual syndrome. *Obstet Gynecol.* 1987;70:533.

40. Ashby C, Carr L, Cook C, et al. Alteration of 5-HT uptake by plasma fractions in the premenstrual syndrome *J Neural Transm.* 1990;79:41.

41. Hrboticky N, Leiter L, Anderson G. Menstrual cycle effects on the metabolism of tryptophan loads. *Am J Clin Nutr.* 1989;50:46.

42. Stone A, Pearlstein T, Brown W. Fluoxetine in the treatment of premenstrual syndrome. *Psychopharmacol Bull.* 1990;26:331.

J. Wurtman's PMS Food Plan*

This food plan is designed to provide protein and other nutrient-rich foods in the early part of the day and carbohydrate-rich snacks and meals during the later part of the day. Although it is not a weight loss menu, all the food was picked to be as low in fat as possible.

Women should be encouraged to take iron supplements through this period, as few of the foods are high in this nutrient. If women do not consume the dairy products listed in the food plan, calcium supplements should be used as well. Calories and carbohydrate contents are given for the portions specified.

For more up-to-date information look on package labels for nutrient and ingredient lists and recently published calorie books.

Finally, this is not an especially nutritious food plan; it should not be followed for more than 7 days; and a vitamin-mineral supplement might be worthwhile taking even during the diet if other nutrients, in addition to iron and calcium, are not being consumed.

*All information derived from Pennington J, *Bowes and Church Food Values of Portions Commonly Used,* 15th ed. Philadelphia: JB Lippincott; 1989.

J. WURTMAN'S PMS FOOD PLAN

Breakfast: This meal should supply between 14 and 20 g of high-quality protein.

Choices:

½ cup part skim milk ricotta cheese	171 kcal, 14 g protein
1 cup 2% fat cottage cheese	203 kcal, 31 g protein
2 cups nonfat yogurt	200 kcal, 18 g protein
1 cup Egg-Beaters egg	100 kcal, 20 g protein
2 poached eggs	160 kcal, 12 g protein
2 cups skim milk (can be chocolate)	300 kcal, 16 g protein

Eat along with:

2 slices toast (any type)	140–160 kcal, 24–28 g carbohydrate
1 bagel (normal size)	163 kcal, 31 g carbohydrate
1 English muffin	140 kcal, 30 g carbohydrate

Add if desired:

1 tablespoon jam or jelly	51 kcal, 13 g carbohydrate
2 cups of cereal (except type with nuts)	
Citrus fruit or juice	110–120 kcal, 25–28 g carbohydrate

Total calories for breakfast will range between 370 and 400 kcal.

Lunch: This meal should supply between 30 and 40 g of protein.

Choices:

Sliced chicken 4 oz.	253 kcal, 33 g protein
Sliced turkey 4 oz.	225 kcal, 34 g protein
Turkey-based luncheon meats	
4 slices pastrami	160 kcal, 20.8 g protein
4 slices turkey roll	166 kcal, 21.2 g protein

Add if desired 1 slice:

Low fat mozzarella cheese	72 kcal, 7 g protein
Tuna fish, canned 4 oz. (light packed) (add diet mayo, if desired)	280 kcal, 28 g protein

Eat along with

2 slices of bread	140 kcal, 24–28 g carbohydrate
or 6″ pita bread	212 kcal, 41 g carbohydrate

Add:

  1 carrot, 1 red or green pepper, or salad bar vegetables: beets,
    broccoli, spinach, alfalfa sprouts.

Add, if desired, one fruit

Eat 1 container nonfat yogurt especially if having luncheon meats to increase protein intake.	100 kcal, 9 g protein

Note: If eating at a restaurant, hot entrees such as fish, chicken, lean beef, seafood, or vegetables/protein combinations like stir-fried chicken and vegetables can be eaten.

Total calories will range from 450 to 600.

Midafternoon to bedtime:

Snacks should be consumed about every 2 hours. Snacks can be substituted for dinner or replace part of dinner. Total snack/meal calories should not exceed 500 to 600, so portion sizes of choices should take this into account.

Snack/Meal Choices

1. Six graham crackers   180 kcal, 33 g carbohydrate

Add if desired:

    2T marshmallow creme, or   90 kcal, 23 g carbohydrate
    Combine marshmallow creme with 4 T chocolate-flavored syrup.
    Crumble one or two graham crackers for texture.   146 kcal, 33 g carbohydrate

2. 1 cup cocoa made with water and,   103 kcal, 22.5 g carbohydrate
    four fig newtons, or   200 kcal, 40 g carbohydrate
    four gingersnaps, or   118 kcal, 22.4 g carbohydrate
    four ladyfingers   158 kcal, 28 g carbohydrate

3. 8 oz of chocolate skim milk, or   158 kcal, 26.1 g carbohydrate
    10 vanilla wafers, or   180 kcal, 30 g carbohydrate
    a box of animal crackers   130 kcal, 21 g carbohydrate

4. ½ cup of instant rice pudding   175 kcal, 60 g carbohydrate

5. ½ cup of instant pudding, chocolate fudge   174 kcal, 31 g carbohydrate

6. One sweet potato   118 kcal, 28 g carbohydrate

7. One large baked white potato   220 kcal, 51 g carbohydrate

8. 1 cup of low-sodium split pea soup, canned, and   159 kcal, 25 G carbohydrate
    15 saltines.   195 kcal, 33 G carbohydrate

9. 1 cup low-sodium vegetable soup, canned, and   79 kcal, 13.2 carbohydrate
    4 breadsticks.   154 kcal, 30 g carbohydrate

10. Two biscuits, and   110 kcal, 14 g carbohydrate
    1 T jelly or jam.   51 kcal, 13 g carbohydrate

11. Three 4″ pancakes, and   171 kcal, 38 g carbohydrate
    1 T honey, or   64 kcal, 17 g carbohydrate
    1 oz of pancake syrup.   103 kcal, 26 g carbohydrate
    Two waffles can be substituted for pancakes.   175 kcal, 29 g carbohydrate

12. Oatmeal, instant with apples and cinnamon, 1 pkg.   134 kcal, 26 g carbohydrate
    Add honey or brown sugar.

13. Chocolate-flavored breakfast cereal, such as Cocoa Puffs, 1 cup   110 kcal, 25 g carbohydrate

14. Sweetened breakfast cereal, like Cap'n Crunch, 1 cup   161 kcal, 32 g carbohydrate

15. Popcorn, microwave, 3 cups   192 kcal, 19 g carbohydrate

CHAPTER 10

Treatment for the Physical Symptoms of Premenstrual Syndrome

Samuel Smith

Emotional symptoms are the most common presenting complaint in premenstrual syndrome (PMS) patients. However, approximately 58% of patients present with moderate to severe emotional and physical symptoms; 5% present with physical symptoms only, and 37% present with emotional symptoms only. The most common physical complaints are headache, cramps, bloating, swelling, backache, and breast tenderness.[1]

This chapter reviews the pathophysiology and treatment of the most common physical symptoms. For ease of discussion, symptoms are categorized as water retention symptoms and pain-related symptoms.

FLUID RETENTION

Pathophysiology

Many women with PMS describe a marked, generalized fluid retention in the premenstrual phase that is associated with symptoms of abdominal bloatedness, breast tenderness, swelling of the extremities, and weight gain. The majority of studies, however, do not demonstrate significant premenstrual water retention and weight gain even in PMS subjects who describe severe bloatedness and swelling.[2] In contrast, a slight increase in body weight in the luteal phase is common,

and generally well tolerated, by many healthy control patients.[3-5]

Several explanations are offered to explain why so many PMS patients describe severe symptoms of water retention, yet fail to demonstrate objective evidence of fluid retention or weight gain.[2-8] It is likely that the swelling observed in the breasts and abdomen result from fluid shifting from the intracellular and/or intravascular compartments to the extracellular fluid compartment. Such a redistribution of body fluid certainly seems possible and is consistent with the lack of correlation between premenstrual mastalgia and documented evidence of fluid retention.[6] In addition, capillary permeability is abnormally increased in some women with PMS who describe bloatedness.[7] Abdominal distention secondary to progesterone-induced intestinal smooth muscle relaxation may also cause the sensation of bloatedness without weight gain. Lastly, altered body perception may account for the symptoms of bloatedness.[8]

Some women with PMS do gain weight and retain salt and/or fluid premenstrually. However, no difference is found between PMS patients and controls with regard to sodium, potassium, or water balance, activity of the renin-angiotensin II-aldosterone axis, or concentrations of atrial natriuretic peptide.[2,9] Dietary indiscretions, such as cravings for carbohydrates, sweets, and salt, may contribute to weight gain or edema in some PMS subjects. Women consuming high sodium–high carbohydrate diets may gain 5 to 10 pounds in 24 hours.[10]

Idiopathic Edema

Some women may actually have idiopathic edema that is inappropriately diagnosed as PMS. Idiopathic edema is characterized by weight gain and edema formation throughout the course of a day. Salt and water are retained during standing and walking, and diuresis occurs with recumbency. Consequently, patients experience swelling of the extremities, tired, achy legs, and carpal tunnel syndrome. In contrast to PMS, the symptoms of idiopathic edema are generally present throughout the menstrual cycle; daily symptom calendars (DSC) can be used to differentiate these two entities.[5]

Diuretic Abuse

Diuretic abuse may also cause edema that can resemble both PMS and true idiopathic edema. Patients who abuse diuretics are frequently overconcerned with their body image. They may take over-the-counter PMS aids in excess or misuse prescription diuretics to control body weight. They may also diet for short periods of time to try to lose weight. If sodium intake is low during the dieting episode, the kidney responds initially with a transient diuresis, but the renin-angiotensin-aldosterone system is soon activated to promote sodium retention. Consequently, when the diet ends, the kidney actively retains sodium and water, weight increases, and the rebound weight gain produces the characteristic symptoms of water retention. Diuretic abuse exacerbates this cycle because diuretics produce a greater reduction in intravascular volume than dieting alone. Chronic activation of the renin-angiotensin-aldosterone system then causes pronounced salt and fluid retention when the diuretics are stopped. When the weight gain occurs, diuretics are restarted, sometimes at higher dosages. Thus, it is essential to question PMS patients about their nutritional habits and diuretic abuse so that this vicious cycle can be recognized and eliminated.[5]

Therapy

Diuretics

Diuretics are among the medications most commonly utilized to treat symptoms of water retention. However, their use should be limited to those women who demonstrate some evidence of premenstrual water retention or weight gain. Nutritional guidance should generally precede diuretic use, because dietary modification can often reduce weight gain sufficiently so that the residual symptoms can be easier to tolerate.

A variety of diuretics have been studied in placebo controlled clinical trials and results are generally favorable with regard to reduction of premenstrual weight gain, edema, abdominal bloatedness, and breast tenderness.[11-14]

Spironolactone has been the most commonly utilized diuretic, usually 25 to 50 mg b.i.d. It is a mild potassium sparing diuretic, acting as an aldosterone antagonist at the level of the distal renal tubules. Spironolactone, and other potassium sparing diuretics, such as amiloride and triamterene, increase the effectiveness of thiazide diuretics and are frequently combined with thiazides. Some examples of potassium sparing diuretic/thiazide diuretic preparations include spironolactone-hydrochlorothiazide (Aldactazide), amiloride HCl-hydrochlorothiazide (Moduretic), and triamterene-hydrochlorothiazide (Dyazide).

By evaluating a patient's symptom calendar, it is possible to identify the menstrual cycle day that water retention and weight gain begin. Diuretic therapy is best initiated at the time of onset of water retention and administered daily until the onset of menstruation, when spontaneous resolution of symptoms usually occurs. Diuretics effectively eliminate disturbing premenstrual weight gain and water retention when they are administered in this fashion.

Diuretics may cause intravascular depletion, electrolyte disturbance, and side effects such as fatigue, headache, irregular bleeding (in the case of spironolactone), and adverse drug interactions. Consequently, it is incumbent on the physician to be very familiar with the diuretics he/she prescribes, use them at the lowest effective dosage in a cyclic manner, monitor electrolytes, BUN, and creatinine intermittently, and generally reserve diuretic use for PMS patients who document premenstrual weight gain on their DSC.

Bromocriptine

Several placebo-controlled clinical trials document the therapeutic efficacy of the dopamine agonist bromocriptine (Parladel) for treating premenstrual fluid retention. Premenstrual mastalgia,[15-17] edema,[15] weight gain,[15,18] abdominal bloating,[15,17,18] and breast size[18] have been shown to improve with bromocriptine therapy. The most common dosage is 2.5 mg b.i.d. in the late follicular and luteal phases, with a range of 1.25 mg to 7.5 mg. The best results were noted in a study where 40% of the subjects demonstrated hyperprolactinemia and/or galactorrhea.[15] Negative results were also obtained in several placebo-controlled clinical trials,[19-21] suggesting that symptoms of fluid retention do not uniformly respond to bromocriptine. In addition, serum prolactin levels in PMS patients are similar to control patients throughout the menstrual cycle.[22]

PMS patients who have breast tenderness, galactorrhea, or hyperprolactinemia are the best candidates for bromocryptine treatment. However, there is no way to accurately predict which patient will respond favorably to bromocriptine. Dose-related side effects are common with bromocriptine. The most commonly reported adverse effects are lightheadedness, dizziness, nausea, nasal congestion, and headache; these are usually tolerable and disappear as the course of therapy continues. It is generally wise to begin at a 1.25 mg dosage and titrate the dosage to 2.5 mg to 5.0 mg daily, since side effects are most common at the initiation of therapy. The author prefers to administer bromocriptine daily throughout the menstrual cycle in contrast to the cyclic late follicular-luteal phase administration described in the controlled clinical trials. Physicians should be cognizant that bromocriptine is an ergot derivative, and is contraindicated in patients with peripheral vascular disease, coronary artery disease, and active liver disease.

Nonsteroidal Antiinflammatory Drugs

Nonsteroidal antiinflammatory drugs (NSAID) are variably successful in placebo-controlled clinical trials for treating premenstrual fluid retention. Mefenamic acid (Ponstel), 250 mg q.i.d., administered during the 4 days immediately preceding expected menstruation significantly reduced breast tenderness, abdominal bloating, and ankle swelling.[23,24] However, improvement was not seen at higher dosages administered for longer duration, 500 mg t.i.d. for 7 to 14 days premenstrually.[25,26] Naproxen sodium (Anaprox), 550 mg b.i.d. for 7 days premenstrually failed to reduce premenstrual water retention or breast tenderness.[27] The benefit of other NSAIDs for fluid retention symptoms has not been studied in a controlled manner.

Jakubowicz et al[28] prospectively treated 80 PMS patients with mefenamic acid, 500 mg t.i.d. for 7 to 14 days premenstrually, for a mean of 13 months. Mastalgia improved in 71% of subjects, and fluid retention significantly improved in 89%. However, there was no placebo control. Side effects usually reported with mefenamic acid include gastrointestinal distress, diarrhea, skin rash, and nausea. Patients need to be informed of the potential for hematologic, renal, and neurologic toxicity. In addition, patients should be informed that the Food and Drug Administration discourages the use of mefenamic acid for more than 7 consecutive days.

Tamoxifen

Tamoxifen[29] and danazol[30–32] are extremely effective treatments for premenstrual mastalgia. Tamoxifen, 10 mg daily from cycle day 5 to 24 inclusive, eliminates severe premenstrual mastalgia in 89% of treated women. Twelve months after the conclusion of a 6-month treatment course, 53% continue to be asymptomatic.[29] Tamoxifen has antiestrogenic and prolactin inhibitory properties, implying that these hormones play a role in the development of premenstrual mastalgia.

Danazol

Danazol (Danocrine) is also extremely effective in reducing premenstrual mastalgia.[30–32] Placebo-controlled clinical trials utilizing dosages of 100 to 200 mg daily demonstrate excellent symptomatic improvement in mastalgia; abdominal bloating, but not fluid retention, and a variety of emotional symptoms are also observed to improve at a 200 mg daily dosage. Similar to tamoxifen, many women have long-lasting improvement in mastalgia after discontinuation of danazol.

Adverse reactions to danazol are common, and dosage dependent. There are more complaints with danazol than with placebo in most published clinical trials, but they tend not be serious at lower dosages. The most commonly reported side effects at dosages of 200 mg or lower are menstrual irregularity, nausea, oily skin, and weight gain. Interestingly, weight loss is observed as frequently as weight gain during low-dose danazol therapy.[30]

It is important that women using lower dosages of danazol maintain effective contraception because danazol can masculinize a female fetus. At dosages of 200 mg daily or lower, most women continue to ovulate. This contrasts with dosages of 400 to 800 mg, which are usually associated with suppression of ovulation. These higher dosages of danazol effectively treat PMS by eliminating ovulation, but are associated with a higher incidence of adverse androgenic and hypoestrogenic side effects.

Exercise

Conditioning exercise is also an effective treatment for premenstrual fluid retention symptoms. Prior et al[33,34] demonstrated that PMS patients who initiated a strenuous running program experienced significantly reduced breast discomfort and fluid retention/bloating symptoms after 6 months of training; anxiety and depression complaints were not improved. Midluteal phase estradiol and progesterone were largely unchanged, but luteal phase length decreased by 1 to 2 days with conditioning exercise.[33,34]

PMS subjects who already exercise strenuously do not seem to derive the same benefit from increasing their level of training as do previously sedentary PMS subjects who begin a new conditioning exercise program.[33,34] Consequently, extremes of exercise are not recommended. Exercise associated hypothalamic amenorrhea may also occur during periods of conditioning exercise. PMS should remit during these periods of amenorrhea, and return when ovulatory cycles are restored. Interestingly, ovulatory athletes who abruptly decrease their exercise training due to injury or vacation frequently report markedly increased fluid retention symptoms during their first nontraining cycle.[33,34]

There is not a precise exercise formula that should be recommended to PMS patients. Generally 20 to 60 minutes of vigorous exercise three or four times weekly reduces physical complaints. The program should begin slowly, so that the patient has a good chance to succeed, develop mastery, and enhanced self-confidence. Gradually, increasing the exercise level will also limit injuries.[33,34]

PAIN

Prostaglandins

PMS is associated with a number of symptoms (abdominal cramps, general achiness, joint pain, headaches, backache) that may be prostaglandin (PG) mediated. PG molecules are ubiquitous and present in nearly every human tissue. They participate in a variety of regulatory processes by interacting and/or modulating the activity of other hormones.

Many of the painful symptoms of PMS resemble symptoms of PG excess. There is ample evidence that PG inhibitors effectively treat the pain component of PMS. As previously mentioned, mefanamic acid, 250 mg q.i.d. for 3 to 4 days premenstrually, reduces breast tenderness.[23,24] Breast size may increase 30% to 40% premenstrually in affected women and be associated with mastalgia. PGE_1 and PGE_2 are found in human breast tissue and may mediate this breast swelling and tenderness; it is suspected that high local estrogen concentrations promote the biosynthesis of PG in the breast.[23,24,35]

Therapy

Nonsteroidal Antiinflammatory Drugs

A longer duration of antiprostaglandin therapy is needed to treat other pain-related complaints of PMS. Naproxen sodium, 550 mg t.i.d., for 1 week premenstrually reduces symptoms of pain more effectively than placebo.[27] Mefanamic acid, 500 mg t.i.d. for 1 week premenstrually reduces symptoms of pain more effectively than placebo.[26] Mefanamic acid, 500 mg t.i.d. for 7 to 14 days effectively relieves lower abdominal/pelvic pain, backache, general aches and pains, and headache in 80 to 100% of women.[28]

A variety of NSAIDs are available for use, although only naproxen sodium and mefanamic acid have been evaluated for PMS therapy. The NSAIDs, as a group, have antiinflammatory, analgesic, antipyretic, and platelet-inhibitory properties.[36] The major mechanism of action of NSAIDs is the inhibition of cyclooxygenase activity, and PG synthesis. NSAIDs are generally well absorbed, highly bound to albumen, and primarily excreted unchanged in the urine. Comparative trials of NSAIDs seldom demonstrate clinically important differences between agents, but variability between patients in efficacy and preference for different NSAIDs is commonly seen in clinical practice.[36]

The most frequent adverse reactions to NSAIDs are gastrointestinal, with dyspepsia being most common.[36] Gastric erosion, peptic ulcerations, and gastrointestinal hemorrhage are much less common, and are usually seen in elderly patients and those with a history of peptic ulcer disease. Renal toxicity is the second major category of side effect.[36] NSAIDS can cause reduced glomerular filtration, acute renal failure, interstitial nephritis, papillary necrosis, chronic renal failure, and hyperkalemia. Patients with preexisting renal impairment and hypovolemia are at greatest risk. There is also the potential for adverse interactions between NSAIDs and a variety of other medications.[36] Of note, diuretics in combination with NSAIDs are associated with an increased risk of renal failure and potassium sparing diuretics in combination with NSAIDs increase the risk of potassium retention and hyperkalemia. Consequently, any PMS patient receiving both medications should have serum electrolytes, blood nitrogen, and creatinine monitored.[36]

Pain-related symptoms begin in the luteal phase and persist until menstruation. NSAID therapy should be initiated just prior to the onset of pain and therapy should continue until menstruation begins. If dysmenorrhea is also a problem, NSAID therapy is continued until menstruation ceases. The particular NSAID agent and its dose should be selected based on the physician's experience and titrated against the patient's complaints. Since therapy is generally given cyclically for 1 to 2 weeks per month, the risk of significant gastrointestinal or renal toxicity is low. Caution must always be advised when diuretics are simultaneously administered, even for short periods. Lastly, patient variability in response to NSAIDs must be taken into consideration; several different NSAIDs may need to be tried before one is found that relieves the cyclic pain of PMS without causing dyspepsia.[36]

Stress Reduction

Stress appears to worsen some of the pain symptoms of PMS, particularly low back pain. Reduction of stress through the elimination or avoidance of personal stresses and the use of relaxation techniques and learned coping strategies is an important component of PMS therapy, one that is frequently overlooked.[37]

MIGRAINE HEADACHES

Pathophysiology

Migraine headaches are recurrent, unilateral, pulsating or pounding headaches generally worsened by physical activity and associated with nausea, vomiting, anorexia, diarrhea, photophobia and/or phonophobia.[38] Migraine attacks may last for 4 to 72 hours and may severely affect a patient's ability to function. "Classic" migraines are usually preceded by transient focal neurologic deficits, the aura, while "common" migraines are not associated with focal neurologic symptoms. Menstrual migraine usually refers to migraines that only occur immediately prior to and during menstruation.[38]

A variety of factors may trigger or worsen a migraine attack. Alcohol, chocolate, aged cheese, and monosodium glutamate are common dietary triggers. Hypoglycemia, physical or emotional stress, fatigue, and lack of sleep are also cited as triggers.[38]

The pathophysiology of menstrual migraine is not entirely clear, but serotonin appears to be an important factor.[38–41] Serotonin is released prior to migraine attacks and stimulates the production of vasodilatory substances that produce the headache. Platelets are the major source of serum serotonin, and reduced platelet serotonin content and abnormal serotonin metabolism are observed in migraine sufferers. Moreover, dihydro-

ergotamine and sumatriptan, selective agonists of serotonin receptors, are effective in aborting migraine attacks.[38–41] Factors other than serotonin may also be important. Disordered sympathetic reactivity,[42] postsynaptic alpha-2 adrenoreceptor hyposensitivity,[43] and impaired central opioid control of the hypothalamic-pituitary–adrenal axis have all been observed.[44] A role for estrogen in migraine is supported by the 3:1 female:male preponderance of migraine, the general improvement noted during pregnancy, and the occurrence of menstrual migraine at a time when serum estrogen concentration is falling.[45,46] The estrogen withdrawal hypothesis of menstrual migraine was proposed by Somerville[46] who suggested that estrogen sensitizes intracranial and extracranial blood vessels to some other factor, and that migraine occurs in susceptible women as estrogen declines premenstrually. This theory is plausible since estrogen is known to affect noradrenergic transmission and prostaglandin synthesis, factors that can initiate the vasoconstrictive phase of migraine.

Evaluation

Evaluation of the patient with menstrual migraine must include a neurologic examination. If any abnormalities are found in the neurologic examination, a more intensive search for other causes of headache must be conducted.[38] Menstrual migraine is diagnosed when a patient has vascular headache limited to the perimenstrual phase of the cycle. Most patients, however, demonstrate migraine headaches throughout the menstrual cycle, often with exacerbation during menstruation.

Treatment

Symptomatic Treatment

Migraine headaches are treated with a combination of vasoconstrictors, analgesics, antiemetics, and sedatives.[38] Sumatriptan is also an effective, well-tolerated treatment for migraine attacks.[39] Severe, protracted attacks may require emergency room care, or even hospitalization; intravenous ergotamine, intravenous hydration, and sedation are currently the mainstay of therapy.[38]

Prophylaxis

NAPROXEN

Several medications are used to try to reduce the frequency of migraine attacks. Naproxen sodium, 250 mg to 550 mg t.i.d., and propranolol hydrochloride, 40 mg t.i.d., are commonly used as migraine prophylaxis.[47] Naproxen inhibits platelet aggregation and prostaglandin biosynthesis. Thus it may act to prevent migraines by preventing platelet aggregation, which is increased in migraine patients. Aspirin at low dosages, 325 mg every other day, also inhibits platelet aggregation, and effectively reduces the frequency of migraine attacks.[40]

Naproxen is associated with a high incidence of gastrointestinal side effects when given continuously, and in one comparative trial propranolol was better tolerated by patients than naproxen, even though efficacy was similar.[47]

ERGONORINE MALEATE

Ergonovine maleate, an ergot derivative with vasoconstrictive properties, is an effective prophylaxis for menstrual migraine. The usual dosage is 0.2 mg t.i.d. to q.i.d. for 3 days, beginning 1 day prior to menstruation. Side effects are usually mild.[48] Long-acting and time-release preparations of dihydroergotamine are also effective for menstrual migraine.[49]

BELLERGAL

Bellergal can prevent menstrual migraine. It is a combination of ergotamine tartrate, bellafoline, and phenobarbital. It is administered b.i.d. for 4 to 7 days beginning just prior to menstruation.[38]

AMITRIPTYLINE

Amitriptyline, 50 to 150 mg q.h.s., is an alternative first-line prophylactic agent. It is particularly effective if stress and tension are considered important triggering factors.[50]

ESTRADIOL

High dosages of percutaneous estradiol effectively reduce the frequency and severity of menstrual migraines.[51] Suppression of cyclic ovarian activity by subcutaneous estradiol implants[51] and percutaneous estradiol gel[52] effectively prevent true menstrual migraine. Ovulation suppression with two 0.1 mg/day transdermal estradiol skin patches (Estraderm, CIBA-Geigy) effectively controls PMS, but has not been specifically evaluated for menstrual migraine.[53] Percutaneous estradiol, 1.5 mg daily beginning 2 days prior to expected onset of migraines, and continued for 7 days, reduces the number of migraine headaches by about 50%, compared to placebo.[54] This author used lower dosages of transdermal estradiol patches, 0.5 to 1.0 mg/day for 7 days perimenstrually, in six patients with menstrual migraine. Five of six responded with at least a 50% reduction in the frequency of attacks (unpublished data). No alterations in menses or significant adverse reactions were reported. These data support Summerville's theory that physiologic withdrawal of estradiol premenstrually is an important trigger for menstrual migraine.

DANAZOL

Danazol, at dosages sufficient to inhibit ovulation and gonadotropin-releasing hormone agonists (GnRHa), eliminates menstrual migraine in many PMS sufferers.[55] GnRHa, however, may cause an initial worsening of migraines as the hypoestrogenic environment is created. Once a chronic hypoestrogenic environment occurs, migraines tend to remit. However, since a long-term hypoestrogenic state is associated with an increased risk of bone loss, GnRH agonist therapy is generally combined with some form of estrogen-progestin replacement. Since migraine sufferers are more susceptible to fluctuations in serum estradiol, transdermal estradiol replacement that creates a steady state estradiol milieu is less likely than oral estrogen replacement to trigger migraine attacks.

STRESS MANAGEMENT

Lastly, menstrual migraine may respond to biofeedback, relaxation techniques, and stress management.[56] These techniques reduce the frequency of migraine attacks and abort impending attacks.[38]

SUMMARY

More than 60% of PMS patients describe disturbing physical symptoms, usually related to fluid retention, pain, or migraine headaches. Treating physical symptoms significantly improves the sense of well-being of patients; improvement of emotional symptoms may also occur, perhaps because of a "domino" effect, or because of shared pathophysiologic mechanisms. Cyclic luteal phase administration of diuretics and NSAIDs is the most effective treatment for fluid retention and pain symptoms, respectively. However, adverse drug interactions must be avoided. Exercise and stress reduction are useful adjunctive measures. The frequency of menstrual migraine headaches can be reduced with a number of prophylactic medications—naproxen, ergots, danazol, and transdermal estradiol, to name a few. Biofeedback, relaxation techniques, and stress reduction are also of help.

REFERENCES

1. Freeman EW, Sondheimer S, Weinbaum PJ, et al. Evaluating premenstrual symptoms in medical practice. *Obstet Gynecol.* 1985;65:500.
2. Vellacott ID, O'Brien PMS. Effect of spironolactone on premenstrual syndrome symptoms. *J Reprod Med.* 1987;32:429.
3. Reid RL, Yen SSC. Premenstrual syndrome. *Am J Obstet Gynecol.* 1981;139:85.
4. Reid RL. Premenstrual syndrome. *Curr Prob Obstet Gynecol Fertil.* 1985;8(2):1.
5. Friedlander MA. Fluid retention: evaluation and use of diuretics. *Clin Obstet Gynecol.* 1987;30:431.
6. Preece PE, Richards AR, Owen GM, et al. Mastalgia and total body water. *Br Med J.* 1975;4:498.
7. Wong WH, Freedman RI, Levan NE, et al. Changes in the capillary filtration coefficient of cutaneous vessels in women with premenstrual syndrome. *Am J Obstet Gynecol.* 1972;114:950.
8. Faratian B, Gaspar A, O'Brien PMS, et al. Premenstrual syndrome: weight, abdominal swelling, and perceived body image. *Am J Obstet Gynecol.* 1984;150:200.
9. Davidson BJ, Rea CD, Valenzuela GJ. Atrial natriuretic peptide, plasma renin activity, and aldosterone in women on estrogen therapy and with premenstrual syndrome. *Fertil Steril.* 1988;50:743.
10. MacGregor GA, Roulston JE, Markander ND, et al. Is "idiopathic" edema idiopathic? *Lancet.* 1971;i:397.
11. Werch A, Kane RE. Treatment of premenstrual tension with metalazone: a double-blind evaluation of a new diuretic. *Curr Ther Res.* 1976;19:565.
12. O'Brien PMS, Craven D, Selby C, et al. Treatment of premenstrual syndrome by spironolactone. *Br J Obstet Gynaecol.* 1979;86:142.
13. Vellacott ID, Shroff NE, Pearce MY, et al. A double-blind, placebo controlled evaluation of spironolactone in the premenstrual syndrome. *Curr Med Res Opin.* 1987;10:450.
14. Hellberg D, Claesson B, Nilsson S. Premenstrual tension: a placebo-controlled efficacy study with spironolactone and medroxyprogesterone acetate. *Int J Gynecol Obstet.* 1991;34:243.
15. Benedek-Jaszmann LJ, Hearn-Sturtevant MD. Premenstrual tension and functional infertility: aetiology and treatment. *Lancet.* 1976;i:1095.
16. Andersen AN, Streenstrup OR, Svendstrup B, et al. Effect of bromocryptine on the premenstrual syndrome: a double-blind clinical trial. *Br J Obstet Gynaecol.* 1977;84:370.
17. Elsner CW, Buster JE, Schindler RA, et al. Bromocryptine in the treatment of premenstrual tension syndrome. *Obstet Gynceol.* 1980;56:723.
18. Graham JJ, Harding PE, Wise PH, et al. Prolactin suppression in the treatment of premenstrual syndrome. *Med J Aust.* 1978;2(suppl 3):18.
19. Ghose K, Coppen A. Bromocryptine and premenstrual syndrome: a controlled study. *Br Med J.* 1977;1:147.
20. Kullander S, Svanberg L. Bromocryptine treatment of the premenstrual syndrome. *Acta Obstet Gynecol Scand.* 1979;58:375.
21. Steiner M, Haskett RF, Carroll BJ, et al. Plasma prolactin and severe premenstrual tension. *Psychoneuroendocrinol.* 1984;9:29.
22. Rubinow DR, Hoban C, Grover GN, et al. Changes in plasma hormones across the menstrual cycle in patients with menstrually

related mood disorder and in control subjects. *Am J Obstet Gynecol.* 1988;158:5.
23. Budoff PW. Use of prostaglandin inhibitors in the treatment of PMS. *Clin Obstet Gynecol.* 1987;30:453.
24. Budoff PW. The use of prostaglandin inhibitors for the premenstrual syndrome. *J Reprod Med.* 1983;28:469.
25. Mira M, McNeil D, Fraser I, et al. Mefanamic acid in the treatment of premenstrual syndrome. *Obstet Gynecol.* 1986;68:395.
26. Wood C, Jakubowicz D. The treatment of premenstrual symptoms with mefanamic acid. *Br J Obstet Gynaecol.* 1980;87:627.
27. Facchinetti F, Fioroni L, Sances G, et al. Naproxen sodium in the treatment of premenstrual symptoms: a placebo-controlled study. *Gynecol Obstet Invest.* 1989;28:205.
28. Jakubowicz DL, Godard E, Dewhurst J. The treatment of premenstrual tension with mefanamic acid: analysis of prostaglandin concentrations. *Br J Obstet Gynaecol.* 1984;91:78.
29. Messinis IE, Lolis D. Treatment of premenstrual mastalgia with tamoxifen. *Acta Obstet Gynecol Scand.* 1988;67:307.
30. Deeny M, Hawthorn R, Hart DM. Low dose danazol in the treatment of the premenstrual syndrome. *Postgrad Med J.* 1991;67:450.
31. Watts JF, Butt WR, Edwards RL. A clinical trial using danazol for the treatment of premenstrual tension. *Br J Obstet Gynaecol.* 1987;94:30.
32. Derzko CM. Role of danazol in relieving the premenstrual syndrome. *J Reprod Med.* 1990;35:97.
33. Prior JC, Vigna Y, Sciarretta D, et al. Conditioning exercise decreases premenstrual symptoms: a prospective, controlled 6-month trial. *Fertil Steril.* 1987;47:402.
34. Prior JC, Vigna V. Conditioning exercise and premenstrual symptoms. *J Reprod Med.* 1987;32:423.
35. Rolland PH, Martin PM, Rolland AM, et al. Benign breast disease: studies of prostaglandin E2, steroids, and thermographic effects of inhibitors of prostaglandin biosynthesis. *Obstet Gynecol.* 1979;54:715.
36. Brooks PM, Day RO. Nonsteroidal antiinflammatory drugs—differences and similarities. *N Engl J Med.* 1991;324:1716.
37. Dickson-Parnell B, Zeichner A. The premenstrual syndrome: psychophysiologic concomitants of perceived stress and low back pain. *Pain.* 1988;34:161.
38. Digre K, Damasio H. Menstrual migraine: differential diagnosis, evaluation, and treatment. *Clin Obstet Gynecol.* 1987;30:417.
39. Subcutaneous Sumatriptan International Study Group: Treatment of migraine attacks with sumatriptan. *N Engl J Med.* 1991;325:316.
40. Buring JE, Peto R, Hennekens CH. Low-dose aspirin for migraine prophylaxis. *JAMA.* 1990;264:1711.
41. Nattero G, Allais G, Lorenzo C, et al. Menstrual migraine: new biochemical and psychological aspects. *Headache.* 1988;28:103.
42. Cavallini A, Micioli G, Sances G, et al. Disordered sympathetic reactivity in menstrual migraine: a cardiopressor and biochemical evaluation. *Func Neurol.* 1989;4:85.
43. Facchinetti F, Martignoni E, Nappi G, et al. Premenstrual failure of alpha-adrenergic stimulation on hypothalamus-pituitary responses in menstrual migraine. *Psychosom Med.* 1989;51:550.
44. Facchinetti F, Martignoni E, Fioroni L, et al. Opioid control of the hypothalamic-pituitary-adrenal axis cyclically fails in menstrual migraine. *Cephalalgia.* 1990;10:51.
45. Welch KMA, Darnley D, Simkins RT. The role of estrogen in migraine: a review and hypothesis. *Cephalalgia.* 1984;4:227.
46. Somerville BW. The role of estradiol withdrawal in the etiology of menstrual migraine. *Neurology.* 1972;22:355.
47. Sargent J, Solbach P, Damasio H, et al. A comparison of naproxen sodium of propranolol hydrochloride and a placebo control for the prophylaxis of migraine headache. *Headache.* 1985;25:320.
48. Gallagher RM. Menstrual migraine and intermittent ergonovine therapy. *Headache.* 1989;29:366.
49. D'Alessandro R, Gamberini G, Lozito A, et al. Menstrual mi-

graine: intermittent prophylaxis with a time-release pharmacological formulation of dihydroergotamine. *Cephalalgia.* 1983;1(suppl):156.

50. Couch JR, Ziegler DK, Hassenein R. Amitriptyline in the prophylaxis of migraine. *Neurology.* 1976;26:121.

51. Magos A, Zilkha KJ, Studd JWW. Treatment of menstrual migraine by oestradiol implants. *J Neurol Neurosurg Psychiatry.* 1983;46:1044.

52. Lignieres B de, Vincens M, Mauvais-Jarvis P, et al. Prevention of menstrual migraine by percutaneous oestradiol. *Br Med J.* 1986; 293:1540.

53. Watson NR, Studd JWW. Use of oestrogen in the treatment of the premenstrual syndrome: a comparison of the routes of administration. *Contemp Rev Obstet Gynaecol.* 1990;2:117.

54. Dennerstein L, Morse C, Burrows G, et al. Menstrual migraine: a double-blind trial of percutaneous estradiol. *Gynecol Endocrinol.* 1988;2:113.

55. Lichten EM, Bennett RS, Whitty AJ, et al. Efficacy of danazol in the control of hormonal migraine. *J Reprod Med.* 1991;36:419.

56. Solbach P, Sargent J, Coyne L. Menstrual migraine headache: results of a controlled, experimental, outcome study of nondrug treatments. *Headache.* 1984;24:75.

CHAPTER 11

Psychotropic Medications as Treatment of Dysphoric Premenstrual Syndrome

Susanna Goldstein and Uriel Halbreich

Behavioral and mood changes are very common during the later phase of the menstrual cycle. These changes are diagnosed as an "illness" or "disorder" based primarily on the severity of impairment in the woman's functioning and her relationships with others.[1] The association between the cyclic hormonal phenomena that are manifested in the menstrual cycle and emotional and behavioral symptoms is intriguing. Gonadal hormones have been shown to significantly influence activity of the central nervous system (CNS) neurotransmitters that affect mood.[2] Even though specific hormonal differences between women with and without premenstrual syndrome (PMS) have not yet been definitely demonstrated, one therapeutic approach to severe and disabling PMS is the elimination of ovulation with gonadotropin releasing hormone agonists or danazol. However, ovulation suppression causes side effects that are unacceptable to many women, and this treatment is usually reserved for more severe cases. A second therapeutic approach utilizes pharmacologic agents proven efficacious in primary psychiatric disorders to treat the emotional and behavioral manifestations of PMS. This chapter reviews the clinical experience accumulated in the treatment of dysphoric PMS with psychopharmacologic medications.

ANTIDEPRESSANTS

Of the multifaceted manifestations of dysphoric premenstrual syndrome, the most frequent one is a syndrome that resembles major depressive disorder (MDD): markedly depressed mood and feelings of hopelessness, anhedonia, easy fatigability, decreased concentration, and other cognitive disturbances as well as changes in sleep and appetite. In the majority of women with dysphoric PMS, the cluster of symptoms is quite similar to atypical depression, with decreased energy, increased sleep, increased appetite, and reactivity of mood. Impulsivity, irritability, and some aggressiveness are also quite prevalent.[3,4] Women with dysphoric premenstrual syndrome were shown to have an increased lifetime prevalence of major depressive disorder and postpartum depression, and women with affective mood disorders have an increased prevalence of premenstrual symptoms.[5]

Biologic Plausibility

Current biological hypotheses on the etiology of affective mood disorders emphasize several neurotransmitter systems, most notably serotonin and norepinephrine. In this context women with PMS were reported to have premenstrual decreased levels of whole blood serotonin[6] and decreased platelet serotonin as compared to women with no PMS. Monoamine oxidase activity was found to be increased premenstrually by some investigators[7] but not by others.[8] Imipramine receptor binding (IMI) in platelets of women with dysphoric PMS was found to be decreased in the beginning of the luteal phase.[9] Women with dysphoric PMS were also reported to have blunted late luteal cortisol response to the serotonergic precursor tryptophan and the serotonergic postsynaptic agonist, m-CPP, indicating a decreased postsynaptic serotonergic response.[10–12] Data on norepinephrine are less conclusive but a premenstrual abnormality of that system is plausible.[11]

Premenstrual depressions may be viewed as a variant of a recurrent time-limited major depression, which might be caused by altered regulation of neurotransmitter-receptor systems, triggered by hormonal changes (which may not be abnormal per se) in vulnerable women.

These associations and the similarities between major depression and dysphoric subtypes of premenstrual changes make antidepressants natural candidates for the treatment of these conditions. Yet, there is very little systematic research on these treatment modalities.

Currently available antidepressants are roughly divided into three categories: heterocyclics (mostly tricyclics but also bicyclics and tetracyclics), monoamine oxidase inhibitors, and the newer "atypical" agents. Heterocyclic antidepressants act mostly by blocking reuptake of norepinephrine and/or serotonin, thus potentiating their action. Monoamine oxidase inhibitors potentiate the action of monoamines by blocking their catabolism. The atypical antidepressants are either more specific, affecting almost exclusively a single monoamine (eg, fluoxetine, which is quite specific to serotonin), or their antidepressant activity is through a yet-unknown mechanism (eg, bupropion).

Heterocyclic Antidepressants

Nortriptyline

Nortriptyline is a tricyclic antidepressant that was given to 11 women[13] with a DSM-III-R diagnosis of late luteal phase dysphoric disorder (LLPDD)[14] who failed to respond to placebo or another medication. When treated with nortriptyline (50 to 125 mg at bedtime in an open trial) for at least 4 weeks preceding the premenstrual period, 8 of the 11 patients were considered re

sponders. Seven patients chose to continue treatment with nortriptyline, maintaining their positive response during the 4- to 8-month follow-up. The investigators noted that some of their patients demonstrated an initial overstimulation in response to the nortriptyline (in a way similar to that reported to occur in some patients with panic disorder, but is uncommonly observed in patients with depressive disorders). To overcome this problem, they recommend initiating the tricyclic medication with a very low dose (10 mg) and increasing it slowly. (Plasma levels of nortriptyline were similar in responders and nonresponders.)

Clomipramine

Another tricyclic antidepressant, clomipramine, was administered by Erikson and colleagues[15] (in a daily dose of 25 to 50 mg for five consecutive menstrual cycles) to five nondepressed women with severe premenstrual irritability and sadness. All subjects reported a dramatic reduction in premenstrual complaints.

Other tricyclic and heterocyclic antidepressants are occasionally mentioned in the literature, mostly as treatment failures with patients with premenstrual dysphoria or depression.

Monoamine Oxidase Inhibitors

Monoamine oxidase inhibitors (MAOI) were found particularly helpful in a subgroup of depressed patients clinically characterized as "atypical," "neurotic," "rejection sensitive," or "dysthymic."[16] The symptoms characteristic of this group, such as hypersomnia, overeating, prominent anxiety disturbances, phobias, hypochondriasis, and panic attacks, along with a highly reactive mood disturbance, are quite prevalent in dysphoric PMS. An acronym proposed by Shader and Greenblatt,[17] TROUBLE, appropriately describes candidates for MAOI treatment and also describes a subgroup of women with dysphoric premenstrual syndromes: T-transient, R-regressive, O-overanxious, U-unstable, B-bulimic, L-labile, E-episodic.

Nevertheless, we are unaware of any reports of treatment of premenstrual syndrome with MAOIs. However, extensive clinical experience with phenelzine (Nardil) and tranylcypromine (Parnate), given in smaller doses during the follicular phase (phenelzine, 15 to 30 mg/day, tranylcypromine 10 to 20 mg/day) and higher doses (usually doubling the dose) in the luteal phase, shows them to be a safe, effective, and well-tolerated treatment. The major drawback of treatment with MAOIs is the requirement to observe a strict tyra mine-free diet. The diet must be thoroughly explained to the patient, and continuing adherence to it should be reinforced as long as the treatment lasts.

New Antidepressants

Fluoxetine

The new generation of antidepressants shows some progress over the previous agents, mainly because of their more favorable side effect profile and higher specificity. The drug that received most attention in this group is fluoxetine. Rickels et al[18] studied 10 women with LLPDD, administering placebo during one menstrual cycle and fluoxetine in the following two cycles (in an open trial). They found significantly greater reductions in premenstrual affective symptoms during fluoxetine treatment than during the placebo cycle. Fluoxetine did not improve somatic symptoms such as breast tenderness and bloating, nor did it have any effect on food cravings. Harrison et al (personal communication, 1990) completed an open study of fluoxetine in patients with LLPDD and concomitant dysthymic disorder, and found that both chronic depression and the LLPDD symptoms were eliminated or alleviated in most cases. Stone et al[19] treated 15 women with confirmed PMS over two menstrual cycles with fluoxetine (20 mg/day) or placebo. Eight of the 9 subjects who received fluoxetine responded favorably to treatment, whereas only 2 of the 6 receiving placebo reported a positive response. All subjects on fluoxetine elected to continue with this treatment after completion of the study. Other published case reports and verbal communications generally confirm the beneficial effect of fluoxetine in LLPPD, including symptoms such as overeating, food craving, and weight gain.[20–22]

We give fluoxetine 20 mg every other day during the follicular phase and increase the dose to 20 mg every day during the luteal phase. Sometimes, twice as much is needed. There are some sporadic verbal reports that patients responded to fluoxetine, which is generally a slow-acting drug, within a few days, but a placebo effect is suspected in these cases. The current enthusiasm for fluoxetine treatment of PMS should be cautiously evaluated, because this drug has been only recently introduced. Our experience is that though it is very efficacious in many patients—at least in some women the efficacy diminishes within 6 to 10 months. This assumed tolerance was observed with several antidepressants in the past. Long-term experience and studies are needed to evaluate this phenomenon in treatment of PMS.

ANXIOLYTICS

A subgroup of women with premenstrual changes experience mostly anxiety symptoms. These symptoms may resemble generalized anxiety disorder: unrealistic or excessive worrying, motor tension such as trembling, twitching, aches, restlessness, and fatigability, autonomic hyperactivity such as shortness of breath, palpitations, and nausea, and exaggerated vigilance such as feeling "keyed up," difficulty in concentrating, and irritability. Other patients may experience discrete panic attacks (attacks of intense fear or discomfort accompanied by a host of symptoms such as dizziness, dyspnea, tachycardia, and sweating). These attacks appear premenstrually in only few women, but more often they appear throughout the menstrual cycle and are more frequent and/or intense in the late luteal phase.

Biologic Plausibility

The current biological hypotheses of the pathophysiology of anxiety focus on the locus ceruleus–noradrenergic system, and the γ-aminobutyric acid (GABA) receptor. The locus ceruleus-noradrenergic hypothesis ascribes the different manifestations of anxiety to chronic or intermittent hyperactivity of the locus ceruleus which "floods" the brain with norepinephrine.[23] The GABA hypothesis stems from the discovery of benzodiazepine receptors that are part of a complex of neuroreceptors which are clustered around the receptor for the inhibitory neurotransmitter, GABA. The benzodiazepines, attached to their receptor, are hypothesized to cause GABA to be more effective by enhancing GABA-induced chloride ion flow into the neuron, thus causing hyperpolarization (which is a more "stabile" state of the neuron) with reduced firing rate.[24,25] At present, the benzodiazepines are probably the most effective drugs for treatment of anxiety in its various forms, but they also have disadvantages, most notably their potential of dependence and abuse.

Premenstrual flare-up or exacerbation of anxiety symptoms or syndromes may be provoked by the hormonal changes inherent to this period in predisposed or vulnerable women.

Alprazolam

For many years, benzodiazepines were the most frequently prescribed drugs in medicine for a wide range of conditions not excluding premenstrual complaints. However, we are unaware of any published reports of this treatment modality except for the relatively new medication, alprazolam. Alprazolam, a triazolobenzodiazepine that was shown to have both antianxiety and antidepressant activity, was the drug used in two placebo-controlled studies: Smith et al[26] studied a group of patients with premenstrual syndrome using a low fixed dose schedule (0.25 mg t.i.d.) and reported improvement in both somatic (bloating, cramps, headaches) and dysphoric symptoms in patients who were on alprazolam. Harrison et al[27,28] studied 30 women with LLPDD in a double-blind crossover design comparing alprazolam with placebo. Medication was started during the luteal phase when symptoms first appeared (6 to 14 days before menses), with 0.25 mg 3 to 4 times daily, and was increased "as needed" up to a maximum of 4 mg/day. At the onset of menses, medication was tapered within 3 to 5 days. In this study, alprazolam relieved premenstrual symptoms better than placebo in most patients. The investigators followed some patients for up to 10 months in an open cyclic treatment and reported no evidence of dependence.

In another study[29] of patients with panic disorder who were successfully treated with alprazolam, premenstrual breakthrough or panic attacks were the first symptoms to reappear during a slow taper of that medication. These patients were then effectively treated by a low dose of alprazolam during the follicular phase and a higher dose during the luteal phase.

Buspirone

Another class of anxiolytic agents has been recently developed. These drugs, exemplified by buspirone, do not interact with the GABA and the benzodiazepine receptors. Rather, buspirone exerts an agonist effect on the serotonergic 5-HT_{1A} receptors[30] that are most prevalent in the dorsal raphe nuclei. Buspirone mimics the effect of serotonin at the 5-HT_{IA} receptors, which reduces neuronal activity from the raphe. Buspirone has the advantages of being nonsedative, not potentiating alcohol, and not causing dependency or having abuse liability. It has the disadvantages of a slow onset of action and decreased or lack of effectiveness in patients previously treated with benzodiazepines.

In one study, buspirone was compared to placebo in a group of women with PMS.[31] An average dose of 25 mg of buspirone or placebo was administered during the last 12 days of the menstrual cycle for three consecutive cycles. Buspirone produced a significantly larger decrease in PMS symptoms than placebo. Both somatic and behavioral and emotional symptoms were reported to be improved.

Our experience with buspirone is quite different. When treatment with 15 mg buspirone was initiated in the midluteal phase, a few days before appearance of symptoms, some women reported increased anxiety, irritability, and restlessness, to a degree that they discontinued the medication and refused to try it again. When treatment with that medication was initiated in the midfollicular phase, the anxiety symptoms were not reported or observed, but in most cases buspirone was not effective premenstrually even in doses of 30 mg/day. The paradoxical midluteal effect might point to a serotonergic hypersensitivity during that period, which is theoretically reasonable and might be of heuristic importance.

MOOD STABILIZERS

Biologic Plausibility

Premenstrual changes may primarily reflect "mood swings." In other words, they may be manifested as a stormy unstable affective state rapidly shifting from depression and withdrawal to irritability and/or elation, hostility, and hyperactivity. These changes may appear in a macro form—women who experience one predominant mood state during each premenstrual period, or more frequently; or they might manifest in a micro form—when the affective states are changing rapidly, several to many times a day, and at times even appear mixed (eg, depression along with increased energy, hyperactivity, and irritability). The first description often closely resembles the mood swings that characterize bipolar disorder, depressed or hypomanic/manic type; while the second situation resembles the bipolar "mixed" or so-called "rapid cyclers."

Lithium

The first line of treatment for bipolar disorder is with the lithium ion. Lithium has multiple neurobiologic effects, but it is not known which one effect is relevant to its therapeutic action. Among others, it affects transmembrane ion pumps, possibly altering the distribution of sodium, potassium, and calcium in the cells. There is no dispute, however, on the effectiveness of lithium as treatment of bipolar disorders, both for the treatment of acute mania and also for prophylaxis maintenance against recurrences. Based on some similarities between bipolar disorders and premenstrual changes, there are several reports of cases and uncontrolled trials[32,33] of lithium as helpful in alleviating PMS.

Positive results were obtained mostly when lithium was begun 10 to 14 days prior to the onset of menses and serum levels were 0.6 to 0.8 mEq/l. However, two controlled studies[34,35] and an uncontrolled one[36] did not supported these positive findings. It appears that other than in a very small and carefully selected group of women who experience a variant of bipolar disorder that cycles with menstruation, lithium is not a very useful treatment for dysphoric PMS. There is another, possibly larger subgroup of women, with primary bipolar disorder who have a premenstrual exacerbation of the illness. Of course, for these patients lithium is indicated.

Some women may benefit from lithium dosage titration along the menstrual cycle, aiming for average higher blood levels for women who exhibit mainly hypomanic/manic features and lower blood levels for women with predominantly depressive symptoms. In both cases a higher oral dose might be needed during the luteal phase, because there are some nonconfirmed case reports of menstrually related fluctuations of plasma lithium levels with lower luteal levels, especially when plasma levels were less than 0.6 to 0.8 mEg/1.[37,38]

Anticonvulsants

More recently, several primarily anticonvulsant drugs were introduced into the psychopharmacological armamentarium as "mood stabilizers."[39] These drugs, mostly carbamazepine, valproic acid, and klonazepam, were empirically found useful in some bipolar patients who did not respond to lithium. These reports led to extensive speculations regarding the mechanism of action of these drugs and whether the anticonvulsant effects are related to their action in affective disorders.

There is limited experience with these "mood stabilizers" in treatment of dysphoric PMS. Theoretically, some clinicians might choose to use them based on the same rationale applied for lithium. Others might refer to the effectiveness of carbamazepine in inhibiting seizures kindled from repeated stimulation of the limbic system, hypothesizing that a kindling-like process is occurring with the repeated cyclic hormonal changes in some vulnerable women.[1,40,41] A small but important subgroup of women has a true premenstrual exacerbation of certain forms of seizure disorders.[42] Some of these women have temporal lobe seizures presenting as altered affective states and behavior. Following electroencephalogram (EEG) confirmation of the diagnosis, the proper anticonvulsant treatment is of course highly effective in such cases.

ANTIPSYCHOTIC MEDICATIONS

The perimenstrual period has been shown to be associated with an increase in severity of psychotic symptoms, particularly in women with psychotic depression.[43] There are also several reports of "periodic psychosis" recurring in association with the menstrual cycle in women with no other psychiatric abnormalities.[44,45] The correct treatment of premenstrual exacerbations of a psychotic illness is with the appropriate antipsychotic drug. Most often the drug of choice is the same that is used for maintenance treatment but in higher doses. In some cases, the symptom profile during the premenstrual psychotic exacerbation may be quite different than during the rest of the cycle, such as a withdrawn, slowed-down apathetic patient who usually is best treated with a nonsedating antipsychotic medication but who may become agitated and insomniac premenstrually. Such a patient may benefit from the addition of a more sedating antipsychotic drug during her premenstrual period only.

The antipsychotics, also called neuroleptics or major tranquilizers, is a group of psychotropic medications differing in chemical structure, but they are all dopamine receptor antagonists. The effects of dopamine receptor blockade at different anatomic sites in the brain putatively produces their therapeutic but also their unwanted effects, such as reversible and irreversible motor disturbances, (eg, tardive dyskinesia and parkinsonism). Consequently, even though the antipsychotic drugs have a fairly large range of indications, their use should be limited to clearly psychotic states, and the dosage should be the minimum needed.

MISCELLANEOUS DRUGS

In recent years, several drugs that were primarily developed and introduced to clinical use for a variety of "nonpsychotropic" indications are finding new applications due to their central nervous system activity. Some of these drugs were actually tried under more-or-less controlled conditions for the treatment of dysphoric PMS.

Fenfluramine

D-fenfluramine releases brain serotonin and blocks its reuptake. Its ability to relieve premenstrual depression and excessive calorie and carbohydrate intake was examined in 17 women.[46] Subjects received 15 mg d-fen-fluramine or placebo twice daily during the luteal phase of six menstrual cycles. D-fenfluramine suppressed premenstrual rise in calorie, carbohydrate, and fat intake significantly better than placebo. Though it decreased premenstrual depression, its influence on dysphoric symptoms was less pronounced.

Beta-Adrenergic Blockers

The beta-adrenergic blockers that are currently in clinical use are competitive antagonists of norepinephrine and epinephrine at the beta-adrenergic receptors. Their primary use is in cardiovascular disorders. A variety of psychiatric uses have been reported although few are well established and none is approved by the Food and Drug Administration (FDA). The beta blockers propranolol and atenolol may significantly reduce symptoms of "performance anxiety" (which is a subtype of social phobia), autonomic symptoms associated with generalized anxiety and panic attacks, as well as impulsive violence in patients with neurological impairment. Although the beta blockers have significant side effects and potentially troublesome interactions with other drugs, they may be indicated and beneficial in a subtype of women with premenstrual changes who exhibit primarily symptoms that appear to be responsive to these drugs. Propranolol (20 mg to 40 mg twice daily during 10 premenstrual days) and atenolol (50 mg daily) were reported to be more effective than placebo in a single patient[47] and atenolol (50 mg daily) was more effective than placebo in a controlled study of 16 women,[48] but the authors did not delineate the symptom profile of these subjects.

Calcium Channel Blockers

Calcium channels are a universal feature of all excitable cells, including neurons. Therefore it is not surprising that a drug that blocks movement of calcium across its channels would have pharmacologic effects on the CNS. However, our limited state of knowledge of emotional and behavioral disease states does not permit a logical selection of a disorder or even symptoms based on molecular mechanism alone. Nonetheless, recent reports suggest the potential usefulness of the calcium channel blocker verapramil in the treatment of mood disorders and particularly mania. Based on the clinical and psychobiological associations between affective disorders and PMS (and pure serendipity), verapramil in dosages of 320 mg/day was reported to be effective for "all affective and cognitive symptoms but not for so-matic symptoms of PMS" in a single patient,[49] while verapramil (50 mg twice daily) given for a cardiac condition improved symptoms of PMS in another single case report.[50]

Clonidine

Clonidine is primary used as an antihypertensive agent whose principal mechanism of action is as an agonist of alpha adrenergic receptors in the CNS. These are predominantly autoreceptors with negative feedback function. Thus, clonidine's net effect is to decrease the activity of central noradrenergic neurons. The psychiatric uses of clonidine are experimental and none has an FDA approval. It suppresses many signs and symptoms of narcotic withdrawal, temporarily blocks panic attacks and generalized anxiety, and seems effective for the treatment of highly treatment-resistant manic episodes. Since all these conditions (withdrawal from endogenous opiates, increased vulnerability to panic attacks, and affective disorder) are associated with premenstrual changes, clonidine appears possible for the treatment of some women with premenstrual syndrome. So far there is only one report of a 4-month study[51] of 24 subjects treated with 17 mg/day of clonidine or placebo. In this study clonidine was significantly more effective and had no side effects.

Naltrexone

A direct link between gonadal steroid secretion and central endogenous opiate activity was repeatedly demonstrated and confirmed.[52] It has been proposed that PMS might be associated with excessive sensitivity to, or increased exposure to, high central levels of endogenous opiates, as well as with the withdrawal of the endogenous opiates when ovarian steroid levels fall.[53,54] The administration of naltrexone, a long-acting narcotic agonist, may act to decrease the magnitude of both the increase and the subsequent decrease of endogenous opiates. In one controlled study,[55] naltrexone (25 mg/day) was given to 20 women with PMS. Naltrexone was "better than placebo" in this study but side effects were serious and included nausea, decreased appetite, dizziness, and fainting.

Bright Light Therapy

Light therapy is not a medication in the pharmacological sense. However, it has been shown to be an effective treatment in some subgroups of affective disorders, mostly those associated with impaired rhythm.[56] The main indication for light therapy is in the treatment of seasonal affective disorder (SAD).[57] Due to the hypothesized rhythm impairment in dysphoric PMS and its presumed association with SAD[2] there has been some rationale for a trial of light treatment in PMS.

Parry et al[47] reported a case history of a patient with LLPDD only in fall and winter months. She was treated with 1 month of "uncontrolled phototherapy" with good results. Next month she was given light and placebo and then light plus melatonin. Melatonin seemed to reverse the therapeutic effects of light. Another study by Parry[58] was a randomized crossover trial of morning versus evening exposure to bright light for 2 hours. This study showed slight improvement with only the evening treatment.

SUMMARY

The treatment of dysphoric PMS is a subject involving many decisions. First, a proper diagnosis is of utmost importance, with a careful differentiation from other possible causes. Once the diagnosis is established, the evaluation of severity might determine the treatment route taken. If pharmacotherapy is chosen, symptomatic treatment might be first tried. The drug of choice is determined according to the symptom profile. In the future, a better understanding of underlying mechanisms will contribute to that decision. With present choices, symptomatic treatment of dysphoric PMS might be preferable to hormonal intervention. We believe, however, that this might change in the very near future.

REFERENCES

1. Halbreich U, Alt IH, Paul L. Premenstrual changes: impaired hormonal homeostasis. *Endocrin Neuropsychiatr Dis.* 1988;6:173.
2. Halbreich U. *Hormones and Depression.* New York: Raven Press; 1987.
3. Halbreich U, Endicott J, Nee J. Premenstrual depressive changes: value of differentiation. *Arch Gen Psychiatr.* 1983;40:535.
4. Halbreich U, Endicott J, Schacht S, et al. The diversity of premenstrual changes as reflected in the Premenstrual Assessment Form. *Acta Psychiatr Scand.* 1982;65:46.
5. Halbreich U, Endicott J. The relationship of dysphoric premenstrual changes to depressive disorders. *Acta Psychiatr Scand.* 1985;71:331.
6. Rapkin AJ, Edelmuth E, Chang LC, et al. Whole blood serotonin in premenstrual syndrome. *Obstet Gynecol.* 1987;70:533.
7. Ashley CR, Carr LA, Cook CL, et al. Alteration of platelet serotonergic mechanisms and monoamine oxidase activity in premenstrual syndrome. *Biol Psychiatr.* 1988;24:225.
8. Rapkin AJ, Buckman TD, Sutphin MS, et al. Platelet monoamine oxidase—B activity in women with premenstrual syndrome. *Am J Obstet Gynecol.* 1988;159:1536.
9. Rojansky N, Halbreich U, Zander K, et al. Imipramine receptor binding and serotonin uptake in platelets of women with premenstrual changes. *Gyn Obstet Invest.* 1991;31:146.
10. Halbreich U. Gonadal hormones and antihormones, serotonin, and mood. *Psychopharmacol Bull.* 1990;26:291.
11. Halbreich U, Rojansky N, Carson S, et al. Gonadal hormones, serotonin, noradrenaline, and mood. *Clin Neuropharm.* 1990;13(suppl. 2):524.
12. Halbreich U, Rojansky N, Wang K. Psychological, hormonal, and neurotransmitter aspects of menstrually-related symptoms. In: Napi G, ed. *Headache and Depression: Serotonin Pathways as a Common Clue.* New York: Raven Press; 1992:191.
13. Harrison WM, Endicott J, Nee J. Treatment of premenstrual depression with nortripyline: a pilot study. *J Clin Psychiatr.* 1989;50:136.
14. American Psychiatric Association: Diagnostic and Statistical Manual III—Revised. Washington DC: APA Press; 1986.
15. Erickson E, Lisjo P, Sundblad C, et al. Effect of clomipramine on premenstrual syndrome. *Acta Psychiatr Scand.* 1990;81:87.
16. Liebowitz MR, Quitkin FM, Stewart JW. Antidepressant specificity in atypical depression. *Arch Gen Psych.* 1988;45:129.
17. Shader RI, Greenblatt DJ. A new axis II diagnosis: TROUBLES. *J Clin Psychopharmacol.* 1984;4:241.
18. Rickels K, Freeman EW, Sondheimer S, et al. Fluoxetine in the treatment of premenstrual syndrome. *Curr Ther Res.* 1990;48:161.
19. Stone AB, Perlstein TB, Brown WA. Fluoxetine in the treatment of premenstrual syndrome. *Psychopharmacol Bull.* 1990;26:331.
20. Jacobson J. Premenstrual syndrome treatments. *J Clin Psychiatr.* 1989;50:393.
21. Metz A. Fluoxetine treatment of premenstrual syndrome. *J Clin Psychiatr.* 1990;51:260.
22. Pies RW. Fluoxetine treatment of premenstrual syndrome. *J Clin Psychiatr.* 1990;51:348.
23. Redmond ED, Huang YH. New evidence for a locus coeruleus—norepinephrine connection with anxiety. *Life Sci.* 1979;25:2149.
24. Tallman JF, Thomas JW, Gallager DW. GABAergic modulation of benzodiazepine binding site sensitivity. *Nature.* 1978;274:383.
25. Pritchett DB, Sondheimer H, Shivers B. Importance of a novel $GABA_A$ receptor subunit for benzodiazepine pharmacology. *Nature.* 1989;338:582.
26. Smith S, Rinehart JS, Ruddock VE. et al. Treatment of premenstrual syndrome with alprazolam: results of double-blind, placebo-controlled, randomized crossover clinical trial. *Obstet Gynecol.* 1987;70:37.
27. Harrison WM, Endicott J, Rablzine JG, et al. Treatment of premenstrual dysphoria with alprazolam and placebo. *Psychopharm Bull.* 1987;23:150.
28. Harrison WM, Endicott J, Nee J. Treatment of premenstrual dysphoria with alprazolam. A controlled study. *Arch Gen Psychiatr.* 1990;47:270.
29. Goldstein S, Halbreich U. Panic disorder and the menstrual cycle. Presented at the Annual Meeting of the APPA, New York, NY, March 1990.
30. Perouka SJ. Selective interaction of novel anxiolytics and 5-hydroxytryptamine$_{1A}$ receptors. *Biol Psychiatr.* 1985;20:971.
31. Rickels K, Freeman E, Sondheimer S. Buspirone in treatment of premenstrual syndrome. *Lancet.* 1989;i:777.
32. DeLeon-Jones FA, Val E, Herts C. MHPG excretion and lithium treatment during premenstrual tension syndrome. *Am J Psychiat.* 1982;139:950.
33. Sletten IW, Gershon S. The premenstrual syndrome: a discussion of its patholophysiology and treatment with lithium ion. *Comprehen Psychiatr.* 1966;7:197.
34. Singer K, Cheng R, Schou M. A controlled evaluation of lithium in premenstrual tension syndrome. *Br J Psychiatr.* 1974;124:50.

35. Mattsson B, von Schoultz B. A comparison between lithium, placebo, and diuretic in premenstrual tension. *Acta Psychiatr Scand.* 1974;255(suppl):75.

36. Steiner M, Haskett RF, Osmun JN, et al. Treatment of premenstrual tension with lithium carbonate—a pilot study. *Acta Psychiatr Scand.* 1980;61:96.

37. Kukopulos A, Minnai G, Nuller-Oerlinghausen B. The influence of mania and depression on the pharmacokinetics of lithium: a longitudinal case study. *J Affect Dis.* 1985;8:159.

38. Conard GD, Hamilton JA. Recurrent premenstrual decline in serum lithium concentrations. Clinical correlates and treatment implications. *J Am Acad Child Psychiatr.* 1986;29:852.

39. Post RM. Mechanisms of action of carbamazepine and related anticonvulsants in affective illness. In: Meltzer HY, ed. *Psychopharmacology: A Generation of Progress.* New York: Raven Press; 1987:567.

40. Post RM, Kopanda RT. Cocaine, kindling and psychosis. *Am J Psychiatr.* 1976;133:627.

41. Rubinow DR, Roy-Byrne P. Premenstrual syndromes: overview from a methodological perspective. *Am J Psychiatr.* 1984;141:163.

42. Backstrom T. The menstrual cycle and epilepsy. *Acta Neuro Scand.* 1976;54:321.

43. Abramovitz ES, Baker AB, Fleisher SF. Onset of depressive psychiatric crises and the menstrual cycle. *Am J Psychiat.* 1982;139:475.

44. Endo M, Daigujl M, Sano Y, et al. Periodic psychosis recurring in association with menstrual cycle. *J Clin Psychiat.* 1978;39:456.

45. Weekes LR, Williams EY. Premenstrual tension associated with psychotic episodes. *J Nerv Ment Dis.* 1952;116:321.

46. Brzezinski AA, Wurtman JJ, Wurtman R, et al. D-fenfluramine suppresses the increased calorie and carbohydrate intake and improves the mood of women with premenstrual depression. *Obstet Gynecol.* 1990;76:296.

47. Parry B, Rosenthal N, Tamarkin L, et al. Treatment of patient with seasonal premenstrual syndrome. *Am J Psych.* 1987;144:762.

48. Rausch JS, Janowsky DS, Golshan S, et al. Atenolol treatment of late luteal phase dysphoric disorder. *J Affect Dis.* 1988;15:141.

49. Deicken R. Verapamil treatment of premenstrual syndrome. *Biol Psych.* 1988;24:689.

50. Price W, Giannini A. Verapamil in the treatment of premenstrual syndrome: case report. *J Clin Psych.* 1986;47:213.

51. Giannini JA, Sullivan B, Sarachene J, et al. Clonidine in the treatment of premenstrual syndrome: a subgroup study. *J Clin Psych.* 1988;49:62.

52. Quigley ME, Yen SSC. The role of endogenous opiates in LH secretion during the menstrual cycle. *J Clin Endocrinol Metab.* 1980;51:179.

53. Halbreich U, Endicott J. Possible involvement of endorphin withdrawal or imbalance in specific premenstrual syndromes and postpartum depression. *Med Hypotheses.* 1981;7:1045.

54. Reid RL, Yen SSC. Premenstrual syndrome. *Am J Obstet Gynecol.* 1981;139:85.

55. Choung C, Coulam C, Bergstralh E, et al. Clinical trial of naltrexone in premenstrual syndrome. *Obstet Gynecol.* 1988;72:332.

56. Lowy AJ, Sack RL, Miller S, Huban TM. Antidepressant and circadian rhythm phase shifting effects of light. *Science.* 1987;235:352.

57. Rosenthal NE, Fack DA, Skwerer RG, et al. Phototherapy for seasonal affective disorder. *Biol Rhythms.* 1988;3:101.

58. Parry BL, Berga SL, Mostofi N, et al. Morning versus evening bright light treatment of late luteal phase dysphoric disorder. *Am J Psych.* 1989;146:1215.

CHAPTER 12

Treatment of Premenstrual Syndrome with Ovulation Suppression

Ken Muse

The premenstrual syndrome (PMS) is virtually unique in being a common ailment about which there is almost no consensus. Fundamental aspects of this illness—its prevalence, pathophysiology, diagnosis, and treatment—remain either disputed or largely unknown. Discovery of the etiology of PMS will allow a focused, rational treatment to be developed; until then, clinicians must rely on empiric therapies, derived by trial-and-error techniques.

Certainly the least debatable point about PMS, and perhaps the simplest foundation on which to build an empiric therapy, is that it is a disease arising from menstrual cyclicity.[1] Various therapies share the rationale that elimination of menstrual cyclicity will abolish PMS symptoms (Table 1). The efficacy of each of these "ovulation suppression" treatments in relieving PMS symptoms has been studied to varying degrees, as have their side effects. In addition, it is recognized that these drugs invoke special risks and side effects due to their creation of a nonphysiologic sex steroid environment.

ORAL CONTRACEPTIVES

Oral contraceptive pills (OCPs) should be the perfect PMS therapy. They suppress endogenous menstrual cyclicity, replace it with constant levels of estrogen and progestin, and provide effective contraception. Surprisingly, little is known about the effects of these commonly prescribed drugs on PMS. In particular, no carefully designed studies have been performed examining the effects of currently available, "low dose" OCPs on well-characterized PMS patients.

Early Studies

Some information can be gleaned from studies done since the 1970s that examined the prevalence of side effects in the general population of women taking OCPs. Although PMS was not evaluated as an entity, many of the individual symptoms studied are promi-

Table 1

Types of Ovulation Suppression Therapies
for Premenstrual Syndrome

Oral contraceptives
Chronic progestin
  Medroxyprogesterone acetate
  (Depo-Provera)
  Levonorgestrel implants (Norplant)
Parenteral estrogen
  Estradiol implants
  Estradiol percutaneous patches (Estraderm)
Danazol (Danacrine)
GnRH agonists

nent in PMS. In 1970, Herzberg and Coppen[2] compared 152 women starting OCPs with 40 women starting barrier contraception. The OCP group recorded a significant decrease in their premenstrual depression, irritability, and dysmenorrhea, with no lasting improvement in fatigue, swelling, or headache. However, some OCP subjects had depression or irritability develop or worsen during the study; these women appeared to have higher levels of depression or other PMS-like symptoms before the study began. In 1971 Herzberg and colleagues[3] studied 218 women starting OCPs and 54 women starting intrauterine device (IUD) use, and reported that depression scores tended to decrease in both groups. Interestingly, women in the OCP group who were unhappy with them and stopped or switched pill use had higher pretreatment scores for depression, "neuroticism," and "premenstrual weepiness" than subjects satisfied with them. Similarly, Fleming and Seager's comparison[4] of 335 OCP users and 179 controls found no difference in the prevalence of depression between the groups, but a third group of 172 ex-users did complain of significantly more depression and "neuroticism."

Some studies have examined very large patient populations. Sheldrake and Cormack[5] studied menstrual cycle-associated symptoms among 3323 university students, of whom 756 were taking OCPs; the latter complained of PMS symptoms slightly less often. Kutner and Brown[6] measured premenstrual depression in 5151 women in the Kaiser Foundation Health plan and noted that pill users had less depression than women who never used them. Depression was less frequent with combination pills than the sequential type, and was lower on pills with increasing progestin dosage. Notably, past users of OCPs had more severe depression than current users or nonusers. (Examining mood changes on different estrogen/progestin therapies, Cullberg[7] also found fewer PMS-like symptoms with high-progestin treatments.)

Two placebo-controlled trials of OCP use have been reported. Silbergeld et al[8] studied eight women using Enovid and placebo for four cycles each in a double-blind, crossover study. As might be expected, Enovid made dysmenorrhea better, swelling and breast tenderness worse, and had mixed effects on emotions: less irritability and anger, no change in depression, and more fatigue and anxiety. Morris and Udry[9] noted that most of the 51 women they studied felt equally worse premenstrually whether they were on OCPs or placebos; only a few women noticed a difference between treatments, with equal numbers of them feeling better or worse on OCPs.

Lower Dosage Oral Contraceptives

Three studies have used a more contemporary concept of PMS in examining the effects of OCP use. Andersch and Hahn's evaluation[10] of 217 established pill users and 595 nonusers found that the former complained of less PMS, except among teenagers, in whom an opposite effect was seen. Graham and Sherwin[11] noted that 101 OCP users and 149 nonusers had the same overall number and severity of all types of symptoms, but classic PMS symptoms (anxiety, depression, fatigue, swelling, impaired social functioning) were milder and of shorter duration in the OCP group. In 1990, Walker and Bancroft[12] studied 122 women who were self-diagnosed as having mild-to-moderate PMS. Daily symptom records for at least 2 months were kept by 35 women well established on monophasic pills, 30 on triphasic preparations, and 57 subjects using barrier methods of contraception. All symptoms showed changes across the menstrual cycle, but except for breast tenderness (which was improved on monophasic pills), the groups were not different with regard to irritability, depression, fatigue, tension, bloating, or libido. (In women starting pills, Bancroft and colleagues[13] had previously found adverse affects on mood more likely on triphasic pills, and among patients with prepill mood problems.)

Extracting clinically applicable information from these disparate studies must be done only with the greatest caution and critical analysis. However, on careful review several noteworthy points emerge. After 20 years of widespread usage, it is obvious that OCPs are not a dramatic cure for PMS, nor do they induce or exacerbate severe PMS in the general population of women. Rather, experience has been that dysmenorrhea, moliminal symptoms, and many premenstrual emotional changes are somewhat decreased (or unaffected) by OCP use. If PMS is very broadly defined, certainly it can be said that OCPs ameliorate it for many women. Use of a monophasic pill with relatively high progestin content is suggested from the limited data currently available.

An opposing trend is also evident. Anecdotally, it has frequently been observed that women with significant PMS say that they "cannot tolerate" OCPs. Some PMS patients try OCPs, feel worse, and change to barrier contraception. When subsequently included as "controls" in the large, cross-sectional studies of OCPs and PMS mentioned above, these women would erroneously make OCPs appear beneficial in treating PMS. An elevated level of PMS-like symptoms has repeatedly been noted in past users of OCPs, when compared to current and nonusers. How OCPs could worsen PMS is unknown, but the pharmacologic levels of estrogen and progestin generated, alternating with one week of placebo therapy each month, may simulate greater-than-normal menstrual cyclicity, enough to aggravate PMS symptoms.

LONG-ACTING PROGESTIN

Despite its demonstrated effectiveness in ovulation suppression and the popular impression that progesterone helps PMS, intramuscular injection of a long-acting progestin preparation (medroxyprogesterone acetate, Depo-Provera) has received almost no attention as a PMS treatment. Keye and DeLia[14] reported a 50% decrease in PMS symptoms in 15 of 20 women treated with medroxyprogesterone acetate, 150 mg every 1 to 3 months. The side effects of this agent (including depression) and its lack of reversibility have probably contributed to the lack of interest in this inexpensive and easily given drug.

Contraceptive implants that release a constant amount of levonorgestrel over 5 years (Norplant) have recently become available. Their effects on PMS are unknown.

PARENTERAL ESTROGEN/PROGESTIN

Estradiol Implants

Sustained-release preparations of estradiol appear to be impressively successful PMS ovulation suppression therapies in the few studies done to date with them. After a retrospective study[15] suggested its effectiveness, Magos and coworkers[16] performed a randomized, prospective, double-blind study in which each of 33 PMS patients had a 100-mg implant of crystalline estradiol inserted deep into the subcutaneous tissue of the anterior abdominal wall. Norethisterone, 5 mg orally per day, was taken for 7 days each month to induce regular menses. A second group was composed of 35 PMS patients undergoing an identical regimen of placebo implantations and pills. Both groups used barrier contraception, recorded their symptoms daily, and were evaluated over 10 months.

After 2 months of therapy, 33 women in the placebo group (94%) noted a significant improvement in their symptoms. However, this waned, and their symptom scores returned to pretreatment levels 4 months later. This placebo response is unusually high, and may be due to the surgical nature of the implant impressing the patients. The estradiol treatment group also noted an impressive improvement in symptoms by 2 months of treatment; unlike the placebo group, though, this improvement persisted throughout the rest of the 10-month study. All symptoms were improved, especially negative affect. Side effects (mastalgia, nausea, weight gain, headache, improved menstrual pattern) were transient and mild, and tended to be similar in both treatment groups.

These investigators subsequently reported a long-term evaluation[17] of this therapy, studying 50 women for 2 to 8 years. They noted impressive relief from depression, bloating, irritability, fatigue, anxiety, and other PMS symptoms, which was maintained over the course of the treatment. The main problem with the therapy was that the cyclic administration of the oral progestin caused PMS-like side effects in 58% of patients; in 24%, these were judged to be severe. Despite changing the dosage or type of preparation, this often remained a problem. These symptoms were judged to be progestin side effects, rather than inadequate PMS relief, because the symptoms followed progestin administration, and did not occur if the progestin was withheld.

Other problems were noted. Eight (16%) of the patients underwent hysterectomy, mainly due to these progestin side effects. Although irregular bleeding was rare, all patients had an increase in uterine size (due to myometrial growth), and 4 were found to have cystic endometrial hyperplasia. Finally, to improve their libido and sense of well-being, 32 of the subjects also had a testosterone implant placed. It is difficult to know the extent to which this therapy affected their PMS symptoms.

Transdermal Estradiol

Although they may affect the patient for up to 2 years after placement, estradiol implants must be replaced every 6 months to maintain anovulatory serum levels of estradiol. To eliminate these minor surgical procedures and to make the therapy more reversible, these authors also investigated the use of transdermal estradiol patches (Estraderm).[18] Forty PMS patients were studied in a randomized, double-blind fashion. The patients wore two 100-µg patches continually, replacing them every 3 days, for 3 months. The patients wore placebo patches for another 3 months; both groups took norethisterone, 5 mg orally, each day for days 19 to 26 each month. Regardless of their initial treatment, all patients noted an improvement in symptoms for the first 3 months. Those on placebo for the last half of the study then had return of symptoms, but women going from placebo to estrogen noted a further improvement in their symptoms (Fig. 1).

In comparing the transdermal patches and the implants to induce anovulation with estradiol, the authors[19] noted that both methods avoid the immediate liver metabolism ("first-pass effect") seen with oral preparations, making the needed dosage less. By having less effect on liver physiology, metabolic side effects from these pharmacologic amounts of estrogen may theoretically be decreased. The constant parenteral absorption leads to less fluctuating serum levels than present with oral medication. Although the transdermal patch is convenient, 10% of women had to discontinue its use due to skin irritation. More importantly, PMS symptoms often appeared when the patch therapy was first initiated (in the first few weeks of the cycle, when they normally are not present). The authors attributed this to the patch rapidly inducing pharmacologic levels of estradiol when first applied; initial absorption from the estradiol implant is slower, and this phenomenon does not occur.

DANAZOL

Danazol, a drug which is commonly used to treat endometriosis, also appears to be an effective PMS ther-

Fig. 1 Mean symptom scores (± SE) for "negative affect" for 40 women wearing estradiol patches and placebo patches for 3 months each. Active treatment to placebo, plain line; placebo to active treatment, open circles; (Reprinted from Watson NR, et al.[18] with permission.)

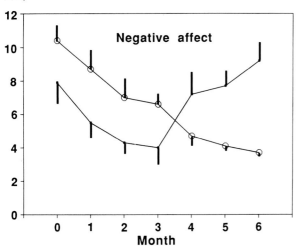

apy. An isoxazol derivative of 17-α-ethinyl-testosterone, the clinical pharmacology of danazol is quite complex.[20] By binding to androgen and progesterone receptors, by inhibiting multiple enzymes involved in ovarian and adrenal steroid synthesis, and by displacing testosterone from its serum binding protein, danazol creates an anovulatory, hypoestrogenic, androgenic milieu. This "pseudomenopause" therapy suppresses ovulation by preventing normal follicular growth, estrogen secretion, and the resulting LH surge, and produces a steady, nonfluctuating hormonal environment.

Controlled Clinical Trials

Gilmore et al[21] studied the effects of danazol, 400 mg/day for 3 months, on 36 PMS patients in a double-blind, randomized, placebo-controlled, crossover fashion. Daily symptom recordings revealed that danazol relieved many PMS symptoms (depression, tension, irritability, mastalgia, swelling, etc.) significantly better than did placebo. Sixteen women failed to complete the study, three due to side effects from the danazol.

Watts and coworkers[22] divided 40 PMS patients into four groups, and gave placebo or danazol at 100 mg/day, 200 mg/day, or 400 mg/day to each for 3 months. By the third month, symptom scores for irritability, anxiety, lethargy, increased appetite, and mastalgia were significantly better on danazol than on placebo, with no improvement in other PMS symptoms. The placebo group showed initial improvement, which largely disappeared by the third month. The authors felt that the 200 mg/day dosage gave optimal symptom relief with fewest side effects, and that the most improvement was seen with mastalgia. A major problem was that 13 women withdrew from the study, citing a combination of side effects from the danazol and failure to obtain PMS symptom relief. These women tended to have higher baseline PMS symptom scores than those who continued the drug.

Other studies have examined the use of danazol tangentially or in a less controlled fashion. In studying the effects of surgical castration and estrogen replacement on PMS, both Casson et al.[23] and Casper and Hearn[24] used danazol in their preoperative evaluations. A dosage of 400 mg/day for several months was given to completely suppress ovarian function. Casson noted that 14 women who had "severe debilitating PMS unresponsive to conventional interventions" saw their symptoms completely eliminated by danazol; symptoms promptly returned on cessation of the drug. Casper placed 5 PMS patients on danazol as a temporary treatment until surgery could be performed; all had "complete resolution" of PMS symptoms while on the drug. Day[25] and Derzko[26] each reported their personal, uncontrolled experience with danazol, and noted positive results, with mastalgia being the most improved symptom. Uniquely, Sarno et al[27] gave danazol, 200 mg/day, or placebo from the onset of PMS symptoms to the onset of menses (luteal phase treatment only) for two cycles each in a double-blind, crossover study. Danazol significantly improved symptoms more than placebo in 11 of 14 patients. No patient reported any drug side effects. All cycles were ovulatory, with no perturbation of the menstrual cycle or its hormones detected. The mechanism for this improvement remains unknown.

Side Effects

Although it is an effective PMS therapy, use of danazol is limited by its expense, side effects, and potential long-term risks. Most patients on danazol experience side effects. Many side effects (depression, weight gain, bloating sensation) mimic PMS symptoms, and are presumably due to danazol's progesterone-like activity. The androgenic side effects are often even more troubling to patients, and include acne, increased sebum production, hirsutism, changes in libido, and deepening of the voice. (These complaints usually disappear after stopping danazol, but the latter effect may be long-lasting.) Hypoestrogenic changes include amenorrhea, menometrorrhagia, hot flushes, and decreased breast size. These symptoms become more distressing at higher dosages, and with longer courses of the drug, making PMS treatment for many months or years especially problematic. Low doses of danazol may allow ovulation and pregnancy; contraception must be carefully practiced to avoid masculinization of a female fetus. Potential long-term metabolic risks include decreased bone mass due to hypoestrogenism, and accelerated cardiovascular disease arising from lowered HDL and increased LDL cholesterol concentrations.

GnRH ANALOGS

Physiology

Gonadotropin-releasing hormone (GnRH) is a small peptide that the hypothalamus secretes, in a pulsatile fashion, into the portal blood which then bathes the pituitary gland. Each "pulse" of GnRH induces a corresponding burst of gonadotropins from the cells in the pituitary (the "gonadotropes") that make follicle stimu-

lating hormone (FSH) and luteinizing hormone (LH). Appropriate gonadotropin stimulation of the ovary, and hence menstrual cyclicity, requires that the GnRH pulses be within a fairly narrowly defined range in terms of their amplitude and frequency (about every 90 minutes). GnRH stimulation outside this window prevents normal menstrual cyclicity, and is a useful therapy for diseases aggravated by the menstrual cycle.

Rather than use GnRH itself, it is more convenient to use one of the many chemically modified versions of GnRH that have been synthesized. These compounds have either agonistic or antagonistic GnRH actions. GnRH antagonists immediately stop gonadotropin secretion; these drugs are just now reaching clinical experimentation, and are not yet studied in PMS. GnRH agonists have been clinically utilized for several years in a variety of gynecologic conditions. They "overstimulate" the GnRH receptor, and for 1 to 2 weeks, an initial "flare" or surge in stimulation is seen in gonadotropin secretion and subsequent ovarian sex steroid production. Paradoxically, a "pseudomenopause" state is then induced by the continued stimulation causing "down-regulation" (decreasing number of GnRH receptors on the gonadotrope), "desensitization" (less FSH and LH released per GnRH stimulus), and other, as yet poorly characterized, mechanisms. The gonadotrope secretes very little normal FSH or LH, instead releasing "gonadotropins" with little or no biologic activity. Without effective stimulation, follicular growth in the ovary ceases, and ovarian sex steroid levels fall to very low, constant levels. This profound "pseudomenopause" is physiologically equivalent to castration, but is rapidly reversible upon cessation of the drug. Equally important, GnRH analogs are very specific. They act only on the gonadotrope, and have no side effects per se. (Of course, symptoms do arise from the low estrogen levels.) Being small peptides, GnRH analogs cannot be taken orally, but daily nasal sprays and subcutaneous injections are available, as are long-lasting depot formulations using intramuscular injections and pellet implants.

Controlled Clinical Trials

Bancroft et al[28] were the first to study the effects of these compounds in PMS. They gave buserelin, 200 µg b.i.d. or t.i.d., intranasally to 14 PMS patients. Most patients improved on therapy, but some worsened. Interpretation of results was made difficult by the large number of extraneous medical problems that occurred during the study (such as cholecystitis, orthopedic and sterilization surgeries, chronic upper respiratory infections), as well as side effects from the agonist (hot flushes, nasal congestion, and so on).

Muse and coworkers[29] studied eight women with severe PMS in a double-blind, placebo-controlled, crossover trial in which, after a cycle of baseline symptom charting to confirm their diagnosis, each subject took 3 months of daily subcutaneous GnRH-agonist (D-Trp[6]-Pro[9]-Net-GnRH) and 3 months of saline placebo. Daily PMS symptom scoring and frequent hormonal evaluations were performed. On placebo therapy, cyclic PMS symptoms persisted and normal menstrual cycle hormone profiles were observed. GnRH agonist administration resulted in an initial stimulation of gonadotropins and sex steroids for 2 weeks, and then constant, menopausal levels of estradiol and progesterone were observed. The luteal phase elevation of PMS symptom scores was abolished, and the noncyclic symptoms observed were similar to the levels seen during the follicular phase of placebo therapy, when the patients said they felt "normal" (Fig. 2). This eradication of PMS symptoms was equally true for both the physical complaints of PMS (breast tenderness and fullness, headache, fatigue, bloating) as well as behavioral ones (irritability, depression, crying spells, nervousness, anger, inability to concentrate, mood swings, increased appetite, craving sweets or salty food). The short duration of the agonist administration (3 months, with the first month being the "flare" response) minimized production of significant side effects from the drug, as well as the patient's realization that it was hormonally different from placebo.

Hammarback and Backstrom[30] subsequently performed a similar study with a larger number of patients. After 2 months of baseline daily symptom recording, 26 women took 3 months of GnRH-agonist and 3 months of placebo in a double-blind, randomized, crossover fashion. The symptoms of feeling swollen, fatigued, cheerful, tense, irritable, depressed, and breast tenderness were evaluated prospectively. Significant improvement was noted on both placebo and agonist therapies, with the GnRH-agonist therapy being significantly better than placebo for each symptom. This is impressive in view of methodologic problems that would tend to minimize a difference between the treatments. The agonist used was buserelin, 400 µg once per day, intranasally. Presumably due to variable nasal absorption and being a relatively low dose of the drug, variable hormonal results were seen: 2 patients were never anovulatory on agonist treatment, and 4 others ovulated at least once during it. Women had about as many menstrual periods on agonist therapy as on placebo, and hypoestrogenic symptoms were rare. Also, 3 subjects were spontaneously anovulatory on placebo therapy. In addition, only 12 of the 23 patients that completed the study had "pure" PMS. They had a higher response rate to agonist treatment (75%) than did the 11 women with "premenstrual aggravation," who had symptoms throughout the menstrual cycle, and of whom only 45% improved on agonist therapy.

Three women dropped out of the study, one due to hypoestrogenic symptoms from the buserelin. Interestingly, two patients withdrew because their PMS symptoms worsened during the first 2 weeks of the active drug, presumably due to the high sex steroid milieu created during the initial "flare" phase of agonist administration.

Limitations of Therapy

From these studies and widespread anecdotal experience, a consensus has formed that GnRH-agonist suppression of ovulation is a very effective treatment for most patients with PMS. Unlike many other PMS thera-

Fig. 2 Mean symptom scores (± SE) for all 15 symptoms, 10 behavioral symptoms, and 5 physical symptoms during GnRH-agonist treatment and placebo treatments; (Reprinted from Muse KN, et al.[29] with permission.)

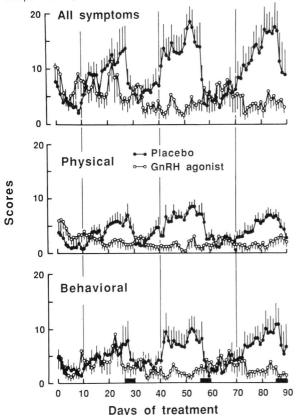

pies, the relief experienced is often proportional to the severity of PMS symptoms before treatment, and to the absence of other diagnoses. The patient with no follicular phase complaints, and classic premenstrual symptoms that prevent a normal work or home life, often claims to be symptom-free as long as GnRH agonist is given, tolerates the side effects of it fairly well, and does not wish to stop the drug. Although poorly studied, PMS symptoms seem to recur on the resumption of menstrual cyclicity.

However, the expense and potential medical risks of GnRH-agonists have severely curtailed their use in PMS. Most patients find agonists to be as expensive as danazol, and can afford only a few months of treatment. The marked hypoestrogenism induces hot flushes in virtually all patients by 2 to 4 months of therapy, and other symptoms (such as vaginal dryness) usually follow. Although these symptoms can be distressing, most patients opt to continue therapy. Concern over accelerating the medical risks found in natural menopause (osteoporosis, atherosclerotic cardiovascular disease, and so on), however, has curtailed the time span over which these drugs are given, usually to 6 months. Although the importance and nature of these risks have yet to be fully defined, a reduction in bone mass due to GnRH agonist-induced hypoestrogenism has been demonstrated after only 6 months of therapy; some recovery of bone mass was seen on return of menstrual cyclicity.[31]

Since PMS lasts for years, the value of an effective therapy that can only be given for a period of months is often questioned. Certainly, patients themselves welcome the respite from symptoms, and a secondary gain is often seen in that the endocrine nature of PMS is reinforced to the patient and her family. This is helpful if they had attributed many of the patient's symptoms to social and personality problems. Similarly, for a variety of reasons (including poorly standardized diagnostic criteria and the time required for lengthy interviews and prospective symptom charting), many physicians are uncomfortable in the evaluation of PMS patients. GnRH-agonist administration may have some value as an aid in diagnosis, in that women with PMS-like symptoms could be "challenged" with a few months of GnRH-agonist therapy. In patients whose symptoms are abolished, the diagnosis of PMS is reinforced (admittedly, a persistent placebo response could be present). Patients whose symptoms continue are unlikely to have PMS. This use of the drug, although sensible, has not been studied to date, and is entirely speculative. Finally, one could speculate that short-term GnRH-agonist administration may be a useful preoperative

adjunct in the surgical therapy of PMS. Casson et al[23] and Casper and Hearn[24] have reported that surgical "ovulation suppression" (bilateral salpingo-oophorectomy and hysterectomy), like "medical oophorectomy" with GnRH-agonist, is an effective therapy for severe PMS. Before undergoing such an irreversible, substantial step, complete suppression of symptoms by agonist would tend to confirm the value of surgical therapy, and vice versa.

Combined GnRH Agonist and Hormone Replacement Therapy

Actually, indefinite treatment of PMS by GnRH agonists may be possible. In the surgical studies cited above, unopposed estrogen therapy was given for months postoperatively, without recurrence of symptoms. In an analogous situation, women obtaining significant relief from PMS on GnRH agonist treatment could, when hypoestrogenic symptoms begin, be given estrogen/progestin replacement in addition to the agonist. Theoretically, this so-called "add-back" therapy could be titrated so that the complications of hypoestrogenism would be prevented, without inducing PMS symptoms.

Mortola and colleagues[32] reported their initial experience with this approach. After 2 months of baseline symptom charting, eight women with severe PMS were given the GnRH agonist histrelin, 100 µg subcutaneously each day, for 6 months. After 2 months of agonist alone, each patient also received four add-back treatments for 1 month each in a randomized, double-blind manner. The four treatments were placebo, conjugated equine estrogens (0.625 mg/day for days 1 to 25), medroxyprogesterone acetate (10 mg/day for days 16 to 25), or a combination of the estrogen and progestin therapies. Confirming earlier studies, histrelin by itself caused a marked decrease in PMS symptoms from baseline levels. Each of the four add-back therapies (including placebo) resulted in a level of symptoms intermediate between baseline and GnRH-agonist alone (Fig. 3). Symptoms on estrogen/progestin combination therapy were significantly lower than baseline levels, indicating the potential feasibility of this add-back regimen as a chronic PMS treatment. However, the elevation of symptoms above that seen with histrelin alone reveals the ability of these regimens to approximate the hormonal milieu necessary to induce PMS symptoms. (The "reverse placebo effect" observed was attributed to the patients' expecting to have symptoms when taking hormonal therapy, and their being aware that they would

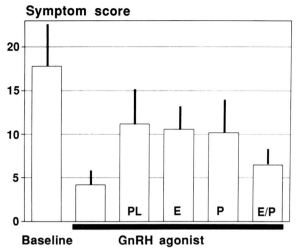

Fig. 3 Mean (± SE) daily luteal phase symptom scores for total PMS symptoms during baseline charting, GnRH-agonist alone, and various "add-back" treatments: PL, placebo; E, estrogen; P, progestin; E/P, combined estrogen/progestin. See text for details. (Reprinted from Mortola JF, et al.[32] with permission.)

be on active drug most of the time.) Although promising, this long-term use of GnRH-agonists in PMS treatment must await further study.

SUMMARY

Ovulation suppression appears to be a successful approach to PMS therapy, with symptomatic relief paralleling the ability of a therapy to reduce sex steroids to as low and as constant levels as possible. Oral contraceptives decrease dysmenorrhea and PMS-like symptoms for the majority of women, but there is evidence to suggest that their constant, pharmacologic sex steroid concentrations actually aggravate symptoms in women with established, severe PMS. Danazol and GnRH-agonist therapies appear much more effective, but their use is limited to the short term by their expense, side effects, and the medical risks associated with chronic hypoestrogenism. Parenteral, physiologic estrogen administration and GnRH-agonist "add-back" therapies have received limited study, but may become successful treatments that can be given as long as the disease lasts.

REFERENCES

1. Hammarback S, Backstrom T. Cyclical symptoms disappeared during anovulation in PMS. *J Psychosom Obstet Gynecol.* 1989;10(suppl 1):157.

2. Herzberg B, Coppen A. Changes in psychological symptoms in women taking oral contraceptives. *Br J Psych.* 1970;116:161.

3. Herzberg BN, Draper KC, Johnson AL, et al. Oral contraceptives, depression, and libido. *Br Med J.* 1971;3:495.

4. Fleming O, Seager CP. Incidence of depressive symptoms in users of the oral contraceptive. *Br J Psych.* 1978;132:431.

5. Sheldrake P, Cormack M. Variations in menstrual cycle symptom reporting. *J Psychosom Res.* 1976;20:169.

6. Kutner SJ, Brown WL. Types of oral contraceptives, depression, and premenstrual symptoms. *J Nerv Ment Dis.* 1972;155(3):153.

7. Cullberg J. Mood changes and menstrual symptoms with different gestagen/oestrogen combinations. A double-blind comparison with placebo. *Acta Psychiatr Scand.* 1972;236(suppl):1.

8. Silbergeld S, Brast N, Noble EP. The menstrual cycle: a double-blind study of symptoms, mood, and behavior, and biochemical variables using Enovid and placebo. *Psychosom Med.* 1971;33: 411.

9. Morris NM, Udry FR. Contraceptive pills and the day-to-day feelings of well-being. *Am J Obstet Gynecol.* 1972;113:763.

10. Andersch B, Hahn L. Premenstrual complaints. II. Influence of oral contraceptives. *Acta Obstet Gynecol Scand.* 1981;60:579.

11. Graham CA, Sherwin BB. The relationship between retrospective premenstrual symptom reporting and present oral contraceptive use. *J Psychosom Res.* 1987;31(1):45.

12. Walker A, Bancroft J. Relationship between premenstrual symptoms and oral contraceptive use: a controlled study. *Psychosom Med.* 1990;52(1):86.

13. Bancroft J, Sanders D, Warner P, et al. The effects of oral contraceptives on mood and sexuality: a comparison of triphasic and combined preparations. *J Psychosom Obstet Gynecol* 1987;7:1.

14. DeLia JE, Keye W. Preliminary report on the effects of depomedroxyprogesterone acetate on premenstrual tension syndrome. In: Abstracts, International Symposium on Premenstrual Tension and Dysmenorrhea, Kiawa Island, South Carolina, 1983.

15. Magos AL, Collins WP, Studd JWW. Management of the premenstrual syndrome by subcutaneous implants of oestradiol. *J Psychosom Obstet Gynecol.* 1984;3:93.

16. Magos AL, Brincat M, Studd JWW. Treatment of the premenstrual syndrome by subcutaneous oestradiol implants and cyclical oral norethisterone: placebo-controlled study. *Br Med J.* 1986;i;292(6536):1629.

17. Watson N, Studd J, Savvas M, et al. The long-term effect of oestradiol implant therapy for the treatment of premenstrual syndrome. *Gynecol Endocrinol.* 1990;4:99.

18. Watson NR, Studd JWW, Savvas M, et al. Treatment of severe premenstrual syndrome with oestradiol patches and cyclical oral norethisterone. *Lancet.* 1989;ii(8665):730.

19. Watson NR, Studd JWW. Use of oestrogen in treatment of the premenstrual syndrome: a comparison of the routes of administration. *Contemp Rev Obstet Gynaecol.* 1990;2:117.

20. Hornstein MD, Barbieri RL. Endocrine therapy of endometriosis: danazol and the synthetic progestins. In: Barbieri RL. *Reproductive Endocrine Therapeutics.* New York: Alan R. Liss; 1988:155.

21. Gilmore DH, Hawthorn RJS, Hart DM. Danazol for premenstrual syndrome: a preliminary report of a placebo-controlled double-blind study. *J Int Med Res.* 1985;13:129.

22. Watts JF, Butt WR, Edwards RL. A clinical trial using danazol for the treatment of premenstrual tension. *Br J Obstet Gynaecol.* 1987;94:30.

23. Casson P, Hahn PM, Van Vugt DA, et al. Lasting response to ovariectomy in severe intractable premenstrual syndrome. *Am J Obstet Gynecol.* 1990;162(1):99.

24. Casper RF, Hearn MT. The effect of hysterectomy and bilateral oophorectomy in women with severe premenstrual syndrome. *Am J Obstet Gynecol.* 1990;162(1):105.

25. Day JB. Danazol and the premenstrual syndrome. *Postgrad Med J.* (suppl 5) 1979;55:87.

26. Derzko CM. Role of danazol in relieving the premenstrual syndrome. *J Reprod Med* 1990;35(1 suppl):97.

27. Sarno AP, Miller EJ, Lundblad EG. Premenstrual syndrome: beneficial effects of periodic, low-dose danazol. *Obstet Gynecol.* 1987;70:33.

28. Bancroft J, Boyle H, Davidson DW, et al. The effect of an LHRH agonist on the premenstrual syndrome: a preliminary report. In: Schmidt-Gollwitzer M, ed. New Developments in Biosciences. 1. LHRH and its Analogues. *Fertility and Anti-Fertility Aspects.* Berlin; Walter de Gruyter; 1985:307.

29. Muse KN, Cetel NS, Futterman LA, et al. The premenstrual syndrome: effects of "medical oophorectomy." *N Engl J Med.* 1984;311:1345.

30. Hammarback S, Backstrom T. Induced anovulation as treatment of premenstrual tension syndrome. A double-blind cross-over study with GnRH-agonist versus placebo. *Acta Obstet Gynecol.* 1988;67:159.

31. Johansen JS, Riis BJ, Hassager C, et al. The effect of a gonadotropin-releasing hormone agonist analog (Nafarelin) on bone metabolism. *J Clin Endocrinol Metab.* 1988;67(4):701.

32. Mortola JF, Girton L, Fischer U. Successful treatment of severe premenstrual syndrome by combined use of gonadotropin-releasing hormone agonist and estrogen/progestin. *J Clin Endocrinol Metab.* 1991;71(2):252A.

CHAPTER 13

The Use of Estrogen in the Treatment of Premenstrual Syndrome

Neale R. Watson and John W. W. Studd

The use of estrogen for the treatment of the premenstrual syndrome (PMS) is contentious if the syndrome is due to relative estrogen excess, as suggested by Frank,[1] or relative progesterone deficiency, as suggested by Dalton.[2] No research has demonstrated an imbalance in these hormones, and no controlled studies have shown progesterone therapy more effective than placebo.[3,4] The etiology of PMS has remained elusive despite considerable research. The mechanism is likely to be a complex interaction between gonadal hormones and neuroendocrine transmitters, with changes in the central nervous system initiated by fluctuating ovarian activity. The importance of ovulation, as first suggested by Studd,[5] is supported by the persistence of cyclic symptoms after hysterectomy if ovarian function is preserved,[6] and by the successful treatment of PMS with agents that suppress ovulation. A number of different treatment approaches have been investigated, initially with estrogens either as a subcutaneous implant[7] and later as a transdermal patch,[8] as described in this chapter or alternatively with GnRH analogs[9] and danazol[10] as described in Chapter 12. Despite having different modes of action on the ovaries, all of these treatments have been shown to be more effective than placebo in the treatment of PMS.

EVALUATION AND DIAGNOSIS OF PREMENSTRUAL SYNDROME

It is now generally agreed that at least 1 month of prospective symptom assessment is essential for the diagnosis of PMS,[11] and it is our practice to confirm the diagnosis with at least 1 month of prospective symptom ratings using the modified Moos menstrual distress questionnaire (MDQ).[12] However, the methods used to evaluate prospectively recorded symptoms are more controversial. In our patients the Moos MDQ is evaluated statistically using Triggs trend analysis as first described by Magos and Studd.[13] This technique takes into consideration the timing of observations, which need not be independent, but when successive observations are dependent as in the premenstrual syndrome, future values can then be predicted with some degree of accuracy. These predictions are calculated using the exponentially weighted averages of the symptom scores. The difference between the predicted and actual score determines the trend, and consistent changes in any one direction "better" or "worse" may be analyzed to see if it reaches statistical significance.

Triggs analysis therefore enables us to define and

measure PMS mathematically. It is then possible to diagnose PMS in an individual patient if the symptoms are shown to exhibit both significant positive and negative trends during one menstrual cycle (Figs. 1 and 2). This technique also allows for the severity of a symptom to be estimated during a menstrual cycle by means of the maximum exponentially smoothed average (ESA) score. The comparison of such scores is useful for the evaluation of the efficacy of different treatments in patients with PMS, as specific end points are generated enabling intergroup comparisons using standard statistical techniques.[13]

ESTROGEN THERAPY

Oral Estrogen

The combined oral contraceptive pill, which effectively suppresses ovulation, would appear to be an ideal treatment for PMS. It is surprising that there has been no prospective placebo-controlled studies of its effect in the treatment of PMS. Reports of dramatic improvements in premenstrual symptoms appeared soon after it was first released,[14] but these were based on anecdotal evidence, and when assessed in controlled studies the evidence was less convincing.[15,16] (See Chapter 12 for a full review).

A possible alternative to the oral contraceptive pill are the natural estrogen preparations, which have been extensively studied for the treatment of menopausal symptoms and have many theoretical advantages to the synthetic estrogens used in the oral contraceptive pill. Since they have much less effect on liver enzymes, clotting factors, and glucose metabolism, they are theoretically much safer in older women.

Both the natural estrogens and the combined oral contraceptive pill have considerable potential for the symptomatic treatment of the premenstrual syndrome. Their efficacy is at present unresolved and underlies the need for prospective randomized placebo-controlled studies. An interesting approach to the use of oral contraceptives is the tricycle or "Ramadan" regimen described by Loudon et al.[17] In this 12-month study, 202 women used the pill continuously for 84 days, followed by 6 pill-free days, before starting on a second 84-day cycle. Women kept a diary card to record pill taking, uterine bleeding, and any side effects for the duration of the study. Analysis of the 196 patients who submitted sufficient data showed side effects were minimal. Approximately 24% complained of some spotting or breakthrough bleeding, but this improved in subsequent cycles; the treatment was otherwise well tolerated. On completion of the study, patients were asked to evaluate the treatment and noted an improvement in both premenstrual and menstrual symptoms. The advantage of this approach in women with PMS is to avoid the drop in hormone levels that occurs during the pill-free week. Previous studies having shown that the cyclical PMS-like symptoms in some women on the pill occur during the pill-free week. This regimen reduces the number of withdrawal bleeds and seems to improve premenstrual symptoms; however, this was retrospectively completed data and the findings have not been prospectively confirmed.[17]

Estradiol Implants

Hormone implants are designed to release a controlled amount of drug into the systemic circulation over a long period, thereby avoiding the peaks and troughs associated with intermittent oral therapy.[18] The active component of the implant is absorbed directly into the systemic circulation, which avoids first pass hepatic metabolism. Moreover, since only 15% to 20% of the total cardiac output is directed to the liver, implants do not demonstrate the bolus effect on liver protein metabolism that occurs with oral estrogen administration. Several different types of estrogen-containing implants have been developed. Currently, small rods containing estrogen are being evaluated as potential contraceptive agents, but the need to remove the rods and unsightly scars have limited their appeal. At present the most widely available implants are the biodegradable fused crystalline pellets marketed by Organon in the United Kingdom.

Technique of Hormone Implantation

The technique of implantation was well described by Greenblatt and Suran[19] and Thom and Studd.[20] It is a simple procedure, requiring only a few minutes, that may be safely performed in an outpatient clinic under local anaesthesia.

The implant is inserted into the subcutaneous fat of the abdominal wall about 5 cm above and parallel to the inguinal ligament. The skin where the implant is to be inserted is cleaned with antiseptic, and 4 ml of 1% lidocaine, with or without ephedrine, is injected along a track to anesthetize the tissue. A superficial 5-mm incision is made in the skin with a small scalpel blade, then a cannula and trochar are pushed through the incision up to the hilt along the track. The trochar is

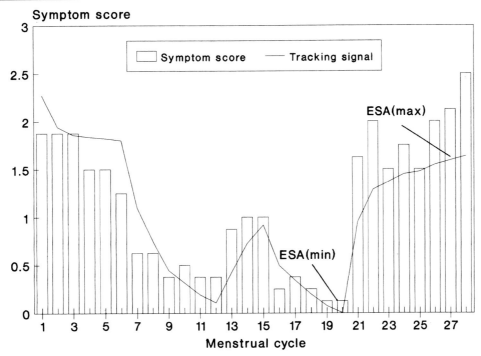

Fig. 1 Trend analysis of symptoms during a menstrual cycle shows significant trends that are diagnostic of PMS. Symptoms are scored on a scale of 0 to 3 depending on the severity of symptoms. ESA (Max), maximum exponentially smoothed average; ESA (Min), minimum exponentially smoothed average. (Adapted from Magos et al. *Am J Obstet Gynecol.* 1986;155:271, with permission.)

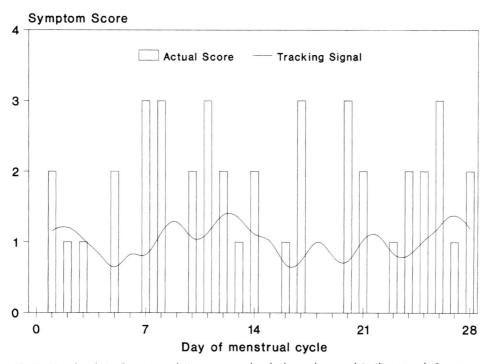

Fig. 2 Trend analysis of symptoms during a menstrual cycle shows absence of significant trends. Symptoms are scored on a scale of 0 to 3 depending on the severity of symptoms. (Adapted from Magós et al. *Am J Obstet Gynecol.* 1986;155:271, with permission.)

then withdrawn and the pellet (or pellets) is loaded into the cannula with forceps. A sterile gallipot is held under the cannula to catch the implant if it should drop out. The pellet is then pushed to the end of the cannula deep within the subcutaneous tissue with the introducer, making sure the hilt of the trochar remains pressed to the skin. The cannula and introducer are then withdrawn and pressure is applied to the wound to prevent bleeding. When hemostasis is achieved a small steristrip is applied to the wound, which is then covered with a dry dressing. The patient is advised to keep the wound dry for at least 24 hours. Complications are rare but include excessive bleeding, which may require the wound to be stitched, and occasional rejection of the implant, probably as a result of infection. In the latter situation it is safe to insert another implant in a different site since a second rejection is extremely uncommon.

Medical Use of Estrogen Implants

The medical use of estrogen implants dates back to 1938[21] when Bishop described their use in the treatment of menopausal symptoms in a 20-year-old girl who had a bilateral oophorectomy for ovarian cysts. Later Greenblatt and Suran[19] described the use of estrogen implants as well as testosterone, progesterone, and deoxycorticosterone implants for the management of a variety of endocrine disorders. In 1969 Emperaire and Greenblatt[22] further extended the indications for estrogen implants when they described their contraceptive efficacy, which they showed was due to suppression of ovulation. They reported that ovulation could be immediately suppressed with a 100-mg implant if it was given early in the menstrual cycle. However, Magos et al.[23] found that in 30% of cases ovarian follicular development, as measured by ultrasound and urinary estrone and pregnandiol concentrations, continued for up to 3 months after insertion of an implant (Fig. 3). In one patient there was both ultrasound and biochemical evidence of follicular rupture and luteinization, which occurred during the second and third cycle after insertion of a 100-mg implant (Fig. 4). Following the initial 100-mg implant the dose of estradiol can be reduced every 6 months to a maintenance dose of 25 mg without any loss of contraceptive efficacy.[24]

This effect on ovulation was further explored by Magos and Studd as a possible treatment for PMS. Initially they treated patients empirically, and have reported the beneficial effects of this approach in a retrospective study.[25] To confirm these initial findings they conducted a double-blind randomized placebo-controlled study.[7]

Sixty-eight patients were entered into the study after the diagnosis of PMS was confirmed by trend analysis of 1 month of daily symptom ratings. Patients were randomized to receive either a 100-mg estradiol implant and 5 mg of norethisterone for 7 days of each cycle or a placebo implant and placebo tablet. During the study the modified Moos menstrual distress questionnaire was completed daily with symptoms rated on a scale of 0 to 3. The 34 symptoms thus obtained were then grouped into 6 adverse symptom clusters (pain, concentration, behavioral change, autonomic reaction, water retention, and negative affect) for analysis, thereby reducing the need for multiple statistical testing. A visual analog scale (VAS) and the general health questionnaire (GHQ) were also completed every 3 months when the women attended the clinic, to assess the women's feelings since their last clinic visit and to screen for any psychiatric morbidity.

The total daily ratings for the pretreatment cycle and every second cycle posttreatment were assessed by trend analysis (Fig. 5), and the VAS and GHQ scores were analyzed by appropriate parametric and nonparametric techniques. The characteristics of the placebo and treatment groups were similar (Table 1). There were no dropouts from the active treatment group, but three women withdrew from the placebo group because they found the treatment had not relieved their symptoms. The adverse symptoms generally improved with both placebo and active treatment, as shown by a fall in mean daily ratings (Fig. 5). However, the benefit from the active implants was sustained and continued to improve with time $(0.0001 < p < 0.05)$, while the initial improvement with placebo implants tended to wane with time and the overall effect never reached significance for any of the Moos MDQ symptom clusters. Comparison of the two treatments showed superiority of the active combination over placebo for all parameters (Table 2). The VAS and GHQ demonstrated similar significant reductions with both treatments but due to the large scatter of data no difference was demonstrable between placebo and active treatment.

Treatment with the implants was well tolerated and side effects were slight and transient. The most common complaints were of mastalgia (estradiol 5, placebo 2), nausea (estradiol 3, placebo 4), weight gain (estradiol 5, placebo 0), and headaches (estradiol 2, placebo 3).

Implants were found to be significantly superior to placebo for treatment of premenstrual symptoms despite an initial placebo response of 94%. The duration

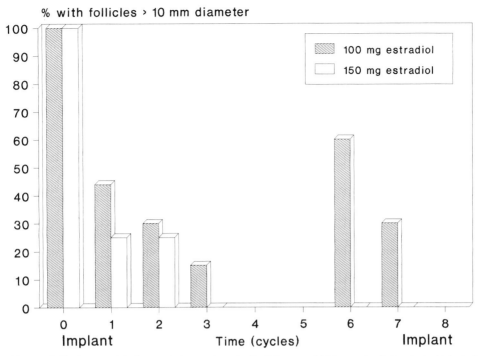

Fig. 3   Follicular growth before and after treatment with 100-mg and 150-mg estradiol implants. (Adapted from Magos et al. *Br J Obstet Gynaecol.* 1987;94:1192, with permission.)

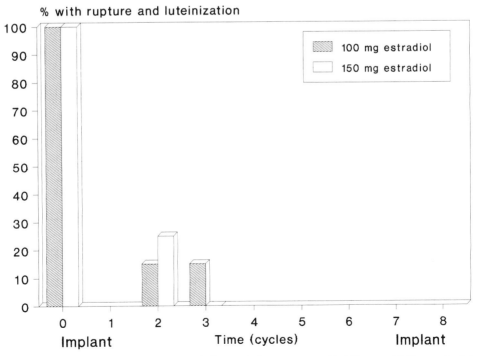

Fig. 4   Follicular rupture and luteinization before and after treatment with 100-mg and 150-mg estradiol implants. (Adapted from Magos et al. *Br J Obstet Gynaecol.* 1987;94:1192, with permission.)

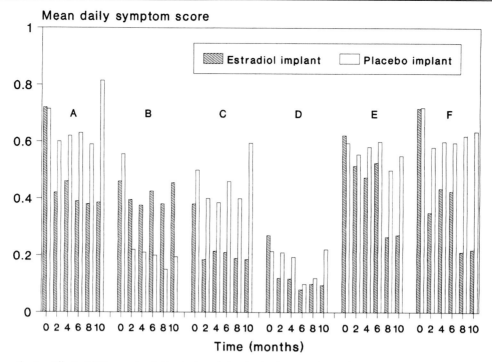

Fig. 5   Effect of 100-mg estradiol implants and placebo implants on the maximum exponentially smoothed symptom scores. (Adapted from Magos et al. *Br Med J.* 1986;292:1629, with permission.)

of this response was variable but returned to pretreatment levels by 6 months and was less marked following administration of further placebo implants. This was not the case with active treatment, as women had a continued further beneficial response to repeated active implants (Fig. 5). The improvement in PMS symptoms in the estradiol-treated group is most likely due to suppression of ovulation. However, the design of the study did not exclude a possible beneficial effect from norethisterone, which was only given to the active implant group. To exclude this possibility, Magos et al in a subsequent study of hysterectomized women treated with estradiol implants showed that norethisterone was associated with a dose-related increase in psychological, behavioral, and physical symptoms.[26]

Transdermal Patches

The estradiol transdermal therapeutic system (TTS) (Estraderm, Ciba-Geigy) is a thin multilayered unit containing a drug reservoir, a rate-controlling membrane, and an adhesive layer. The reservoir contains a high dose of 17-β-estradiol, the main estrogen produced by the ovary (Fig. 6). The rate of delivery of drug is determined by the surface area of the patch. They are commercially available in the United Kingdom in three sizes, 5, 10, and 20 cm², which release 25, 50, and 100

μg of estradiol per day, respectively.[27] Previous studies had shown the patches to be effective in the treatment of menopausal symptoms including hot flushes, sleeping disturbances, irritability, and impaired concentration.[28] We therefore decided to study the effects of estraderm patches initially on ovulation, and then for the treatment of premenstrual syndrome.

Clinical Trials

The initial study was to assess if a dose of two 100-μg estradiol patches changed every 3 days was effective in suppressing ovulation. This dose was selected so as to achieve plasma estradiol levels of greater than 600 pmol/l, which previous studies have shown is the lowest plasma level of estradiol necessary to suppress ovulation. Ten patients with regular 27- to 30-day menstrual cycles were randomly recruited from the Premenstrual Syndrome Clinic at Dulwich Hospital after obtaining informed consent. Patients completed a daily symptom and menstrual chart for the duration of the study. Ovulation was monitored in the patients over four menstrual cycles by alternate day ultrasound and measurement of four plasma progesterone levels taken on day 21 of each 28-day cycle. The first month of the study was without any treatment to confirm that the patients were ovulating normally. From the first day of menstru-

Table 1

Characteristics of Patients before Treatment with Estradiol Implants. Values are Means
(SD in parentheses)

	Estradiol Group		Placebo Group	
Number of patients	33		35	
Age	35.1	(3.5)	35.9	(5.0)
Married	26		24	
Duration of PMS	3.8		3.1	(2.8)
Length of menstrual cycle	27.3	(2.5)	27.6	(2.7)
Duration of symptoms	3.8	(4.4)	3.1	(2.8)
Previous treatment for PMS	30		32	
Weight (kg)	57.9	(6.5)	58.9	(9.1)
Menstrual distress questionnaire:				
Number of symptom clusters with trends	4.5	(1.5)	4.7	(1.5)
ESA (max)	1.15	(0.4)	1.17	(0.5)
ESA (min)	0.14	(0.1)	0.14	(0.1)
Mean daily score	0.56	(0.2)	0.58	(0.3)
100-mm Visual analog scale	84.9	(13.0)	84.2	(14.6)
General health questionnaire:				
Mean score	17.2	(15.0)	15.6	(13.2)
Score > 12	16		19	

Table 2

Changes in Total Menstrual Distress Questionnaire Scores with Treatment. Results Expressed as Mean Difference
between Pretreatment and Posttreatment Scores for Each Symptom[a]

	n	Estradiol Group	n	Placebo Group	R	Z	p
ESA (max)							
0–2	30	0.5312	30	0.300	815	1.47	< 0.2
0–4	23	0.422	25	0.175	510	2.10	< 0.02
0–6	14	0.458	10	−0.023	81	—	< 0.01
0–8	9	0.705	8	0.162	48	—	< 0.01
0–10	9	0.651	5	0.005	19	—	< 0.01
ESA (min)							
0–2	30	0.033	30	−0.036	809	1.56	< 0.2
0–4	23	0.043	25	−0.068	484	2.64	< 0.02
0–6	14	0.047	10	−0.035	95	—	< 0.01
0–8	9	0.092	8	−0.008	57	—	< 0.01
0–10	9	0.103	5	−0.064	24	—	< 0.01
Mean daily score							
0–2	30	0.252	30	0.115	821	1.38	< 0.2
0–4	23	0.206	25	0.035	495	2.41	< 0.02
0–6	14	0.236	10	−0.030	79	—	< 0.01
0–8	9	0.388	8	0.030	47	—	< 0.01
0–10	9	0.378	5	−0.084	18	—	< 0.01

[a]Changes in total MDQ scores with treatment. Wilcoxon's sum of ranks test for between groups comparison of treatment effect. (Reprinted from Magos AL et al. *Br Med J.* 1986;292:1629, with permission.)

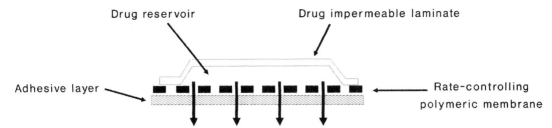

Fig. 6   Cross-sectional view of an Estraderm patch.

ation in their second cycle, patients were treated with two 100-μg estradiol patches, which were changed every 3 days for the remaining 3 months of the study. When the patches were changed, a different site on the buttock or anterior abdominal wall was used to prevent skin irritation.

Follicular growth and luteinization occurred in all 10 women in the pretreatment month and in 1 patient during the first month of treatment as demonstrated by an ultrasound measurement of a follicle over 10 mm in diameter and by progesterone assay of greater than 15 pmol/l (Table 3). Ovarian activity was suppressed in the other patients from the start of treatment and subsequently in all patients for the remaining 2 months of treatment. This study established that two 100-μg TTS patches every 3 days were rapidly effective in suppressing ovulation, when treatment was started on the first day of menstruation.[29] These findings demonstrate a potential for estraderm patches as contraceptives, but they need to be confirmed in a larger study, specifically directed at establishing the duration of their efficacy, especially if patients forget to change their patches.

The next study was undertaken to assess the efficacy of this anovulatory dose of transdermal estrogen for the treatment of PMS. Forty patients with the diagnosis of PMS confirmed with at least 1 month of prospective daily symptom ratings were recruited into a randomized double-blind placebo-controlled study after obtaining informed consent. The use of two 100-μg estradiol patches every 3 days was assessed under double-blind, placebo-controlled conditions over 6 months with a single cross-over at three months. The placebo was identical to the active patches except they did not contain 17-β-estradiol. All patients began treatment on the first day of menstruation and received norethisterone 5 mg from day 19 to 26 after the start of treatment to ensure a regular withdrawal bleed. Daily symptom ratings were recorded by the patients for the duration of the study using the modified Moos MDQ. The GHQ was also completed at the start of the study and again at 3 and 6 months after starting treatment to exclude any patients with psychiatric morbidity, and to assess any potential differences between the two treatments.

Triggs trend analysis of the prospective symptom ratings showed a significant improvement with active treatment for the six negative Moos symptom clusters (Table 4). Initially the improvement occurred for both active and placebo treatments and at 3 months there was no difference between the two groups. However after the crossover at 3 months the symptoms of the placebo-treated group tended to return to baseline,

Table 3
Effects of Transdermal Estradiol Patches on Ovulation[a]

	Pretreatment	First month	Second month	Third month
Number who ovulated	10			
Number who menstruated	10	1	None	4 Spotting
Mean estradiol nmol/l (range)	0.37	0.58	1.1	0.62
	(0.2–0.5)	(0.2–0.9)	(0.2–2.9)	(0.3–0.8)
Mean progesterone nmol/l (range)	30.1	2.6	0.4	0.4
	(13–81)	(0.2–7.4)	(0.1–1.0)	(0.1–0.9)

[a]Progesterone concentration in patient who ovulated was 34 nmol/l. (Reprinted from *Br Med J.* 1988;297:900, with permission.)

Table 4
Changes in Menstrual Distress Symptom Clusters Scores[a]

| | Maximum Exponentially Smoothed Average Scores (ESA max) | | | | | |
| | Group I Active–Placebo (Mean Difference) | | | Group II Placebo–Active (Mean Difference) | | |
	3 Months	6 Months	p	3 Months	6 Months	p
Pain	2.880	0.062	< 0.005	0.868	3.403	< 0.05
Concentration	4.732	0.183	< 0.005	2.416	4.681	NS
Behavioral change	3.249	− 0.77	< 0.001	1.641	3.838	< 0.05
Autonomic reaction	3.201	− 0.55	< 0.001	1.641	3.838	< 0.05
Water retention	4.059	− 1.47	< 0.01	3.889	6.828	< 0.01
Negative affect	4.059	− 1.47	< 0.001	3.889	6.828	< 0.05
Arousal	− 0.49	0.881	NS	0.067	− 0.14	NS
Control	− 0.55	0.583	NS	0.072	− 0.18	NS

[a] 3 and 6 month scores subtracted from pretreatment ESA max scores. A positive score is therefore an improvement. NS, not significant. (Reprinted from *Lancet.* 1989;ii:730, with permission.)

whereas those in the active group continued to improve[8] (Figs. 7–9) Analysis of the GHQ between groups and within groups showed no statistical differences, probably as a result of the wide scatter of data.

The main side effect of treatment is the development of cyclical symptoms similar to PMS in some patients when taking the progestogen (Figs. 10–12). These symptoms are much less severe and occur for a shorter period than their initial presenting symptoms. If they become troublesome they can be reduced by halving the dose or decreasing the duration of norethisterone; changing to a different progestogen is also useful. Occasionally these side effects are sufficiently severe as to justify either a hysterectomy or stopping treatment.[30]

These are side effects of progestogens and not symptoms of untreated PMS, because they are dose related, do not occur if they are omitted for a cycle, and resolve after hysterectomy when cyclical progestogens are no longer necessary. The symptoms caused by these synthetic progestogens are analogous to PMS, suggesting a possible role for progesterone in the etiology of this condition. Magos et al[26] reported these symptoms in hysterectomized patients on estrogen replacement therapy and cyclical progestogens, suggesting it as a model for PMS.

Comparison of Routes of Administration

Percutaneous administration of estrogen either by transdermal patch or pellet implantation has advan-

tages over oral therapy since it avoids first pass liver metabolism. Virtually all estrogen absorbed after oral administration passes through the liver, where up to 60% is metabolized.[31] Percutaneous estrogen passes straight into the systemic circulation, initially avoiding the liver, and only a small and diluted proportion of the absorbed estrogen will pass through and be metabolized by the liver with each circuit around the body. Therefore, when the percutaneous route of administration is used a smaller dose of estrogen can be used to achieve a specific biological effect.

Deleterious effects on liver metabolism occur with all orally administered estrogens. The synthetically derived estrogens ethinyl-estradiol and mestranol used in the oral contraceptive pill produce adverse changes in renin substrate,[32] clotting factors[33,34] and alter the metabolism of carbohydrates[35] and lipids.[36,37] These alterations are believed to contribute to the increased mortality from strokes and myocardial infarction among pill users.[38,39,40] Paradoxically this increase is not seen with long-term estrogen use in hormone replacement therapy, despite an increase of risk factors in this age group.[37] This difference may be due to the increased potency of the synthetic estrogens or a specific side effect of synthetic estrogen. Thom et al[40] reported no alterations in the clotting and fibrinolytic system with natural estrogens, but significant increases in platelet aggregation and plasminogen concentration with ethinyl-estradiol. These findings were in agreement with the earlier work of Notelovitz and Greig[41] who found simi-

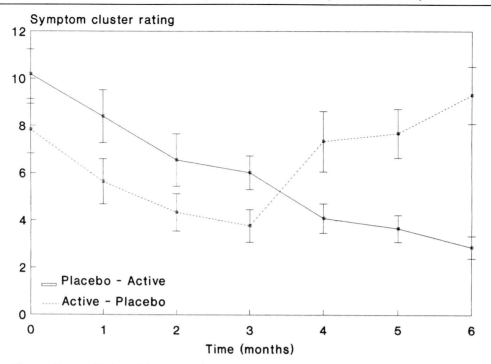

Fig. 7   Change with time of the Menstrual Distress Questionnaire (MDQ) symptom cluster for negative affect.

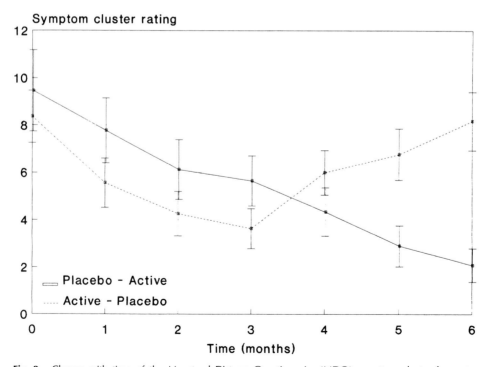

Fig. 8   Change with time of the Menstrual Distress Questionnaire (MDQ) symptom cluster for water retention.

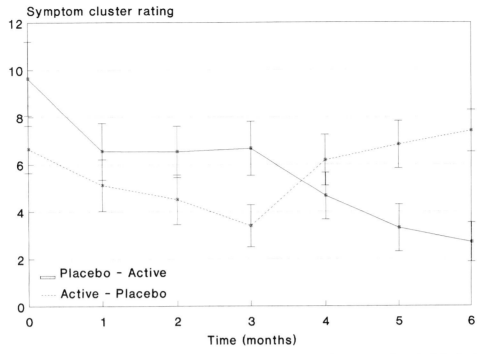

Fig. 9 Change with time of the Menstrual Distress Questionnaire (MDQ) symptom cluster for behavioral change.

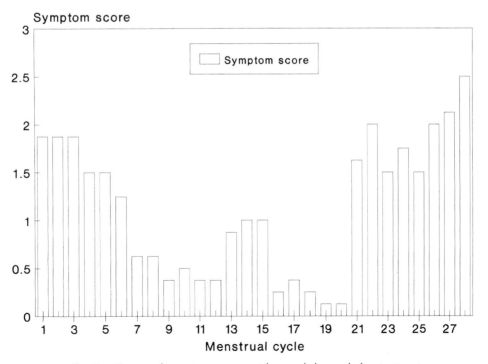

Fig. 10 One-month symptom assessment for mood changes before treatment.

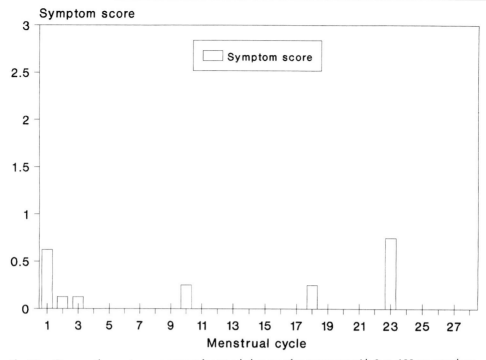

Fig. 11   One-month symptom assessment for mood changes after treatment with 2 × 100 μg estraderm patch.

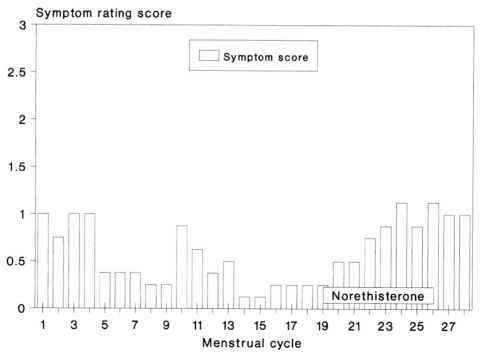

Fig. 12   One-month symptom assessment for mood changes after treatment with 2 × 100 μg estraderm patch and 5 mg norethisterone for 7 days.

lar differences between natural and synthetic estrogens. The Boston Collaborative study[42] found no increase in the incidence of thrombotic episodes in women taking hormone replacement therapy (HRT), although Gow and MacGillivray[43] reported a 16% incidence of thrombosis in menopausal women treated with the synthetic estrogen mestranol. This effect on clotting factors in women using oral contraceptives appears to be related to the estrogen dose.[44] The type of heart disease in women using the pill may well be thrombotic in nature, whereas in menopausal women the disease process is more likely to be atherogenic. The safest route of administration in premenopausal women is therefore likely to be by the percutaneous route, as this minimizes any potential thrombotic effects.

Side effects of the Estraderm patches include an exacerbation of symptoms in a small proportion of patients during the initial week of therapy, which is normally when PMS symptoms would be expected to improve. It is sufficiently common for us to warn patients before treatment and stress the need to persevere for at least 1 month. The rapid rise in estradiol levels that occurs with patches could explain these findings and supports the hypothesis that change in the levels of gonadal hormones is the precipitating cause of premenstrual symptoms. This effect has not been reported with estradiol implants, from which the absorption of estradiol is more gradual. However this may also be due to not evaluating patients on implants during this phase of treatment; Magos et al[7] in their implant study first assessed the symptoms in the second month after implantation when symptoms were unlikely to be present.

With patches, 10% of women developed skin irritation severe enough to stop treatment, although less severe symptoms were more common.[8] The incidence of irritation in patients using patches for HRT is slightly lower[45] but in these studies they were only using one patch. The problems of irritation may often be reduced by advising patients to move the patch each day and by leaving the adhesive side of the patch uncovered for a few minutes before application to allow the surface alcohol to dissipate. The current development of newer smaller patches that use different flux enhancers is likely to reduce these problems.

The absorption from the patch is less constant than from the subcutaneous implant,[46] which would explain our clinical observation that in the long-term, patients are generally better with implants. However, the implants have a prolonged duration of action requiring a degree of commitment from patients and their doctors, which makes them only suitable for long-term treatment of PMS. We have shown that they continue to be effective in the long-term, but the incidence of progestogenic symptoms is high. In 50 patients treated for 2 or more years, 5 required a hysterectomy for progestogenic symptoms and 2 for menorrhagia due to prolonged estrogen stimulation causing myometrial hypertrophy.[29]

Implants have recently been reported to lead to tachyphlaxis when used for postmenopausal estrogen replacement therapy. Patients with tachyphlaxis develop symptoms of estrogen deficiency despite high plasma estradiol levels, and they return for repeat implants at decreasing intervals.[47] Tachyphlaxis is very uncommon in our experience. Of 1388 patients regularly treated with estradiol implants, 38 had an estradiol level of greater than 1750 pmol/l when they returned with a recurrence of symptoms. Fifteen of these patients had been treated for PMS for a mean of 5.5 years, and of these 9 had been diagnosed as suffering from depression, unresponsive to antidepressants prior to starting on implants. It appears from these figures that tachyphlaxis occurs most commonly in women with a previous psychiatric history and that a similar pattern is seen in those women treated for menopausal symptoms.[48] It is our experience that a pharmacological dose of estrogen has a tonic effect on mood, which may allow some patients to safely stop any antidepressants or tranquillizers that they are taking prior to treatment.[49]

SUMMARY

Oral contraceptives have a potential role in treating PMS in younger women, but there are few properly controlled placebo studies.[50] In addition, most women present with PMS after age 30, when there is an increased risk of cardiovascular disease with oral contraceptive use. Percutaneous estrogens as used for the treatment of the menopause are a more logical approach. The estraderm patch is ideal for a woman who has not completed her family or in the patient apprehensive of estrogen treatment, since therapy can be readily discontinued. The erratic absorption and skin irritation that occurs with the current patch may be reduced with the new smaller patches under investigation. Progestogen-containing patches may reduce the incidence of progestogenic side effects that occur with oral therapy.

The only report of long-term treatment of PMS has been with subcutaneous estradiol implants, which continued to be effective for at least 5 years after first administered.[29] It is an effective contraceptive, ideal for the older woman who needs birth control at an age when oral contraceptives are unacceptable.

REFERENCES

1. Frank RT. The hormonal basis of premenstrual tension. *Arch Neurol Psychiat.* 1931;26:1053.

2. Dalton K. *The Premenstrual Syndrome and Progesterone Therapy.* London: Heinemann; 1977.

3. Maddocks S, Hahn P, Moller F, et al. A double-blind placebo-controlled trial of progesterone vaginal suppositories in the treatment of premenstrual syndrome. *Am J Obstet Gynecol.* 1986; 154:573.

4. Andersch B, Hahn L. Progesterone treatment of premenstrual tension—a double-blind study. *J Psychosom Res.* 1985;29:489.

5. Studd JWW. Premenstrual tension syndrome. *Br Med J.* 1979;1: 410.

6. Backstrom T, Boyle H, Baird DT. Persistence of symptoms of premenstrual tension in hysterectomised women. *Br J Obstet Gynaecol.* 1981;88:530.

7. Magos AL, Brincat M, Studd JWW. Treatment of the premenstrual syndrome by subcutaneous oestradiol implants and cyclical norethisterone in the treatment of premenstrual syndrome. *Br Med J.* 1986;292:1629.

8. Watson NR, Studd JWW, Savvas M, et al. Treatment of severe premenstrual syndrome with oestradiol patches and cyclical oral norethisterone. *Lancet.* 1989;ii:730.

9. Muse KN, Cetel NS, Futterman LA, et al. The premenstrual syndrome: effects of "medical ovariectomy." *N Engl J Med.* 1984; 311:1345.

10. Watts JF, Butt RW, Logan Edwards R. A clinical trial using danazol for the treatment of premenstrual tension. *Br J Obstet Gynaecol.* 1987;94:30.

11. Magos AL. Premenstrual syndrome. *Contemp Rev Obstet Gynaecol.* 1988;1:80.

12. Moos RH. The development of a menstrual distress questionnaire. *Psychosom Med.* 1968;30:853.

13. Magos AL, Studd JWW. Assessment of menstrual cycle symptoms by trend analysis. *Am J Obstet Gynecol.* 1986;155:271.

14. Goldzieher J, Moses LE, Ellis L. Study of norethindrone in contraception. *JAMA.* 1962;180:359.

15. Graham CA, Sherwin BB. The relationship between retrospective premenstrual symptom reporting and present oral contraceptive use. *J Psychosom Res.* 1987;31:45.

16. Cullberg J. Mood changes and menstrual symptoms with different gestagen/estrogen combinations. A double-blind comparison with placebo. *Acta Psychiatr Scand.* 1972; 236(suppl):1.

17. Loudon NB, Foxwell M, Potts DM, et al. Acceptability of an oral contraceptive that reduces the frequency of menstruation: the tri-cycle regimen. *Br Med J.* 1977;2:487.

18. Watson NR, Studd JWW. Management of the menopause. *Clin Endocrinol.* (in press).

19. Greenblatt RD, Suran RR. Indications for hormone pellets in the therapy of endocrine and gynecological disorders. *Am J Obstet Gynecol.* 1949;57:294.

20. Thom MH, Studd JWW. Procedures in practice—hormone implantation. *Br Med J.* 1980;1:848.

21. Bishop PMF. A clinical experiment in oestrin therapy. *Br Med J.* 1938;1:939.

22. Emperaire JC, Greenblatt RB. L'implantation de pellets d'oestradiol dans la contraception. *Gynecol Pract.* 1969;20:327.

23. Magos AL, Collins WP, Studd JWW. Effects of subcutaneous oestradiol implants on ovarian activity. *Br J Obstet Gynaecol.* 1987;94:1192.

24. Greenblatt RD, Asch RH, Mahesh VB, et al. Implantation of pure crystalline pellets of estradiol for contraception control. *Am J Obstet Gynecol.* 1977;127:520.

25. Magos AL, Collins WP, Studd JWW. Management of the premenstrual syndrome by subcutaneous implants of oestradiol. *J Psychosom Obstet Gynaecol.* 1984;3:93.

26. Magos AL, Brewester E, Singh R, et al. The effects of norethisterone in postmenopausal women on oestrogen replacement therapy: a model for the premenstrual syndrome. *Br J Obstet Gynaecol.* 1986;93:1290.

27. Sitruk-Ware R. Transdermal delivery of steroids. *Contraception.* 1989;39:1.

28. Laufer LR, De Fazio LJ, Lu JKH, et al. Estrogen replacement therapy by transdermal estradiol administration. *Am J Obstet Gynecol.* 1983;146:533.

29. Watson NR, Studd JWW, Riddle AF, et al. Suppression of ovulation by transdermal oestradiol patches. *Br Med J.* 1988;297:900.

30. Watson NR, Studd JWW, Savvas M, et al. The long-term effects of estradiol implant therapy for the treatment of premenstrual syndrome. *Gynecol Endo.* 1990;4:99.

31. Leivertz RW. Pharmacology and pharmacokinetics of estrogens. *Am J Obstet Gynecol.* 1987;156:1289.

32. Mandel FP, Geola FL, Lu JKH. Biological effects of various doses of ethinyl-estradiol in postmenopausal women. *Obstet Gynecol.* 1982;59:673.

33. Meade TW. Oral contraceptives, clotting factors and thrombosis. *Am J Obstet Gynecol.* 1982;142:758.

34. Poller L, Thomson JM, Thomson W. Oestrogen/progestogen oral contraceptive and blood clotting: a long-term follow-up. *Br Med J.* 1971;4:648.

35. Wynn V, Doar JWH. Some effects of oral contraceptives on carbohydrate metabolism. *Lancet.* 1966;ii:715.

36. Burkman RT, Robinson JC, Kruszon-Morgan D, et al. Lipid and lipoprotein changes associated with oral contraceptive use: a randomized clinical trial. *Obstet Gynecol.* 1988;71:33.

37. Bradley DD, Wingard J, Pettiti DB, et al. Serum high-density lipoprotein cholesterol in women using oral contraceptives, estrogens and progestins. *N Engl J Med.* 1978;299:17.

38. Stadel BV. Oral contraceptives and cardiovascular disease (Part 2). *N Engl J Med.* 1981;305:672.

39. Vessey MP, Mann JI. Female sex hormones and thrombosis. *Br Med Bull.* 1978;34:157.

40. Thom M, Dubiel M, Kakkar VV, et al. The effect of different regimens of oestrogen on the clotting and fibrinolytic system of the postmenopausal woman. *Front Horm Res.* 1978;5:192.

41. Notelovitz M, Greig HBW. Natural estrogen and anti-thrombin III activity in postmenopausal women. *J Reprod Med.* 1976;16:87.

42. Boston Collaborative Drug Surveillance Programme. Oral contraceptives and venous thromboembolic disease, surgically confirmed gall-bladder disease and breast tumors. *Lancet.* 1973;i:1399.

43. Gow S, MacGillivray I. Metabolic, hormonal, and vascular changes after synthetic oestrogen therapy in oophorectomised women. *Br Med J.* 1971;2:73.

44. Böttiger LE, Boman G, Eklund G, et al. Oral contraceptives and thromboembolic disease: effect of lowering oestrogen content. *Lancet.* 1980;i:1097.

45. Utian WH. Transdermal estradiol overall safety profile. *Am J Obstet Gynecol.* 1987;156:1335.

46. Stanczyk FZ, Shoupe D, Nunez V, et al. A randomized comparison of nonoral estradiol delivery in postmenopausal women. *Am J Obstet Gynecol.* 1988;159:1540.

47. Ganger K, Cust M, Whitehead Ml. Symptoms of oestrogen deficiency associated with supraphysiological plasma oestradiol concentrations in women with oestradiol implants. *Br Med J*. 1989; 299:601.

48. Garnet T, Studd JWW, Henderson A, et al. Hormone implants and tachyphylaxis. *Br J Obstet Gynaecol*. 1990;97:917.

49. Studd JWW, Watson NR. Oestrogens and depression. In: Belfort P, Pinotti JA, Eskes TKAB, eds. *Advances in Gynecology and Obstetrics*. Vol 6. The Proceedings of the XIIth World Congress of Gynecology and Obstetrics, Rio de Janerio, October 1988;297.

50. Graham CA, Sherwin BB. A prospective treatment study of premenstrual symptoms using a triphasic oral contraceptive. *J Psychosom Res*. 1992;36:257.

CHAPTER 14

Progesterone Therapy for Premenstrual Syndrome

Ellen W. Freeman

Although progesterone suppository therapy is the most widely used treatment for premenstrual syndrome (PMS), controlled studies of its effectiveness have failed to demonstrate that it is better than a placebo. With the recent production of micronized progesterone for oral administration, and the consistent lack of effectiveness reported for progesterone suppositories, proponents of progesterone treatment for PMS have shifted from suppository to oral administration as the treatment of choice. It is clear that administration of oral progesterone can produce high plasma levels of progesterone, and it is theoretically possible that bioavailability of its metabolites may differ with the mode of administration, thereby altering symptom response. However, the present evidence from placebo-controlled studies of the effectiveness of oral progesterone in reducing symptoms of PMS is insufficient, although studies in progress may develop a clearer picture.

This chapter reviews the rationale for and clinical trials of progesterone in PMS treatment, focusing on information from placebo-controlled studies. The final sections evaluate the current status and unanswered questions engendered by the dominant role that progesterone therapy has played in PMS treatment.

THE HORMONE PROGESTERONE

Progesterone is a C-21 steroid hormone, secreted from the ovaries with a small contribution from the adrenal. Natural progesterone is synthesized and commercially available in the United States for pharmacologic use.

Progesterone has a normal cyclicity in the menstrual cycle. Reproductive-age women have a progesterone production of 2 to 3 mg/day in the follicular phase, increasing to 20 to 30 mg/day in the luteal phase. Plasma levels of progesterone in the follicular phase are less than 1 ng/ml, increasing to 5 to 10 ng/ml in the luteal phase. A plasma level of progesterone over 3 ng/ml is reliable evidence of ovulation.[1]

During pregnancy, increasing amounts of progesterone are produced, first by the corpus luteum and, after the twelfth week of pregnancy, by the placenta. At term, plasma levels of progesterone range from 100 to 400 ng/ml, a huge increase from nonpregnant levels.

Progesterone binds to its specific receptors to induce its progestational effects. It also interferes with the activity of other hormones through competitive inhibition of enzyme binding sites, exhibiting antiestrogenic and antiandrogenic activity and antimineralocorticoid effects.

The primary functions of progesterone are to promote development of the endometrium and the maintenance of pregnancy. Progesterone inhibits gonadotropin secretion from the anterior pituitary, stimulates breast alveolar development, limits uterine contractility during pregnancy, and promotes sodium and water excretion. An immunosuppressant role has been suggested for progesterone.[2] Progesterone has a role in parturition, although little is known about the specific functions of the greatly increased levels of steroids produced throughout pregnancy.[1]

Progesterone has a rapid effect (in milliseconds) on nerve cell membrane activity in the brain, with specific effects depending on the cell or organ system examined.[3] Metabolites of progesterone have hypnotic and sedative properties.[4,5] Four of the six metabolites known to have hypnotic or sedative effects in animals were identified in postmenopausal women following administration of 400 mg of oral progesterone.[6]

Routes of Administration

Until recently, the clinical use of natural progesterone was circumscribed by its short half-life and rapid inactivation by the liver following oral ingestion. However, with the development of micronized progesterone, it appeared that significant absorption and endometrial effects followed oral administration,[7–12] and that absorption could be further improved by both the particle size and the vehicle of administration.[13]

Luteal phase plasma progesterone concentrations are easily reached with vaginal, rectal, oral, and sublingual routes of administration of progesterone, with peak levels attained in 1 to 5 hours depending on dose and mode of administration.[11] However, the rate of progesterone absorption appeared quite variable in the same subjects and also between different subjects using the same dose of progesterone and the same or different routes of administration.[11] In another dose–response study of progesterone in normal cycling females, luteal phase levels of plasma progesterone were readily achieved, but term pregnancy levels (ie, > 100 ng/ml) were not attained until a dosage of 1200 mg oral progesterone was administered, and then only in some subjects.[14] Again, the rate of absorption was quite variable in the same subjects as well as between subjects on the same dose of progesterone. A "plateau" effect in progesterone absorption has been suggested. Following a 400-mg suppository dose, smaller increments in plasma

progesterone were observed compared to a 200-mg dose,[15] and others reported similar results in plasma progesterone levels with repeated administration of 200- and 400-mg progesterone suppositories in cycling women.[16,17] An unexpected result of suppression of luteal estradiol production suggested that administration of progesterone suppresses endogenous production of progesterone, although how natural progesterone might interfere with luteal function is unclear.[15]

Synthetic Progestins

The short half-life and rapid inactivation of progesterone with oral administration limited its clinical usefulness and led to the development of the progestins. These synthesized, closely related progesterone compounds are widely available in the contraceptive formulations and a number of other gynecologic medications. They have the same basic chemical composition as progesterone, but have differences in radicals and shape of the benzene rings that alter transport and binding properties.

There are numerous identified characteristics of the progestins that are important in specific therapies, but they also have unwanted side effects and hold risks of birth defects for the fetus. Dalton argued that progestins have no place in PMS treatment because they are not equivalents of natural progesterone,[18] but the small placebo-controlled studies that have been conducted[19–21] found results similar to those for natural progesterone, that is, an overall beneficial effect of treatment but no significant differences between the progestin (dydrogesterone) and placebo.

RATIONALE FOR PROGESTERONE THERAPY

That the ovarian hormones whose levels normally fluctuate over the menstrual cycle should be the source of PMS has been an unproven hypothesis for many years. Since progesterone has the greatest concentration in the luteal phase, a deficiency in progesterone levels was postulated as the cause for luteal phase problems and symptoms,[22,23] with progesterone administration advocated to correct the deficiency.

However, measurements of progesterone levels in women with PMS failed to find consistently low levels of progesterone. A recent study measured progesterone daily for 2 months in 18 women with PMS and found that high luteal phase plasma progesterone levels positively correlated with severity of PMS.[24] Moreover, the attempt to link the negative affective symptoms of PMS with declining progesterone levels in the second half of the luteal phase contradicts observations that the symptoms frequently begin to appear in the early luteal phase when progesterone is increasing to its peak level.

Further contradictions to the progesterone deficiency hypothesis are findings that some physical symptoms appeared to worsen with progesterone treatment, thereby implicating progesterone as a cause of some negative mood changes and physical symptoms associated with PMS.[25,26] Worsening symptoms were also observed with the addition of progestins to estrogen therapy for PMS[27] and to postmenopausal replacement therapy.[28]

A reduced progesterone-estrogen ratio (low progesterone and raised estradiol levels) was argued as the rationale for progesterone therapy in the influential publications of Dalton.[18] Some evidence for reduced progesterone ratios in the midluteal phase in women with PMS was found,[29,30] but whether this is an etiologic factor in PMS requires further confirmation, especially in view of the pulsatile release of progesterone and the complexity of their interactions with other hormones. Dalton more recently argued that the etiology of PMS lies not in the total but in the free hormonal levels, and that it may lie "anywhere along the pathways from the cerebral cortex, along the hypothalamic-pituitary-ovarian axis to the progesterone receptors in the tissue cells, but it appears that the progesterone transport mechanism Sex Hormone Globulin Binding (SHGB) is involved in all cases of severe premenstrual syndrome."[18]

Sedative-Hypnotic Effects

Large doses of progesterone would be expected to produce pharmacologic effects related to its central activity in brain function. It was suggested that since progesterone had a direct sedative effect on the central nervous system,[31] progesterone therapy might relieve the irritability and aggressiveness that are characteristic of PMS.

Progesterone in high doses has long been known to have sedative-hypnotic effects in animals.[4] Intravenous administration of 250 to 500 mg progesterone in women induced sleep.[32] Although vaginal suppository treatment of PMS has not been reported as sedating, clinical reports of oral micronized progesterone in treatment of PMS,[33] premature labor,[34] postmenopausal replacement therapy,[8] and in pharmacokinetic studies[10] all reported drowsiness as a side effect.

Recently, 3-alpha-hydroxy-5-alpha-pregnane-20-one, a metabolite of progesterone, and the analogous 3-alpha-5-alpha reduced metabolite of deoxycorticosterone (DOC) were reported as potent enhancers of γ-aminobutyric acid (GABA) transmission by binding to the GABA receptor complex at or near the barbiturate binding site.[35] Direct application of progesterone to rat brain preparations significantly enhanced GABAergic transmission.[36] Since the enzymes necessary for the reduction reaction are present in brain, gut, and liver, and DOC is itself a metabolite of progesterone after oral administration,[9] oral administration of progesterone could lead to significant elevation of progesterone, DOC, and their 3-alpha and 5-alpha reduced metabolites in blood and the central nervous system. Potentiation of GABAergic transmission by these metabolites could account for the reported relative sedative properties of progesterone. Alternatively, progesterone's effects on premenstrual symptoms might be due to other hormonal effects on the hypothalamic–pituitary–ovarian axis.

CLINICAL EVALUATION OF PROGESTERONE THERAPY

In recent years, a number of placebo-controlled studies of progesterone therapy for PMS have been conducted, with none showing more effectiveness for progesterone suppository treatment than for placebo.

Progesterone Suppository

In the largest study of progesterone suppository treatment ($n = 168$ randomized to treatment in a double-blind crossover design),[37] premenstrual symptoms were not significantly improved by progesterone compared with placebo in any measure used in the study, including daily symptom reports maintained throughout treatment, clinician evaluation of improvement, and patient global reports of symptom severity, relief, and disruption of daily activity. No symptom cluster or individual symptom differed significantly between progesterone and placebo treatment.

Since previous criticisms of progesterone studies indicated that dosage was inadequate, doses of 400 mg and 800 mg progesterone were used in the first and second months of treatment, respectively. Symptoms significantly decreased when the same treatment (either placebo or progesterone) was administered for the second month at an increased level of two suppositories. However, these decreases occurred for both progesterone and placebo and therefore were not due to additional active medication. Although parity was cited as affecting the dosage required,[18] there was no measurable effect of parity on treatment response.

Increasing progesterone dose beyond 800 mg did not seem to be warranted based on the evidence that increments of serum progesterone were already minimal with vaginal doses of 400 mg.[16] In an earlier study, we found that serum progesterone levels, measured before and after administration of 400-mg progesterone suppositories in a subgroup of study participants, were consistent with those in other reports,[15,38] but had a highly significant negative correlation between the duration of treatment and the increase in serum progesterone level from baseline (the longer the treatment, the less the increase). All subjects studied absorbed the progesterone and had basal progesterone levels compatible with a functioning corpus luteum.[16] Others similarly suggested a threshold effect in the concentrations of progesterone produced by progesterone suppository administration.[15,17]

Although a number of medical history and background variables were significantly related to the severity of PMS, none had a significant effect on treatment response when examined as covariates of progesterone treatment.[37] These included most notably the fluctuations in response during the washout period and the level of postmenstrual symptoms (complete absence compared with low or minimal postmenstrual symptoms). Other factors that were significantly related to the severity of PMS but had no relationship with progesterone treatment response included pretreatment depression (assessed at the postmenstrual time), pretreatment anxiety (assessed at the premenstrual time), physical symptom levels (assessed at washout baseline), dysmenorrhea, and parity.[37]

Other background, medical, psychological, and historical variables that were examined in the study had no significant effects on either severity of PMS or treatment response.[37] These included duration of symptoms, age at first symptoms, daily stress rating, history of major depressive disorder, age, marital status, employment, education, race, height:weight ratio, mother with PMS, family history of mental illness, and family history of alcoholism.

The number of women who completed the study ($n = 121$) provided statistical power of 95% to detect a 15% improvement over placebo in PMS symptoms.[37] These results indicated that it is unlikely that progesterone suppository therapy has a clinically significant therapeutic effect for relief of total symptoms or any single symptom of PMS as defined in this study.

Another recent study compared progesterone, placebo, and behavioral psychotherapy in a 6-month parallel design, with subjects randomly assigned to one of the three treatments and the progesterone and placebo treatments double-blinded.[39] Progesterone dosage was 200 mg suppository b.i.d. At the 3- and 6-month assessments, approximately half the subjects showed some improvement in total premenstrual symptom scores recorded in daily diaries, but there were no significant differences between treatments.

Other indicators in the study also failed to support treatment effectiveness.[39] Overall, compliance was poor, with only 36% of the women continuing treatment for 6 months. Progesterone was less tolerated than placebo, with more subjects dropping out of treatment earlier and fewer wanting to continue after 6 months. Forty-eight percent of the subjects taking placebo wanted to continue placebo after 6 months, compared to only 20% of subjects taking progesterone ($p < .03$). However, women taking placebo reported more side effects, including menstrual cycle changes. Neither progesterone nor the behavior therapy as administered in this protocol appeared better than placebo treatment.

The results of these recent studies were consistent with all previous controlled studies of vaginal or rectal administration of progesterone.[17,25,26,40–42] Maddocks et al administered 200-mg progesterone vaginal suppositories b.i.d. to 20 women for three cycles each of progesterone and placebo.[17] Symptom reports completed by the subjects every 3 days showed no significant differences between progesterone and placebo treatment. This study also investigated progesterone content and absorption, comparing the polyethylene glycol base used in the study with two other free fatty acid bases. Progesterone suppositories with a polyethylene glycol base had the highest peak concentration in serum progesterone (14.6 ± 1.9 ng/ml at 12 hours) and maintained the highest levels of serum progesterone from 6 to 24 hours after suppository administration, although there was little difference in progesterone levels before 6 hours.

Richter et al administered 400-mg progesterone suppositories to 22 women in a crossover design of 4 months duration with random assignment to four treatment sequences.[26] There was no significant difference in the subjects' reports of relief compared between progesterone and placebo. The subjects' monthly relief ratings, daily symptom reports, and overall ranking of the four treated cycles all showed the same results. Of interest in this study was the suggestion that those with higher symptom scores were more likely to report relief with progesterone therapy, while those who preferred the placebo cycles experienced worsening of symptoms with progesterone treatment. It appeared that women with high premenstrual scores for symptoms of irritability, depression, and increased appetite were the most likely to have relief with progesterone therapy.

Andersch and Hahn administered 100-mg progesterone suppositories b.i.d. in the luteal phase to 15 women with moderate to severe premenstrual symptoms in a double-blind crossover trial of 2 months.[40] The women significantly improved with progesterone and placebo, with no significant difference between the two treatments.[40] Vandermeer et al used 200-mg progesterone suppositories b.i.d. in the luteal phase, administered rectally, in a crossover trial of 4 months.[41] There was no significant difference between progesterone and placebo treatment in the psychological, somatic, or total symptoms recorded daily by the patients.[41] Hormonal measures on the first day of menses showed that plasma progesterone levels were high (39 ± p nmol/1) and significantly greater during progesterone-treated than placebo-treated cycles. Sampson conducted two crossover trials of progesterone suppositories of 2 months each during the luteal phase, one using 200 mg progesterone and one using 400 mg progesterone.[25] This study also showed no significant difference between progesterone and placebo in either daily symptom reports or retrospective assessment by the subjects. There was some evidence that progesterone induced physical symptoms at the 400-mg dose.[25]

Intramuscular Progesterone

Smith administered 50 mg progesterone intermuscularly every other day from day 19 to 28 of the cycle and compared four treatment regimens: progesterone, progesterone plus spironolactone, spironolactone, and placebo. Of 14 subjects, three did better with progesterone, three were worse with progesterone, and eight showed no differences between progesterone and placebo.[42] Plasma levels of progesterone, measured throughout treatment, were unrelated to therapeutic benefit or lack of it.

Oral Progesterone

The only controlled trial to suggest benefit of progesterone compared to placebo was that of Dennerstein et al who treated 23 women in a 4-month crossover trial using micronized progesterone administered orally— 100 mg AM, 200 mg PM for the last 10 days of the cycle.[33] Statistically significant differences in favor of progesterone were reported for 2 of 10 symptoms charted daily (swelling of the abdomen, arms, legs, and hot flushes) and for 2 of 8 Moos menstrual distress questionnaire symptom clusters, water retention and a control factor. These few differences led to speculation that the oral administration of progesterone may be effective in reduction of PMS symptoms, but it is important to underscore that most of the assessed symptoms were not improved and there was no overall difference between the two treatments.

Progestins in PMS Therapy

The progestin dydrogesterone (6-dehydro-retroprogesterone) was evaluated in placebo-controlled, double-blind crossover trials in PMS treatment.[19,20] Both were 4-month studies and administered dydrogesterone 10 mg b.i.d. for 14 days on cycle days 12 to 26. Both studies found an overall beneficial effect of treatment but no significant differences between dydrogesterone and placebo. Sampson et al. also found that dydrogesterone-treated patients had an increase in frequency of breast tenderness, menstrual cycle changes, headache, and nausea, but showed a decrease in the severity and number of days of menstrual pain, a known effect of dydrogesterone.[19]

A third study evaluated dydrogesterone in a single-blind placebo-controlled crossover design.[21] The 6-month study administered dydrogesterone 10 mg b.i.d. for 14 days on cycle days 12 to 26. The results of clinician assessment showed that 72% of the subjects improved, but only 21% improved only on dydrogesterone; 24% improved on placebo and maintained on dydrogesterone, 12% improved on dydrogesterone and maintained on placebo, and 15% improved on all treatment cycles. Side effects were increased breast tenderness and menstrual cycle changes. Of interest is that dydrogesterone treatment lowered plasma progesterone levels by about 17% ($p < .01$), and that subjects reported improvement rather than worsening of their symptoms, thereby contradicting the progesterone deficiency theory as the cause of PMS.

Other studies examined dydrogesterone in open trials and reported improvement for PMS symptoms.[43,44] The possibility that suppressed rather than augmented progesterone levels are associated with symptom reduction was also suggested in a report of estradiol implant therapy for PMS, where 45% of the subjects experienced return of PMS symptoms when the progestin (norethisterone, 5 mg) was administered for 7 to 10 days each month.[27] Similar results were found in postmenopausal replacement therapy when symptoms occurred with the progestin (lynestrenol, 5 mg) administered to induce withdrawal bleeding.[28]

Other progestins were examined in PMS treatment and none found the progestin better than placebo, although studies were small and some were in combination with other hormones and/or medications. The placebo-controlled studies include medroxyprogesterone acetate (Provera), 2.5 mg t.i.d. for 10 days before menses,[45] ethisterone, 25 mg b.i.d. and dimethisterone, 5 mg t.i.d. for 9 days before menses,[46] norethisterone, 5 mg b.i.d. for 10 days[47] and 7.5 mg for 10 days.[48] In the study of Appleby et al,[46] it is noteworthy that not only was the progestin little better than placebo, but much less effective than either chlorothiazide or meprobamate in reducing PMS symptoms. Furthermore, although all the women had four treatments, few responded to more than one, suggesting the efficacy of active medication for specific symptom clusters of PMS.

A randomized, placebo-controlled double-blind study in which cyclical oral norethisterone was used to ensure regular withdrawal bleeding in conjunction with estradiol patches (2 × 100 µg) to suppress ovulation[49] found significant improvement in 5 of 6 symptom clusters (Moos menstrual distress questionnaire) and 6 of 10 symptoms assessed daily in the last 3 months following the crossover of medications. In the first 3 study months, there was no significant difference between active medication and placebo. The only reported side effects were skin irritations that resulted from the patches. Although the primary mode of action in this study was estradiol to suppress ovulation and not the progestin, it is significant that symptoms abated with the clear suppression of ovulation and that symptoms were not reported during the administration of the progestin. However, unexpected symptoms of PMS appeared during early therapy in the weeks following menses, suggesting that fluctuating estrogen levels also have a role in PMS symptoms.

Side Effects of Progesterone

The side effects of progesterone appear to be minimal on the basis of information from treatment effectiveness studies and clinical experience. The minor side effects cited by Dalton,[18] who reported the longest use of progesterone therapy, were those associated with the mode of administration (vaginal or anal soreness, diarrhea or flatulence associated with suppositories, soreness or abscess at the needle site with injections) and alterations in menstrual cycle length that can be corrected by the timing of the progesterone dose.

None of the studies of progesterone therapy reported serious adverse effects for the doses and length of time studied. Side effects experienced in the largest controlled study of progesterone suppository treatment were predominantly menstrual changes, bloating and weight gain, breast tenderness, and vaginal/rectal irritation or rash.[37] Notably, however, side effects did not significantly differ between progesterone and placebo treatments, including the most frequent side effect of menstrual changes, which were reported by more women during placebo-treated cycles.

There are no long-term clinical studies of the safety of natural progesterone administered as treatment for PMS, and therefore there is no FDA approval for this use. On the other hand, it is the most widely prescribed medication for PMS, and Dalton has found no serious side effects and no carcinogenic effects associated with natural progesterone. She has prescribed progesterone therapy for more than 40 years and reported monitoring 19 women who had continuous progesterone therapy for over 15 years, and 120 women who had continuous progesterone therapy for 5 years.[18] No side effects of natural progesterone have been reported in regard to lipids profile, coagulation factors, and blood pressure in studies of oral micronized progesterone administered daily in hormonal replacement therapy.[50]

Criticisms of Clinical Trials of Progesterone Therapy

Proponents of progesterone therapy argued that failure to respond indicated either an incorrect diagnosis or incorrect dosage.[18] They contended that results of clinical trials were inconclusive, since small samples may not allow detection of statistically significant effects. Dosage regimens were too low, too late, or unadjusted for parity, and there was lack of quality control in progesterone suppositories.[51,52] Other criticisms were that study patients were not representative of women with PMS, particularly in terms of possible predisposing factors such as depression or their motivation for treatment in a study protocol. More recently, sustaining factors of PMS were cited as having insufficient attention in progesterone effectiveness studies, as, for example, the postulated need to maintain a steady blood sugar level to enable progesterone receptors to utilize progesterone.[52]

The accumulating evidence belies the arguments. It is clear that many women significantly improved with progesterone therapy, but factors other than progesterone alone contributed to the symptom reduction. Numerous factors examined as covariates of treatment showed no effects on treatment outcome.[37] Progesterone suppositories in dosages up to 800 mg daily during the luteal phase of the cycle did not appear to have an effect significantly greater than a placebo, even in a sample size sufficient to detect a 15% difference between progesterone and placebo with 95% power.[37] This suggests that any effect of progesterone administered in the luteal phase is too small to be clinically relevant for women meeting the current criteria for a PMS diagnosis.

CURRENT STATUS OF PROGESTERONE THERAPY FOR PMS

There is no controlled study evidence that either natural progesterone, administered in suppository form during the luteal phase, or the closely-related progestins are more effective than placebo in PMS treatment. Nonetheless, some clinical programs described success in using progesterone therapy for PMS,[18,53] and many women as well as clinicians maintain their strong advocacy of this treatment. The current emphasis among adherents of progesterone therapy is on its oral administration, using 100- to 300-mg capsules of natural micronized progesterone. This is supported by one placebo-controlled study with arguable findings that oral progesterone reduced some symptoms of PMS.[33] Other controlled studies of the effectiveness of oral progesterone are in progress.

Natural progesterone appears to be a benign treatment without major side effects, although information on its long-term use rests on the clinical reports of medical practitioners. There are no long-term research safety data on progesterone in PMS therapy, and consumers should know that this use of progesterone consequently does not have FDA approval. However, the greatest problem in continuing to advocate progesterone treatment for PMS is not the risks or side effects of progesterone, but its impediment to developing treatments with proven effectiveness and to gaining knowledge of the causes of PMS when the ill-supported belief in the efficacy of progesterone treatment is maintained.

UNANSWERED QUESTIONS IN PROGESTERONE THERAPY

While it is clear that progesterone is not an effective treatment for PMS overall, there may be a subgroup, albeit a very small one, with a more specific response to progesterone. Possible reasons for a beneficial response of some women could lie in hormonal actions or in other unidentified characteristics of women who report moderate to severe PMS.

While progesterone deficiency does not appear to be a cause of PMS, both the possible sedative and anxiolytic effects of progesterone metabolites and the interactions of progesterone with hormones other than those of the reproductive system are insufficiently studied. It is particularly puzzling why there has not been more evidence of anxiolytic or sedating effects of progesterone, which might reduce the well-known irritability-tension-anxiety cluster of PMS symptoms. Possibly progesterone doses are not high enough to produce sufficient levels of the progesterone metabolites that produce these effects. Perhaps a threshold effect for progesterone levels, which occurred with repeated administration of progesterone suppositories at plasma progesterone levels far below those reached in term pregnancy, impedes attaining levels needed to reduce anxiety or induce sedation.

Evidence that progesterone[54] and progestins[19,49,55] relieved PMS symptoms when administered to suppress ovulation suggests that the success of progesterone therapy requires doses and timing to induce an antiovulatory effect. Sampson reviewed clinical cases of PMS treated with progesterone and concluded that "only when the cycle was disrupted was there usually, but not always, an improvement in symptoms."[56] However, the generally recommended procedures for progesterone therapy in PMS have been to administer progesterone only during the luteal phase of the cycle. In line with this approach, the reported placebo-controlled studies administered progesterone only after ovulation, and consequently have not answered the question of the effectiveness of progesterone in doses to suppress ovulation.

Evidence that progestins produce PMS symptoms when administered in conjunction with estrogen raises questions of the extent to which progesterone causes at least some of the symptoms of PMS, thereby confounding treatment results. Possibly the changing progesterone levels have a trigger function that signals other hormonal or psychological changes of PMS, but there has been little study of hormones other than the sex steroids in relation to symptoms of PMS.

Large symptom variability in PMS samples may obscure very small treatment effects, but this has theoretical more than practical significance, since such small effects would not be clinically meaningful. The recent attempts to develop firm diagnostic guidelines for a PMS diagnosis are producing more consistent samples, particularly in terms of symptom severity and swing related to menses and differentiation from other psychiatric conditions, but the heterogeneity of symptoms remains substantial. It must be recognized that a great range of nonspecific symptoms can meet the current criteria for PMS, and also that the individual variations in predisposing, precipitating, and sustaining factors of PMS are extremely large, making it difficult to elucidate any single treatment approach for this complex and poorly understood disorder.

SUMMARY

The complexity of the endocrine system makes it simplistic to say that progesterone does or does not affect PMS symptoms. The successful advocacy of progesterone therapy over the past two decades brought vastly increased awareness of PMS among women and clinicians and stimulated greatly improved guidelines for its diagnosis. Now it is time to recognize the limitations of progesterone therapy, evaluate other treatments, and examine other hormonal relationships to understand PMS.

REFERENCES

1. Speroff L, Glass RH, Kase NG. *Clinical Gynecologic Endocrinology and Infertility.* 4th ed. Baltimore: Williams & Wilkins; 1989.
2. Siiteri PK, Febres F, Clemens LE, et al. Progesterone and maintenance of pregnancy: is progesterone nature's immunosuppressant? *Ann NY Acad Sci.* 1977;286:384.
3. Maxson WS. The use of progesterone in the treatment of PMS. *Clin Obstet Gynecol.* 1987;30:465.
4. Selye H. Correlations between the chemical structure and the pharmacological actions of the steroids. *Endocrinology.* 1942;30:437.
5. Heuser G. Induction of anesthesia, seizures, and sleep by steroid hormones. *Anesthesiology.* 1967;28:173.
6. Arafat ES, Hargrove JT, Maxson WS, et al. Sedation and hypnotic effects of oral administration of micronized progesterone may be mediated through its metabolites. *Am J Obstet Gynecol.* 1988;159:1203.
7. Whitehead MI, Townsend PT, Gill DK, et al. Absorption and metabolism of oral progesterone. *Br Med J.* 1980;280:825.
8. Lane G, Siddle NC, Ryder TA, et al. Dose dependent effects of oral progesterone on the oestrogenised postmenopausal endometrium. *Br Med J.* 1983;287:1241.
9. Ottoson UB, Carlstrom K, Damber JE, et al. Serum levels of progesterone and some of its metabolites including deoxycorticosterone after oral and parenteral administration. *Br J Obstet Gynecol.* 1984;91:1111.
10. Maxson WS, Hargrove JT. Bioavailability of oral micronized progesterone. *Fertil Steril.* 1985;44:622.
11. Chakmakjian ZH, Zachariah NY. Bioavailability of progesterone with different modes of administration. *J Reprod Med.* 1987;32:443.
12. Padwick ML, Endicott J, Matson C, et al. Absorption and metabolism of oral progesterone when administered twice daily. *Fertil Steril.* 1987;46:402.
13. Hargrove JT, Maxson WS, Wentz AC. Absorption of oral progesterone is influenced by vehicle and particle size. *Am J Obstet Gynecol.* 1989;161:948.
14. Freeman EW, Weinstock L, Rickels K, et al. A placebo-controlled study of effects of oral progesterone on performance and mood. *Br J Clin Pharmac.* 1992;293.
15. Glazener CA, Bailey I, Hull MGR. Effectiveness of vaginal administration of progesterone. *Br J Obstet Gynecol.* 1985;92:364.
16. Myers ER, Sondheimer SJ, Freeman EW, et al. Serum progesterone levels following vaginal administration of progesterone during the luteal phase. *Fertil Steril.* 1987;47:71.
17. Maddocks S, Hahn P, Moller F, et al. A double-blind placebo-controlled trial of progesterone vaginal suppositories in the treatment of premenstrual symptoms. *Am J Obstet Gynecol.* 1986;154:573.
18. Dalton K. *The Premenstrual Syndrome and Progesterone Therapy,* 2nd ed. Chicago: Year Book Medical Publishers, Inc.; 1984.
19. Sampson GA, Heathcote PRM, Wordsworth J et al. Premenstrual syndrome. A double-blind cross-over study of treatment with dydrogesterone and placebo. *Br Med J.* 1988;153:232.
20. Dennerstein L, Morse C, Gotts G et al. Treatment of premenstrual syndrome: a double-blind trial of dydrogesterone. *J Affective Disord.* 1986;11:199.
21. Kerr GD, Day JB, Munday MR et al. Dydrogesterone in the treatment of the premenstrual syndrome. *Practitioner.* 1980;224:852.
22. Israel RS. Premenstrual tension. *JAMA.* 1938;110:1721.
23. Greene R, Dalton K. The premenstrual syndrome. *Br Med J.* 1953;1:1007.
24. Hammarback S, Damber JE, Backstrom T. Relationship between symptom severity and hormone changes in women with premenstrual syndrome. *J Clin Endocrinol Metab.* 1989;68:125.
25. Sampson GA. Premenstrual syndrome: a double-blind controlled trial of progesterone and placebo. *Br J Psychiatry.* 1979:135:209.
26. Richter MA, Haltvick R, Shapiro SS. Progesterone treatment of premenstrual syndrome. *Curr Ther Res.* 1984;36:840.
27. Magos AL, Collins WP, Studd JWW. Management of the premenstrual syndrome by subcutaneous implants of oestradiol. *J Psychosom Obstet Gynecol.* 1984;3:93.
28. Hammarback S, Backstrom T, Holst J, et al. Cyclical mood changes as in the premenstrual tension syndrome during sequential estrogen-progesterone postmenopausal replacement therapy. *Acta Obstet Gynecol Scand.* 1985;64:393.
29. Facchinetti, F, Nappi G, Petraglia F, et al. Oestradiol/progester-

one imbalance and the premenstrual syndrome. *Lancet.* 1983;ii:1302.

30. Varma TR. Hormones and electrolytes in premenstrual syndrome. *Int J Gynaecol Obstet.* 1984;22:51.

31. Herman WM, Beach RC. Experimental and clinical data indicating the psychotropic properties of progestagens. *Postgrad Med J.* 1978;54(suppl 2):82.

32. Merryman W, Boiman R, Barnes L, et al. Progesterone "anesthesia" in human subjects. *J Clin Endocrinol Metab.* 1954;14:1567.

33. Dennerstein L, Spencer-Gardner C, Gotts G, et al. Progesterone and the premenstrual syndrome: a double-blind crossover trial. *Br Med J.* 1985;290:1617.

34. Erny R, Pigne A, Prouvost C, et al. The effects of oral administration of progesterone for premature labor. *Am J Obstet Gynecol.* 1986;154:525.

35. Majewska MD, Harrison NL, Schwartz RD, et al. Steroid hormone metabolites are barbiturate-like modulators of the GABA receptor. *Science.* 1986;232:1004.

36. Smith SS, Waterhouse BD, Chapin JK, et al. Progesterone alters GABA and glutamate responsiveness: a possible mechanism for its anxiolytic action. *Brain Res.* 1987;400:353.

37. Freeman EW, Rickels K, Sondheimer SJ, et al. Ineffectiveness of progesterone suppository treatment for premenstrual syndrome. *JAMA.* 1990;264:349.

38. Nillius SJ, Johannson EDB. Plasma levels of progesterone after vaginal, rectal, or intramuscular administration of progesterone. *Am J Obstet Gynecol.* 1971;110:470.

39. Corney RH, Stanton R, Newell R, et al. Comparison of progesterone, placebo, and behavioral psychotherapy in the treatment of premenstrual syndrome. *J Psychosom Obstet Gynecol.* 1990;11:211.

40. Andersch B, Hahn L. Progesterone treatment of premenstrual tension. *J Psychosom Res.* 1985;29:489.

41. Vandermeer YG, Benedek-Jaszmann LJ, VanLoenen AC. Effect of high dose progesterone on the premenstrual syndrome. *J Psychosom Obstet Gynecol.* 1983;2:220.

42. Smith SL. Mood and the menstrual cycle. In: Sachar EF, ed. *Topics in Psychoendocrinology.* New York: Grune & Stratton, Inc.;1975:19.

43. Taylor RW. The treatment of premenstrual tension with dydrogesterone. *Curr Med Res Opin.* 1977;4:35.

44. Day JB. Clinical trials in the premenstrual syndrome. *Curr Med Res Opin.* 1979;6:40.

45. Jordheim O. The premenstrual syndrome. *Acta Obstet Gynecol Scand.* 1972;51:77.

46. Appleby BP. A study of premenstrual tension in general practice. *Br Med J.* 1960;1:391.

47. Ylostalo P, Kauppila A, Puolakka J, et al. Bromocriptine and norethisterone in the treatment of premenstrual syndrome. *Obstet Gynecol.* 1982;59:292.

48. Coppen AJ, Milne HB, Outram DH. Dytide, norethisterone and a placebo in the premenstrual syndrome: a double-blind controlled comparison. *Clin Trials J.* 1969;Feb:33.

49. Watson NR, Studd JWW, Savvas M, et al. Treatment of severe premenstrual syndrome with oestradiol patches and cyclical oral norethisterone. *Lancet.* 1989;ii:730.

50. Sitruk-Ware R, Bricaire C, DeLignieres B, et al. Oral micronized progesterone. *Contraception.* 1987;36:373.

51. Dalton K. Trial of progesterone vaginal suppositories in the treatment of premenstrual syndrome. *Am J Obstet Gynecol.* 1987;156:1555.

52. Mackenzie N, Holton W. Premenstrual syndrome and progesterone suppositories. *JAMA.* 1991;26.

53. Norris RV. *Premenstrual Syndrome.* New York: Fawson Assoc; 1983.

54. Dalton K. *The Premenstrual Syndrome and Progesterone Therapy.* London: William Heinemann Medical Books; 1977.

55. Keye WR. Medical treatment of premenstrual syndrome. *Can J Psychiatry.* 1985;30:483.

56. Sampson GA. Endocrine treatments for premenstrual syndrome: principles and clinical evaluation. In: Brush MG, Goudsmith EM, eds. *Functional Disorders of the Menstrual Cycle.* London: John Wiley & Sons Ltd.; 1988.

CHAPTER 15

Group Psychotherapy for Premenstrual Syndrome

Kathleen Ulman

In the past few decades much scientific attention has focused on investigating both the etiology and treatment of premenstrual symptoms. While the exact etiology is still not understood, much information on the physical aspects of premenstrual syndrome (PMS) has become available. As a result, in the medical field PMS is generally accepted as a real physical phenomenon, with no single treatment proven effective for all symptoms. Psychological correlates of PMS are less well understood. The premenstrual hormonal changes influence some women's moods and psychological functioning and in turn are thought to be influenced by a woman's overall psychological state. As in all medical conditions, menstruation occurs in the context of cultural beliefs that influence a woman's menstrual experience.

This chapter describes a psychological approach to evaluating and treating women with premenstrual symptoms in groups. This model seeks to explore and work with the complexity of physical, psychological, and social factors that impinge on each individual woman to produce distressing premenstrual symptoms. There is a short discussion of the overall rationale for this approach followed by a detailed description of the evaluation process, formulation of a treatment plan, and implementation of the group program, including two case examples.

GROUP THERAPY

Psychological Treatment of Medical Conditions

Recently, we have seen increasing evidence to support the idea proposed some time ago by Dunbar[1] that emotional functioning and general level of stress may contribute to the onset and course of various illnesses.[2,3] Helz and Templeton,[2] in their review of psychological factors and diabetic control, conclude that stress may influence the course of the illness by interfering with treatment compliance and by direct effects on neuroendocrine function. Godkin et al[3] found a correlation between a diagnosis of cervical cancer and interviewer-rated hopelessness at the time of biopsy.

Psychological interventions are related to decreased exacerbations of chronic illnesses[2,4] and increased longevity.[5] Effective interventions range from traditional psychotherapy, which explores unconscious conflicts and feelings, to cognitive therapy that addresses the impact of frequent thought patterns on emotional functioning, to behavioral therapy which seeks to change particular behaviors that are thought to exacerbate symptoms. Templeton[6] reports the stabilization of diabetic control as a result of intensive psychotherapy in a woman whose insulin requirements were grossly erratic. Spiegel et al[5] found increased survival rates in breast cancer patients who underwent group psychotherapy. Behavioral stress reduction techniques such as relaxation were found to improve diabetic control in some patients.[2] Whatever the theoretical bias, most psychological interventions with medically ill patients are based on the rationale that psychological and physiological functioning are interrelated, each influencing the other. It is thought that internal conflicts and stress will weaken the immune system and render a patient more susceptible to illness. In turn, a medical illness will diminish an individual's internal sense of order and control over her life, interrupt her usual coping style, and simultaneously diminish her self-esteem. The recovery process and medical management of an illness are impeded by internal conflicts and the diminished self-esteem and decrease in positive attitude the patient brings to the process. Psychological interventions are aimed at increasing self-esteem, developing a sense of internal control over an individual's life, reducing conflicts, and teaching stress reduction.

The usefulness of group counseling for medical problems has long been established.[7-9] Studies of the effects of support groups for asthma, weight loss, and cardiac problems have demonstrated increased self-care and compliance with medical regimens, decreased hospital stays, increased longevity, and increases in positive attitude.[9]

The need for relatedness to others, a long-understood idea in psychological treatment, has recently been integrated into medical understanding of illness. The isolation and withdrawal characteristic of depression increases an individual's distress. Groups offer a unique experience for individuals with medical problems. They address isolation and decreased self-esteem in ways that individual counseling cannot. Meeting and interacting with others who share the same problem diminishes isolation and a sense of defectiveness. This interaction is curative. The patient is faced with others who share her symptoms and struggles in a supportive, accepting environment. In a group, it is difficult to hold on to the belief that one is alone with suffering. In addition, the positive regard of group members and the opportunity to help others enhances a woman's sense of worth and effectiveness. Group therapy offers all members a chance to learn about how they are experienced by others and how they experience others. This provides for correction of distortions in self-image that individuals bring to social interactions. For example, an individual may believe that she is valued only when she concerns herself with others' problems and overextends

herself. In a group she will have an opportunity to learn that the group members will not turn away from her when she does not overextend herself for another group member. In fact, they most likely will encourage her to take care of herself and point out the other member's responsibility for herself.

Group interventions for medically ill patients are structured in various ways, ranging from one session groups in hospital and outpatient settings to long-term groups with a fixed membership. Most have been found to be efficacious.[10] Outpatient medical groups most frequently use a model of a didactic presentation followed by an open ended discussion either in an open, drop in setting or a short-term setting with a fixed membership.

Psychological Treatment of PMS

As stated previously, the exact etiology of PMS is not yet understood. Generally PMS is considered by many to be a medically based condition that impacts psychological functioning. However, women with PMS report more intense mood and behavior changes than patients with most medical conditions. Several approaches to understanding and treating PMS have been offered, ranging from a descriptive psychiatric approach,[11] to one of medical management,[12] to a stress model.[13] These approaches all conceptualize PMS as a physiologically based phenomenon in a psychological context. They see PMS as influenced by stress level, physical state, personality, and interpersonal relationships, and recommend supportive psychological interventions as part of the overall treatment.

As with all medical conditions, PMS exists in a social context. In our society, any medical condition that is believed to impair rationality, such as epilepsy or PMS, is feared. Women have been socialized to repress their anger. Women who express their anger are often criticized and avoided. Women report that they feel ashamed of their irrational and angry premenstrual feelings and believe they would be shunned if others knew how they felt.

The use of group therapy for PMS is in keeping with the current state of knowledge related to treatment of medical conditions. Among patients with medical problems, women with PMS are unusually vulnerable to a sense of defectiveness, isolation, and shame. This vulnerability may be due in part to the shame of the irrationality and anger experienced by these women, and in part due to the continued existence of the menstrual taboo in our society that considers menstruation unclean and something to be avoided. In addition, our culture has been highly influenced by the psychoanalytic view that menstrual complaints are not physiologically based, but rather are the result of unconscious conflicts related to femininity.

Groups offer women with PMS a unique opportunity to share experiences with other women, overcome the sense of isolation and shame, understand their experiences and feelings more fully, and obtain support to initiate self-care measures. Several investigators found that women received benefits from participating in PMS groups.[14–16] I also have found group treatment to be beneficial for women with PMS in effecting changes in self-esteem, body image, and symptom management.

GROUP TREATMENT PROGRAM FOR PMS

Goals

My overall goals for working with women with premenstrual symptoms are to help them become more observant of the connections among their behavioral, physical, and emotional responses, and to understand and accept their bodies as they are, so they may make changes that will decrease their premenstrual distress. Through this process of understanding and accepting her physical and emotional changes across the menstrual cycle, a woman gains a fuller understanding of herself.

Women frequently say that they feel in control premenstrually until they suddenly explode at their family. They do not experience distress in their relationships at other times of the month and are not aware of any subtle changes in their mood or sense of physical comfort previous to the explosion. As we work together over the course of the group sessions, the women often become aware of the onset of premenstrual changes leading up to the explosion. They learn that at a particular point in their cycle they begin to feel increasingly uncomfortable physically, feeling tense and/or tired, and they simultaneously experience irritable, depressed, or angry feelings. The women may have suppressed these feelings because they considered them unacceptable. They also learn that conflicts and tensions exist in their family relationships throughout each month, but that when they are in the preovulatory phase of the cycle and feel better physically and emotionally, they are less tense, react less impulsively, and are able to overlook the conflicts. They also may learn that, as the premenstrual physical changes occur, they feel more

dependent, needy, and less sure of themselves. These factors have interacted to produce unpredicted behavior.

Women need the freedom and encouragement to explore all sides of themselves, including the feelings and behaviors that are less culturally accepted for women, such as rage, aggression, and resentment. This kind of self-exploration often involves the recognition of vulnerable and shameful sides of oneself. Many women with severe PMS feel isolated from other women because of the differences between their symptoms and those of women with mild PMS. Meeting other women who have had similar experiences often reduces shame and isolation.

Group Leader

As stated previously, groups offer an ideal setting to deal with vulnerability and shame, to correct distorted views of the self, as well as provide the encouragement and motivation to make changes that are often difficult. This type of self-exploration is done best in a safe setting, which requires a trained therapist who can provide the necessary boundaries to create a sense of safety. The power of groups to produce change through sharing and self-exploration cannot be taken lightly. Many feelings and vulnerabilities can be stirred up in groups. A trained group therapist is essential to manage the interactions.

Structure of Group

Because my goal is to provide a setting in which women can learn didactic information about PMS, meet other women with similar experiences, reduce a sense of shame and isolation, and do some in-depth self-exploration, I prefer a time-limited group with a fixed membership. My groups meet for 10 sessions. Each session is 1 ½ hours long; they start and end on time. This time gives the members a framework within which to set goals and accomplish some changes. The small number of sessions helps to mobilize energy and the will to change. The length of the group extends longer than two normal cycles, with the hope that each member will go through two premenstrual phases while in group. The membership is fixed and does not exceed eight persons. Members are asked to keep all group information confidential, and to participate in the group as best they can. Also, in the pregroup interview I tell prospective members that they do not have to reveal everything immediately but may proceed at their own pace. Each member is expected to attend all sessions.

A sense of safety and trust develops optimally in group when there is predictability and continuity. This depends on the leader's maintenance of an unchanging stance in the group and on the members' regular attendance. Women become important to each other as sources of support and as persons who reflect acceptance back to the patient. The group itself becomes a place to bring and share painful and overwhelming feelings with people who can be counted on. When a member is absent, it impedes the sense of safety and continuity for the remaining members.

Each session is a mixture of didactic presentation, sharing, and exploration. The exploration aspect is somewhat structured in that I usually address each particular member regarding her experiences during the week. As the group proceeds, I let the conversation flow and am less directive. I do not promote the development of negative group processes, but rather focus on the similarities between the experiences of group members and promote group cohesiveness as one would at the start of a long-term therapy group. I acknowledge negative issues such as conflicts between group members only if they threaten to interfere with the group. I pass over much interpersonal material that would be dealt with in long-term groups.

All new PMS patients meet at least once individually with me for evaluation. The goals of the initial interview are: (1) to perform an overall psychiatric evaluation including a psychiatric, social, and family history, (2) to gather information on the history and severity of PMS symptoms and have the patient start prospective charting of daily symptoms, (3) to assess appropriateness for group treatment, (4) to come to an agreement with the patient about the treatment plan and, (5) to set the stage for active participation and self-exploration by the patient.

Psychiatric Evaluation

The first step is to do an overall psychiatric evaluation. This is of prime importance in working with any patient complaining of PMS because of the frequent overlap between PMS and depression[11] and the generality of many PMS complaints that might obscure other medical or psychiatric problems. PMS is often the first phase of the development of a more general depression.[11] Some women who are experiencing general psychological problems unrelated to the menstrual cycle, such as anxiety disorder, adjustment reactions, or depression, identify themselves as having PMS. For these women, having a biologically-based explanation for their symptoms is the most acceptable diagnosis.

In the first part of the evaluation, I investigate the woman's main complaint. I ask the woman to phrase her request for help with her PMS. I carefully pay attention to the wording of her initial complaint and the ways she asks for help. This approach gives me information regarding the patient's hopes, expectations, and motivations. It helps me assess whether she is expecting to be an active participant in her care or whether she wants something to be done for her. Frequently, a woman requests a test to determine which hormone is "out of balance." She experiences the onset of her symptoms as so sudden and disconnected from the rest of her life, and considers the accompanying feelings of irritability, depression, or rage so foreign to her, she is convinced that only a chemical change in her body could produce such changes and only a chemical intervention could correct them. Some women request medical treatment because they fear that any health professional who offers psychological treatment must believe their symptoms are "all in their heads." Often these women are seeking validation for their experience. They want someone to say "I believe this comes over you suddenly, feels out of your control, and I do not consider you weak or crazy." Some women request help in gaining a sense of control of their symptoms. These women see themselves as active participants in their care regardless of whether they receive medication. They often have been in psychotherapy for other reasons. In this part of the interview I take extremely careful detailed information regarding current PMS symptoms and obtain details of a woman's functioning in the remainder of her cycle. I try to obtain a full picture of this woman's premenstrual experience.

Next I obtain detailed information on any current or past psychiatric symptoms, including details of past depressions. The psychiatric history of family members is also helpful. Data show that many women who are diagnosed with PMS have had past episodes of depression.[11] If a woman has had a depression in the past, this can be used as one indicator that the PMS symptoms may expand into a general depression and that antidepressants may be needed in the future. I also obtain a complete menstrual history including physical and psychological symptoms, starting with menarche, and ask about any difficult experiences related to menstruation. I inquire as to the meaning of menstruation to the patient and to her family. In addition, I ask for details of the first recognition of PMS symptoms and the development of the symptoms over the years. I also ask about sexual history and past incidents of sexual assault.

Any information that gives me an understanding of the general context of a woman's life is of interest to me. This includes any recent changes in the patient's life such as relationships, job, health, or losses. These changes may have an influence on PMS symptoms.

During this phase of the interview I try to put current symptoms in a context and answer the question "Why is this person coming for help now?" The answer to this one question can elucidate much about the patient's motivation and expectations. Most often there has been about 2 to 6 months of symptoms that feel out of control, with a recent episode that has felt frightening to the woman. It may have been sudden suicidal thoughts, unexpected crying, or a behavioral explosion such as yelling or throwing things. As much detail as possible should be gathered about this experience of loss of control.

A brief social and family history helps to form a fuller picture of the patient and gives a context in which to understand the meaning of her symptoms and her coping styles. In the course of inquiring about these areas, sometimes new information related to recent life changes comes up.

As part of the initial interview, I do a routine mental status evaluation assessing current functioning such as sleep, appetite, energy level, concentration, cognitive functioning, quality of associations, eye contact, affect in session, and mood to rule out depression, anxiety disorders, a thought disorder, or delusional thinking. Any underlying psychiatric disorder needs to be treated along with PMS. I also collect information regarding reported differences in sleep, appetite, energy level, mood, and cognitive functioning between a woman's premenstrual phase and other phases of her cycle. At this time I also note the current phase of the menstrual cycle for this woman.

In addition to the above mentioned information, I inquire as to lifestyle patterns such as nutrition, exercise, methods and frequency of relaxation, and experience of stress in various areas. Improved nutrition, exercise, and stress reduction have been found to help ameliorate PMS symptoms.[17-19] I am particularly interested in how a woman cares for herself and others. How much responsibility does she have for others, how much time does she have for herself, and what is the quality of her close relationships? Are there any people in her life on whom she can depend when she feels tired or overwhelmed and how does she use them?

Usually I see a woman for one initial interview before making a plan. However, if a woman is in crisis or has an unusually complicated history, I see her twice. After gathering the relevant information, I give the patient a chart on which to record PMS symptoms all month. This is presented as a tool to learn more about the

intensity, timing, and frequency of symptoms. Any observations concerning the relationship of symptoms to other events made by the patient herself, instead of the clinician, become more easily integrated into the patient's understanding of herself. I recommend she return in a month after charting for one cycle.

Formulating a Treatment Plan

Throughout the interview I organize the information to evaluate whether the patient currently has a major depression, bipolar disorder, anxiety disorder, or an adjustment disorder instead of or in addition to PMS. Once all the information is gathered, the relationship between a woman's PMS, general psychological functioning, and the context of her life can be assessed and a treatment plan can be formulated.

Sometimes, in recounting details, the patient sees that the progression of symptoms point to the onset of an overall depression, as well as the existence of PMS. In this case, medication may be considered as well as psychotherapy. In some instances, a woman has had significant symptoms with no evidence of their cycling with the menstrual cycle. Often the patient comes to realize this as she recounts her story. Here I will recommend an evaluation for antidepressant medication and psychotherapy. However, if the patient maintains the view that she has PMS and displays serious psychopathology, I recommend she chart her symptoms for a month and return the next week for further exploration of her symptoms. I also recommend that she consider an evaluation for medication soon. At this point I do not challenge her belief that she has PMS. Usually when such a patient charts her symptoms over several cycles, it becomes evident that the symptoms are not cyclical. By that time I have met several times with the patient, have established a relationship with her, and we have begun to address other areas of concern. My goal is to meet with the patient as long as needed to redefine her problem and to obtain appropriate treatment.

For most patients the picture is more ambiguous. Many women who come for help have clear cycling of symptoms as well as serious stressors. Some patients who seek help for PMS are already in psychotherapy and sometimes on medications such as tranquilizers or antidepressants. If there are clear symptoms, such as anxiety and tension or depression, which might be treated by antidepressants or tranquilizers, I refer the woman for a medication evaluation. Other women appear to have clear PMS and no other stress in their lives. For both of these types of patients the question I ask myself throughout the interview is "Is she appropriate for a group and is she interested?" Some women rule themselves out immediately because of a fear of groups, an unwillingness to commit to 10 sessions, or scheduling problems. Others rule themselves out because they wish to be treated only with medication, in spite of the lack of clear treatable symptoms, and are unwilling to be a partner in their treatment. For these women, I set up an individual contract, review nutritional information, and have them return in a month to 6 weeks. About half of these women cancel or do not come for their follow-up appointment. These often include those women who showed no interest or curiosity in learning to participate in the management of their symptoms. Others may not have returned because they obtained all the information they needed in one session and found they could carry out the necessary changes on their own.

For the remainder of women, I rule out prospective group members as one would rule out members for any short-term psychotherapy group. Excessively paranoid, hostile, unusual, and bizarre individuals are usually not appropriate and may initially alienate and frighten other members and drive them away. Difficulties in interpersonal relationships prevent these women from working, over a short period of time, with other group members on the agreed on tasks. Many of the women who come to PMS groups want to see themselves as normal in every way except for their PMS. Patients with a history of serious psychosis, bizarre behavior, or violence frighten other group members and disrupt an outpatient PMS group. These more disturbed patients can be helped with their PMS symptoms individually. If there were a sufficient number of these more disturbed patients with disruptive or violent behavior, they could be seen together in a PMS group.

Group Preparation

Once I have determined a patient is appropriate and willing to participate, I review the group agreement. This is an essential ingredient to the success of any group, particularly a short-term group. Patients are very anxious about a group experience and find clearly defined expectations relieving. Also, these guidelines give the therapist a framework within which to function. This agreement outlines the structure of the group and expectations of the patients. I tell group members that they are expected to attend all 10 sessions, come on time, pay for all 10 sessions regardless of absences, participate as best they can in all sessions, and maintain confidentiality.

CASE EXAMPLES

Two case examples of typical PMS group patients are presented here and later discussed in terms of their progress in each group session.

The first case example is Brenda, a 40-year-old married woman with children. She is a serious, conscientious, perfectionistic woman who works part time and expects herself to run her home well and be in control of all her responsibilities. She is friendly, outgoing, and liked by people at work and in her community. She considers herself normal psychologically and has never been in psychotherapy. Her main complaint is that she wakes up one morning each month feeling like a different person. She feels tense, uncomfortable, and everything irritates her, and at the same time she feels overwhelmed and unable to carry out her daily schedule. It takes enormous effort to speak and interact with others, let alone be pleasant. She would like to stay in bed for the next few days until her period starts. She has never canceled any obligation because of PMS. Recently her husband learned he may be laid off from his management job due to the economy. Brenda would then have to work full time just to pay basic expenses. She feels she has had mild PMS for many years but has experienced more intense symptoms over the past 2 years and has felt out of control for the past 2 months. Several years ago she read some books on PMS and was able to manage her symptoms with some lifestyle changes. She decided to seek help because during the past 2 months she felt out of control of her behavior when she was premenstrual. On one occasion, when her son was sick and both she and her husband had important meetings at work, she precipitated a fight with her husband. Instead of discussing the problem to find a solution, she felt hopeless and overwhelmed, yelled at her husband in ways uncharacteristic of her, and threw a dish against a wall, something she had never done before.

The second case is that of Donna, a 33-year-old married woman with no children. She works as a lawyer in a prominent firm in her city. She had two previous major depressions and took antidepressants with a good response. She also was in psychotherapy for a short time after the last depression and found it helpful. However, she terminated treatment as soon as her serious symptoms diminished. She was not interested in further exploration as to the psychological correlates of her depression. In the past 4 months, when premenstrual, she has experienced extreme lethargy, joint pain, tearfulness, difficulty concentrating, and suicidal ideation. For the remainder of the month, her functioning is somewhat dysthymic, but does not include any of the premenstrual behavior. Donna seeks treatment because she is frightened by her suicidal ideation and cannot stand the lethargy that interferes with her job performance. She is thinking of returning to psychotherapy, but fears this means that her depression has returned.

Procedure for Each Group Session

The First Group Session

The first session starts with a review of the group format, including the time of the meeting, specific dates for the 10 meetings, agreement of confidentiality, agreement to pay bills, goals of the group program, and agreement to participate in each group. I outline the goals of the group program as the creation of a setting for women to: (1) learn more about the timing, intensity, and frequency of their premenstrual symptoms, (2) to understand the relationship of their responses to other lifestyle patterns, and external and internal events, and (3) to explore ways that they might ameliorate their symptoms. Over the course of the first few sessions, each woman is expected to define in more detail her own goals. Then I encourage each woman to describe briefly the PMS symptoms that brought her into treatment. The degree of detail is left up to the individual woman. I hand out more daily symptom charts and ask the women to bring them in each week. I then encourage each woman to discuss her experience of charting and what she has learned about her symptoms. To help each woman begin to define her goals for the group, I have the members fill out a self-assessment form, derived from one used to assess stress. It divides PMS symptoms into three categories—behavioral, psychological, and physical (see Appendix I). Each woman rates the severity of her PMS symptoms in each category and adds up these ratings so that she ends up with a score for each category. Most women who attend these groups find that their most severe symptoms cluster in the psychological category. Each woman then identifies particular symptoms from the daily charts or self-assessment forms that she would like to work on decreasing over the course of the group. I ask each woman to observe these symptoms or behaviors over the next week and note her progress and the types of feelings, behaviors, and events that might make them worse or better. For the remaining time, usually 15 to 30 minutes, I open up the group to a discussion of the women's histories, experiences, and feelings about their symptoms. At this time I try to give permission for the expression of any feelings about PMS.

Brenda found that her symptoms fell mostly in the psychological category, but she also had some physical and behavioral symptoms. Her highest score was on irritability. She chose this as her target symptom to decrease over the course of the group program. Donna's symptoms were evenly distributed between the three categories. She chose her lethargy and joint pain as her target symptoms to decrease. She felt her suicidal ideation was too overwhelming to take on at this point. Both Brenda and Donna expressed the wish to find ways to decrease the intensity of their PMS symptoms and to restore stability to their functioning over their menstrual cycle. Both expressed a sense of loss of control that they could not push themselves to perform as they had in the past.

The Second Week

At the start of the second session I review the daily charts and encourage continued record keeping. I focus the discussion on observing symptoms and on connecting the most severe symptoms with time of cycle, diet, stress, and other events. I then review the goals that each woman outlined at the initial group, inquire as to each member's progress, and encourage each woman to explore what might help or impede her progress. Then each woman fills out a self-assessment form for stress which evaluates a woman's responses to her PMS symptoms (see Appendix II). I ask each woman to rate how frequently she engages in particular behaviors in response to her PMS symptoms. The behaviors are grouped according to whether they are external solutions, such as taking a pill or smoking a cigarette, or whether they are internal solutions such as doing deep breathing, thinking of a joke, or calling a friend. In reviewing the options listed on the form, each woman usually comes across constructive options she has not thought of using, such as telling a joke or listening to music. I then have each woman pick several behaviors she would like to decrease, and at least one that she would like to add to her usual response pattern. I then repeat the open-ended discussion described in the first session.

Both women kept daily charts. Brenda had a reasonable week in that all went smoothly at work and at home. She observed her outgoing and optimistic feelings and wondered how she could remember them at her worst premenstrual times. Brenda decided to decrease her compulsive eating, which she does only premenstrually, and to try instead to practice yoga to reduce tension. Donna had a difficult week. She was premenstrual and lacked the energy to do daily charting. She thought about not coming to this group as she was very tired and cried all the way to the group. She felt too ashamed to cry in front of the group members and feared she would not be able to control herself. Donna decided to decrease her alcohol intake and increase the time she spends reading, watching TV, and being with friends.

The Third Week

At the start of the third session I again review the daily charts and encourage the women to discuss the patterns that emerge in the course of record keeping. I also focus the discussion on understanding the exacerbation of symptoms that did occur, and encourage the women to think about possible precipitants or events that may have diminished symptoms. I then start a discussion of the goals each member outlined at the two previous sessions and encourage each woman to look at what behaviors she has changed and what may have impeded her carrying through with her stated goals. At this session I introduce a third self-assessment stress questionnaire that focuses on the cost to the woman of the stress reducing coping strategies she chooses. As in the second questionnaire, the concept is introduced that some strategies such as taking tranquilizers or drinking alcohol may increase stress. For the last half of the session I promote an open-ended discussion of recent PMS symptoms and strategies to deal with them. In the course of the discussion I listen for and encourage the expression of feelings of loss of control, shame, and anger.

At the third session Brenda reported that she was preparing for her upcoming premenstrual week by getting all the food on which she might binge out of the house. However, because of her busy schedule, she was unable to find time to arrange a yoga class. The group discussed this with her and encouraged her to find the time to set up the class. In the open discussion, Brenda mentioned a sense of shame and loss of control. She did not relate specifics of her previous behavior that brought her into the group. In the past week Donna had her worst premenstrual days. In spite of tearfulness and suicidal thoughts, she called an old friend. However, she was unable to eliminate alcohol completely. Donna discussed the shame associated with her previous depressions and ways the current premenstrual times remind her of the past.

The Fourth Week

For the first half of the fourth session a nutritionist discusses nutritional aspects of PMS management. She discusses the rationale for decreasing the intake of caf-

feine, alcohol, salt, and sugar. She then recommends a well-balanced diet of protein and complex carbohydrates with frequent small meals. At the request of many group participants, the nutritionist reviews the nutritional research on vitamin therapy and recommends only a multivitamin. The group is then opened up to questions. This is a popular section of the group experience. Many women who seek help have poor nutritional habits and little understanding of their nutritional needs. For the remainder of the session, group members review the daily charts and individual goals. Again, the discussion focuses on the successes and obstacles each woman encounters in trying to change her behavior.

At this session Brenda discusses her premenstrual cravings for sweets and her struggle to keep her overall food intake in control. After briefly reviewing Brenda's eating habits with her, the nutritionist recommends that she eat frequently and not skip meals to protect herself from decreased blood sugar and food cravings. She also recommended that she eat a balance of protein and carbohydrates at each main meal. Donna described her difficulties in discontinuing caffeine and alcohol intake. The nutritionist recommended decaffeinated warm drinks and fruit juices as alternatives.

The Fifth Week

At this session I review the biology of the menstrual cycle. I present standard diagrams of the normal hormonal changes over a monthly cycle and show a diagram of the changes in the ovary with the development of the corpus luteum and the simultaneous changes in the uterine lining. Many adolescents and women do not understand the monthly changes that accompany the menstrual cycle. Diagrams and pictures are useful. After the presentation, I encourage the group members to discuss in detail their experience with the changes in their bodies over the menstrual cycle. For those who have difficulty in expressing these experiences in words, I encourage them to draw (at home) their images of themselves, their abdomen, or their uterus at various stages of their cycle and tell us about the drawings at the next group. With some groups, I encourage the members to draw in the group sessions. The purpose of this is to encourage the members to think about and to express their bodily sensations so they become recognizable and available to be modified either through relaxation, use of imagery, or stress reduction techniques. The last half of the session is a general discussion with a focus on bodily sensations and their relation to each individual's goals and behaviors.

Brenda reported that she had never thought about her physical sensations, aside from noticing the tension and general discomfort. As she thought about it, she described her abdomen as larger and tighter than usual, and as protruding excessively. She pictured her uterus as inflamed and irritated. During the remainder of the month, she is unaware of her uterus and forgets she has one. Donna stated that, similar to the rest of her body, her abdomen felt very heavy when she was premenstrual. She pictured her uterus as a heavy ball of dough impeding her productivity.

The Sixth Week

For the first half of the sixth week I introduce the concept of physical relaxation and exercise as antidotes to a sense of stress. I discuss progressive relaxation and aerobic exercise as two methods to relieve the sense of intense tension many women describe. I then introduce deep breathing as a third method of physical relaxation and teach it to the group. We discuss which method appeals to each group member and I encourage them to incorporate at least one into their daily schedule. For the remainder of the time the group members review their experiences of the previous week in terms of their worst symptoms and goals.

Brenda chose the deep breathing, because she had started yoga classes and learned to breathe slowly and deeply. She told the group that she had become more aware of the constant muscle tension in her body and discussed the methods she had learned to relax. Through the encouragement of the yoga teacher, she had stopped pushing herself in every task and had begun to think about doing what felt comfortable for her. Donna chose walking as a means of relaxation. She stated that she found the activity and rhythm of it soothing. She also found that walking on the city streets where she could see people reduced her sense of isolation.

The Seventh Week

At the start of the seventh session I review the daily charts and each woman's progress on behavior changes. I also encourage the members to anticipate any difficulties in the upcoming week due to each woman's particular position in her cycle or because of upcoming stressful situations. I then open up the discussion to issues of shame and anger and encourage the members to discuss the sense of feeling "crazy" that many women experience each month. I encourage them to discuss the particular difficulties many women have

when their premenstrual time coincides with other stresses such as family celebrations, work deadlines, and holidays. Often these are times when the group members behave in ways that they find unacceptable and shameful. Although I have encouraged expression of these feelings before, this is a good point in the life of the group to have an extended discussion of these difficult feelings. The women have been together for 7 weeks and have begun to feel comfortable with each other. I have worked to create an atmosphere of acceptance and empathy.

Brenda told the group of the episodes that brought her into the group and discussed her sense of shame about her behavior. Others shared similar stories. Brenda also discussed how frightening her premenstrual anger had been for her because she characteristically puts her angry feelings aside. Donna discussed her previous depressions and stated that her premenstrual symptoms remind her of these painful times. Others discussed occasional premenstrual suicidal feelings.

The Eighth Week

For the first half of the eighth session, I focus on reviewing the information presented in the sixth week on relaxation and exercise. First we discuss each member's experiences with introducing one of these methods into her daily schedule. I then lead the group in doing deep breathing together. Individuals need to review this more than once to feel competent to do it on their own. The remainder of the group is spent reviewing daily charts and progress toward goals. As there are only two more groups, I invite group members to consider where they are in reaching their goals. If individuals have difficulty in changing aspects of their behavior, schedules, or relationships that are aggravating their premenstrual symptoms, I encourage them to think about entering long-term psychotherapy to understand and work with their self-defeating patterns. I also recommend appropriate follow-up for those who have delineated other problems, such as alcohol and drug addictions, eating disorders, marital difficulties, or vocational problems. At the end of this group I remind the members that the group ends after two more group meetings. I encourage some recognition that this group of people is special for the members and that its ending will be a loss for them.

Brenda reported that she had been attending yoga class regularly and felt better physically. She was eating a well-balanced diet but still was binging on sweets when premenstrual. She described ways that she planned to continue to work on this problem. She discussed her realization that she and her husband expected too much from her. Both had been under stress due to his job change and had been working on ways to rearrange job sharing at home. As a result of the group, Brenda is talking more to her husband. Donna discussed her improved diet and her significant decrease in alcohol intake. She found that she was less lethargic premenstrually since these changes. She is able to keep up with her walking most days and finds it helps her to feel more energetic. When she feels particularly suicidal, walking is helpful. She reported that she was considering joining a long-term psychotherapy group to deal with her low self-image and recurrent depression.

The Ninth Week

At the start of the ninth session I briefly review the nutritional information presented by the nutritionist at the fourth session and invite a discussion of the group members' experiences. Here I reintroduce a discussion of each woman's physical experience of herself over the menstrual cycle, and I inquire about images and drawings. This helps to give visual and verbal expression to physical and emotional experiences that had previously felt unformed and out of control. For the remainder of the session, the group members discuss goals and future plans.

Brenda discussed the fact that she had been experiencing less premenstrual tension throughout her body, including her abdomen, since starting yoga. She felt more flexible and relaxed. Donna stated that her image of her uterus had changed from a ball of dough to a hollow ball. Both reported feeling encouraged by their ability to maintain the diet and exercise changes they had chosen.

The Tenth Week

At the beginning of the final session I remind the members that this is our last session. I then encourage the members to review the topics we covered and encourage them to discuss those aspects of the program that are more and less helpful to them. We then review each member's progress toward her goals and discuss her follow-up plans if appropriate. We then take time to say good-bye.

Both Brenda and Donna reviewed their feelings of success related to sustaining the changes. Brenda still felt tense and, at times, overwhelmed premenstrually, but used the deep breathing to help relax. When confronted with angry feelings toward her husband she removed herself from the situation until she understood what she was feeling and felt in control of her behavior. She then returned to talk to her husband. Donna discussed the fact that she continued to feel ill and depressed premenstrually, but that the elimination of alcohol and the addition of exercise had allowed her to function better. She discussed the fact that she was looking forward to group therapy.

SUMMARY

Most group members find the PMS groups helpful and stay for all 10 sessions. Occasionally members drop out because of lack of motivation to continue to work on changing behavior, or sometimes due to schedule changes.

During the course of the 10 weeks, most members make changes in at least one behavior pattern that has aggravated their PMS. Many use the time to make several changes in behavior patterns, and in the course of doing so, feel better about themselves. Taking responsibility for managing their premenstrual symptoms in consultation with health professionals becomes a model for changes in other areas of health care and of their lives. They find that they can use the detailed techniques learned in the analysis of the relationship between PMS symptoms, internal and external events, and behavior to understand and change other behaviors. Group members also report decreased shame, increased self-esteem, and a sense of relief at knowing other women who have similar premenstrual feelings of loss of control. Most women who come to PMS groups consider themselves normal women who only behave irrationally when premenstrual. Through open discussion, the women become more tolerant of the less rational sides of themselves. In putting these "crazy" unacceptable feelings into words and images and sharing them with other women, the group members feel more in control of these feelings, and thus more accepting of themselves.

REFERENCES

1. Dunbar HF, Wolfe TP, Rioch JM. Psychiatric aspects of medical problems. *Am J Psych.* 1936;93:649.
2. Helz JW, Templeton B. Evidence of the role of psychosocial factors in diabetes mellitus: a review. *Am J Psych.* 1990;147:1275.
3. Godkin K, Antoni MH, Blaney PH. Stress and hopelessness in the promotion of cervical intraepithelial neoplasia to invasive squamous cell carcinoma of the cervix. *J Psychosom Res.* 1986;30:67.

4. Karasu TB. Psychotherapy of the medically ill. *Am J Psych*. 1979; 136:1.

5. Spiegel D, Bloom JR, Kraemer HC, et al. Effect of psychosocial treatment on survival of patients with metastatic breast cancer. *Lancet*. 1989;ii:888.

6. Templeton B. Psychotherapeutic intervention in insulin resistance: a case report. *Diabetes*. 1967;16:536.

7. Pratt JH. The tuberculosis class: an experiment in home treatment. In: Rosenbaum and Berger, eds. *Group Psychotherapy and Group Function*. New York: Basic Books; 1963.

8. Ibrahim MA, Feldman JG, Sultz, HA, et al. Management of myocardial infarction: a controlled trial of the effect of group psychotherapy. *Int J Psychiatry Med*. 1974;5:253.

9. Lonergan EC. *Group Intervention: How to Begin and Maintain Groups in Medical and Psychiatric Settings*. New York: Jason Aronson, Inc.; 1985.

10. Goodman, B. Group therapy for medically ill patients. In: Halperin, DA, ed. *Group Psychodynamics: New Paradigms and New Perspectives*. Chicago: Year Book Medical Publishers; 1989.

11. Endicott J, Halbreich U, Schacht S, et al. Affective disorder and premenstrual depression. In: *Premenstrual Syndrome: Current Findings and Future Directions*. Washington: American Psychiatric Press; 1985;3.

12. Devalon, ML, Bachman JW. Premenstrual syndrome: a practical approach to management. *Postgrad Med*. 1989;86:51.

13. Sommer B. Models of menstrual stress. In: Dan AJ, Graham EA, Beecher CP, eds. *The Menstrual Cycle. Vol. I: A Synthesis of Interdisciplinary Research*. New York: Springer Publishing Co.;1980:26.

14. Walton J, Youngkin E. The effect of a support group on self-esteem of women with premenstrual syndrome. *J Obstet Gynec Neonatal Nurs*. 1986;16:174.

15. Gise, LH. Group approaches to the diagnosis and treatment of the premenstrual syndromes. In: Halperin DA, ed. *Group Psychodynamics: New Paradigms and New Perspectives*. Chicago: Year Book Medical Publishers; 1989.

16. Kirkpatrick MK, Brewer JA, Stocks B. Efficacy of self-care measures for perimenstrual syndrome. *J Adv Nurs*. 1990;15:281.

17. Prior JC, Vigna Y. Conditioning exercise and premenstrual symptoms. *J Reprod Med*. 1987;32:423.

18. Abraham GE. Nutritional factors in the etiology of the premenstrual tension syndrome. *J Reprod Med*. 1983;28:446.

19. Golub, S. *Periods: From Menarche to Menopause*. Newbury Park, California: SAGE Publications; 1992.

STRESS QUESTIONNAIRE 1
SYMPTOM CHECKLIST

Each of us experiences stress in different ways. It is useful to see in which areas your stress symptoms predominate: physical, emotional, or behavioral. This helps you understand yourself better, develop more awareness, and make the best use of the techniques you learn.

Circle the appropriate number after each item, then total up your score for each section.

0 = never   2 = sometimes

1 = rarely   3 = often

Physical symptoms

Headaches 0 1 2 3
Indigestion 0 1 2 3
Stomach pain 0 1 2 3
Back pain 0 1 2 3
Tension in neck or shoulders 0 1 2 3
Racing heart 0 1 2 3
Sweaty palms 0 1 2 3
Difficulty sleeping 0 1 2 3
Tiredness 0 1 2 3
Restlessness 0 1 2 3
Dizziness 0 1 2 3
Ringing in ears 0 1 2 3

    Total = _____

Emotional symptoms

Crying, sad 0 1 2 3
Feeling overwhelmed 0 1 2 3
Nervous, anxious 0 1 2 3
Angry 0 1 2 3
Bored—can't find any meaning to things
  0 1 2 3
Lonely 0 1 2 3
Can't stop worrying 0 1 2 3
On edge—feeling ready to explode 0 1 2 3
Can't laugh 0 1 2 3

Unhappy for no particular reason 0 1 2 3
Powerless to change things 0 1 2 3
Easily upset 0 1 2 3

    Total = _____

Behavioral symptoms

Smoke excessively 0 1 2 3
Grind teeth while sleeping 0 1 2 3
Trouble thinking clearly 0 1 2 3
Drink alcohol excessively 0 1 2 3
Forgetful 0 1 2 3
Difficulty making decisions 0 1 2 3
Bossiness 0 1 2 3
Compulsive eating 0 1 2 3
Thoughts of running away 0 1 2 3
Critical of others 0 1 2 3
Compulsive gum chewing 0 1 2 3
Can't seem to get things done 0 1 2 3

    Total = _____

Totals: Physical _____
       Emotional _____
       Behavioral _____

STRESS QUESTIONNAIRE 2
STRESS REDUCTION INVENTORY

We all have various ways of relieving stress. Some of these are primarily external, when we rely on things outside of ourselves. Others are internal, when we rely on our own inner resources. Circle the appropriate number after each item and total up your score on each.

0 = never 2 = sometimes

1 = rarely 3 = often

External

Take tranquilizers   0   1   2   3

Take caffeine
   (coffee, tea, colas, chocolate)   0   1   2   3

Smoke   0   1   2   3

Eat compulsively   0   1   2   3

Chew gum   0   1   2   3

Use recreational drugs   0   1   2   3

Take aspirin or other over-the-counter pain relievers
   0   1   2   3

Have an alcoholic drink   0   1   2   3

   Total = _____

Internal

Meditate   0   1   2   3

Exercise (aerobic)   0   1   2   3

Spend a short time breathing deeply or enjoying a
   fantasy   0   1   2   3

Think of something funny, tell a joke,
   or use humor in any way   0   1   2   3

Stretch or do yoga exercises   0   1   2   3

Confide in a friend   0   1   2   3

Try to see the situation differently   0   1   2   3

Use deep muscle relaxation   0   1   2   3

Take a walk   0   1   2   3

   Total = _____

CHAPTER 16

Surgical Therapy of Premenstrual Syndrome

Heather Shapiro and Robert F. Casper

Frank described in 1931 roentgen treatment to the ovaries for women with "indescribable tension from seven to ten days preceding menstruation" who have "a desire to find relief by foolish and ill considered actions."[1] He reported good results and concluded that, "in the severest cases of this nature temporary or permanent amenorrhea is the proper treatment." However, he cautioned against its liberal use because of the consequences of the symptoms of the menopause.

Following these early findings little attention was directed toward induction of menopause as a treatment for premenstrual syndrome (PMS). Although surgical ablation of the ovaries would seem a logical progression from Frank's pioneering work, it was not described in the literature until recently. Now the role of surgery in the management of PMS is being reevaluated. The procedure of hysterectomy and bilateral salpingoophorectomy has been called "the ultimate solution" for PMS.[2] This chapter reviews the role of surgical castration and related treatments in the management of PMS.

INDUCED AMENORRHEA WITH PRESERVATION OF OVARIAN FUNCTION

It has been hypothesized that PMS is more a manifestation of a psychological process than a syndrome with an organic basis, and that menstruation merely serves as a marker for all that is associated with being female. Johnson states "PMS is an appropriate symbolic representation of conflicting societal expectations that women be both productive and reproductive."[3] Backstrom et al[4] examined premenstrual symptoms in seven women undergoing hysterectomy with preservation of ovarian function. He hypothesized that if premenstrual tension was triggered by the anticipation of menses, that in the absence of menses, it would disappear. The diagnosis of PMS was confirmed by prospective charting for 1 month prior to surgery. All women developed tension, irritability, and depression during the 7 to 10 days premenstrually and had no persistent symptoms during the rest of the cycle. At the time of surgery (timed to be in the luteal phase), the corpus luteum was enucleated so that the woman would not be able to anticipate the date of her next period. Ovarian cyclicity was assessed by twice weekly 12-hour urine samples for total estrogen and pregnanediol. The nadir of the pregnanediol level was used to mark the end of the luteal phase. After the surgery, cyclic ovarian activity persisted, as indicated by the changes in estradiol and pregnanediol excretion. Prospective charting was carried out for 2 months following surgery. Following hysterectomy, in the presence of ovulation, the women continued to experience cyclical changes in mental and physical symptoms, despite the absence of the marker of menstruation.

Silber et al[5] also assessed PMS symptoms in hysterectomized women with intact ovaries. Premenstrual tension was assessed retrospectively prior to surgery, and prospectively following surgery. Ovarian cyclicity was followed by daily urine for luteinizing hormone (LH) and daily saliva for progesterone. All patients were ovulatory during the study period. There were continued symptoms after surgery, but they were diminished in nature. This diminution was felt to reflect the difference in reporting rather than an absolute difference in the symptoms. In addition, recent evidence suggests that some women may experience early ovarian failure following surgery.[6] This, along with the problems inherent in a retrospective review, may account for the lessening of symptoms following simple hysterectomy. Despite its weaknesses, the work of Silber et al[5] demonstrated that absence of menses does not obliterate the symptoms of the premenstrual syndrome.

Although the etiology of PMS is unknown, prostaglandins may contribute to PMS symptoms, and one may expect PMS to decline with a decrease in uterine prostaglandin synthesis. Although no significant change in PMS was found with hysterectomy,[4,5] one study[7] suggests that laser ablation of the endometrium may have a beneficial effect on PMS. Lefler reviewed his experience with laser ablation of the endometrium in eighteen patients.[7] A preoperative PMS score was assigned based on recall. The symptoms were recorded as present or absent; severity was not quantified. Of the 10 symptoms, 3 (pelvic cramping, pelvic aching, and sharp pelvic pain) were menstrually related but not PMS related. In follow-up questioning at 3 and 6 months, the median score dropped from 7 to 2. The improvement appeared to correlate with the degree of endometrial ablation. Lefler concluded that PMS symptoms were related to events or products from the uterine cavity rather than endocrine factors, since there was a postoperative improvement without an alteration of the hormonal status. The fact that there was no prospective charting, the symptom constellation that was used was not the standard for diagnosing PMS, the severity of the symptoms were not quantified, and the placebo effect was not taken into consideration makes the conclusion that laser ablation improves PMS very tenuous.

An interesting etiology for PMS was suggested by Toth et al.[8] They noted that infertility patients with PMS reported an improvement in their symptoms after treatment with doxycycline. Based on this observation, he hypothesized that a compromised ovarian and/or endometrial function due to bacterial infection exists. He then conducted a prospective, randomized, double-blind trial, and found that PMS decreased after treatment with doxycycline. If an infectious etiology to PMS does exist, then hysterectomy or laser ablation, by removing the source of infection, may in fact be therapeutic. This is highly speculative at the present time.

In summary, a number of factors may explain an apparent improvement in PMS in the studies described above. The pain and discomfort associated with menstruation may contribute to emotional distress in the premenstrual period so that removal of menstruation may reduce PMS, but not eliminate it. The decrease in endometrial prostaglandin release by hysterectomy or laser ablation of the endometrium may reduce menstrual symptoms, which may improve the ability to cope with PMS. The surgical removal of the uterus may compromise the ovarian blood flow and decrease ovarian function or result in anovulation in some women, such that premenstrual syndrome is improved. Finally, the improvement of symptoms with hysterectomy was not proven to be caused by a preconceived idea about menstruation.

MEDICAL ABLATION
OF OVARIAN FUNCTION

Whatever the exact etiology of PMS, there is general agreement that hormonal fluctuation throughout an ovulatory menstrual cycle is facilatory and that PMS disappears with cessation of ovarian function. However, inhibition of ovarian function brings with it other medical problems and treatment decisions. Currently, there are two methods of reversible ovarian suppression, GnRH analogs and danazol.

GnRH Analogs

Three controlled trials on the use of GnRH analogs in the treatment of PMS are published.[9,10,11] The first was reported by Muse et al. in 1984.[9] In a single-blinded crossover study, eight patients were given either a GnRH agonist or placebo by daily subcutaneous injection for 90 days. By daily blood sampling, it was shown that there was a fall in LH, follicle-stimulating hormone, (FSH), estradiol (E_2), and progesterone (P) in the treatment group and continuing ovarian cyclicity in the placebo group. Concomitant with the ovarian function was the presence of PMS symptoms. The luteal phase PMS score in the treatment group fell to less than that of the pretreatment follicular phase value. The difference in the treatment and placebo group PMS score was statistically significant. Although the average E2 with the GnRH agonist was 19 pg/ml, only one patient complained of hot flushes and none discontinued the trial because of adverse effects.

The results with an intranasal GnRH-agonist (buserelin) were less favorable.[10] Of 20 women who started the trial, 10 dropped out within 2 months because of worsening symptoms or severe side effects. Endocrine function was measured by thrice weekly urine pregnanediol and total estrogen. There was no overall reduction in urinary estrogen levels during treatment. Forty percent of the women continued to menstruate. Symptoms were decreased, but they still continued to be greater in the second half of the cycle. There was a trend toward less improvement in the group who maintained menses, but this was not statistically significant. Only 5 patients were given placebo in an apparently nonrandomized fashion. Placebo was given in each case after the treatment. Two women had a return of symptoms prior to any evidence of ovulation. These results are difficult to interpret because of the design of the study. The results are less dramatic than those of Muse et al[9] because the patients' ovarian function was not always suppressed and the placebo effect was not well accounted for. When buserelin was able to depress ovarian function, it appeared that PMS was ameliorated. These results also suggest that a subgroup of women may experience worsening of their PMS with a dose of GnRH agonist that fails to ablate ovarian function.

Hammarback and Backstrom[11] studied 26 women in a double-blind crossover study using intranasal buserelin. A dose of 400 mg of buserelin was used. Three women did not complete the study, 2 because of exacerbation of PMS and 1 because of hot flushes. Blood samples for estradiol and progesterone were taken once weekly. Four of 23 patients showed ovarian cyclicity after 3 months. There was no overall difference in the estradiol levels between the two groups. The authors could not demonstrate differences in the plasma levels of estradiol between the patients who did or did not become significantly improved by the GnRH agonist. Nonetheless, there was a significant improvement in symptoms in the treated group compared to placebo.

From these studies it can be concluded that PMS can be treated with GnRH agonists. GnRH agonists suppressed ovarian activity and lowered estradiol levels,[9] although not consistently.[10,11] The result is probably dose dependent. Decreased estrogen levels are associated with side effects that may cause significant patient noncompliance.[9] GnRH agonists also appear to provoke PMS in some women.[10,11] This may be due to

the initial hyperestrogenic and subsequent hypoestrogenic state that is provoked.[12] The absence of ovulation was documented in almost all cases, less often with the lower dose of drug. There was a better correlation between the presence of ovulation and PMS occurrence than between estradiol level and PMS in two of the studies.[9,10] This finding supports the theory that ovulation is a prerequisite for PMS to occur.

Danazol

The mechanism of danazol action on ovarian cyclicity is not entirely clear. However, danazol is known to suppress gonadatropin release and to inhibit ovarian function. Danazol was used in three studies in order to assess its efficacy in the treatment of PMS. In a study by Watts et al[13] patients received either 100, 200, or 400 mg of danazol or placebo per day. There was a 30% dropout rate among the danazol users compared to 10% in the controls. Serum progesterone levels and symptoms of breast pain, irritability, anxiety, and lethargy were assessed on a weekly basis. At a dose of 400 mg, all became anovulatory, but not all became amenorrheic. It appears that some symptoms improved with certain doses, and overall there was an increase in the symptom-free periods with danazol compared to placebo in those patients who remained on the treatment.

Sarno et al[14] gave either 200 mg danazol or placebo from the time of symptom onset until menses. LH, FSH, E2 and P were measured in the midluteal phase. Eleven of fourteen patients reported an improvement in their symptoms, but none was symptomfree. There was no difference in any of the hormone levels between groups. In light of the hormonal status in this study, it is difficult to understand the mechanism of action of danazol. Ovulation was not prevented; there was no hypoestrogenism or hypogonadotrophism. It is possible that the improvement in PMS is due to a direct central effect of danazol to improve feelings of well-being, possibly mediated through the androgenic effects of danazol.

Derzko[15] studied danazol use for treating PMS in a noncontrolled trial. Danazol was given in a dose up to 200 mg twice daily, titrated to symptom relief. Hormonal status was not assessed. Although 85% reported some or good improvement, there was a high incidence of side effects. Thirty percent of the patients withdrew from the study because of depression. The best results were in those who complained of mastalgia, and the worst in those who complained of depression and anxiety. Without knowledge of the ovarian steroid levels, it is not possible to draw any conclusions about the relationship between danazol, ovarian suppression, and PMS from this chapter.

Medical suppression of ovarian function and amelioration of PMS is possible in most cases with relatively high doses of a GnRH agonist or danazol. Without reaching castration levels of ovarian steroids with treatment, the results may vary. Since the average age of PMS patients is the early thirties, a practical treatment modality must be be applicable for 15 or 20 years. Neither GnRH agonists nor danazol, as they are presently used, would be acceptable for such long-term therapy.

SURGICAL ABLATION OF OVARIAN FUNCTION

With the accumulated evidence of a link between ovarian function and PMS and the uncertainty about long-term medical ovarian suppression, surgical castration as a treatment option for PMS has been considered. In 1987, it was stated that "alleviation of premenstrual symptoms, especially those associated with premenstrual syndromes" may be a consideration in favor of oophorectomy at the time of hysterectomy.[16] In 1990, almost 60 years after Frank's pioneering work, the first scientific papers on the role of ovariectomy in the treatment of PMS were published.[17,18]

Clinical Studies

Casson et al[17] reported on the outcome of 14 patients with severe PMS. The major symptoms were psychological rather than physical. The women were treated with danazol in a dose that induced amenorrhea. All had elimination of PMS symptoms while taking danazol, and all had return of symptoms with the cessation of the treatment. Weight gain and muscle cramps were the most common side effects of the danazol, and these were described as minor in comparison with the PMS. Ovariectomy and concomitant hysterectomy was then offered. Hysterectomy was performed to simplify hormone replacement therapy and to avoid the risk of recurrence of PMS by the addition of cyclic progestin.[19] Postoperatively patients received conjugated equine estrogen at 1.25 mg daily. All PMS symptoms resolved following the surgery. The daily physical and psychological scores were virtually identical on danazol and postoperatively (Fig. 1). There were no intraoperative or postoperative complications described.

The patient profile in this study is noteworthy. The 14 patients were selected from 485 who were assessed in this tertiary care center during the same period. The average age was 35.1 years. The average number of previous consultations for PMS was 2.6. The average number of treatments and the average number of months of treatment in the clinic before surgery were 3.8 and 19, respectively. The patients who required surgical management for PMS, therefore, represented a small minority (less than 3%) of the patient population. The PMS symptoms were primarily psychological and severe. Seventy-one percent had recurrent premenstrual suicidal ideation. The number of patients who received danazol without relief or received relief but decided against ovariectomy is not stated. Nonetheless, these women clearly represent a very small, severely affected group, in keeping with the conclusion of the authors that a surgical solution to PMS should be considered only as a "last resort."

In another study,[18] we examined the effect of surgically induced menopause in fourteen patients with severe PMS whose average age was 38.4 years. The average duration of symptoms was 9.4 years. The women used a mean of 2.8 different medical treatments without significant improvement. Six of the 14 had suicidal ideation or had attempted suicide in the past. Twelve of the women or their partners had had permanent sterilizations. The diagnosis of PMS was confirmed by prospective charting of symptoms for two consecutive cycles. The women also had psychological assessments of quality of life and mood profiles, one in the follicular phase and one in the premenstrual phase of the cycle. Danazol (100 mg q.i.d) was used as a temporary treatment in five women while waiting for surgery. All had complete resolution of PMS symptoms during this ovarian suppression.

All 14 women agreed to surgical therapy for their PMS which, in 13 women, consisted of total abdominal hysterectomy and bilateral salpingo-oophorectomy. One woman had had a previous hysterectomy, and her surgery involved bilateral salpingooophorectomy only. All surgeries were uneventful and the postoperative courses were uncomplicated except for two cases of urinary tract infection. The surgery was followed by continuous administration of estrogen replacement therapy without progestin. At 6 months, a repeat evaluation of prospective rating scale scores and psychological measures was performed.

The prospective rating scale scores, 6 months postoperatively, were no longer compatible with a diagnosis of PMS (Fig. 2), and were not different from those of a group of normal women. The Profile of Mood States was significantly improved after surgery compared to

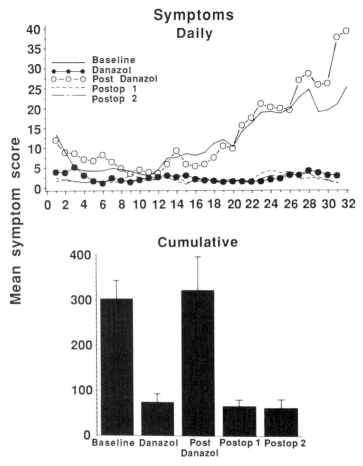

Fig. 1   Mean daily (upper panel) and monthly cumulative (lower panel) symptom scores for 14 women with severe PMS. Baseline (solid line), danazol treatment (closed circles), post-danazol (open circles), and 2 postoperative months (dotted lines) are represented. Day 0 is first day of menses for spontaneous cycles or start of calendar month for danazol and postoperative cycles. (Reprinted from Casson P, et al[17], with permission.)

the preoperative luteal phase mean. Whereas the indicators of quality of life in the Overall Life Satisfaction ratings preoperatively were low, in both the follicular and luteal phase, the 6-month postsurgery ratings of Overall Life Satisfaction were significantly higher than the presurgery ratings. Quality of life scores were comparable to the mean rating of a large North American sample.

In both the above studies daily oral estrogen replacement was used. It has been suggested that there is an advantage to transdermal estrogen replacement in these patients, presumably because it provides less fluctuation in the estrogen levels.[19] However the results with oral estrogen indicate that estrogen replacement by any route in doses adequate to relieve hot flushes will not result in return of PMS.

HORMONE REPLACEMENT THERAPY AND PMS

In postmenopausal women, Hammarback et al[20] compared the effects of estrogen replacement with or without lynestrenol, a synthetic progestin, on cyclic mood changes. Eight of eleven women in the estrogen alone group, and seven of eleven in the estrogen and progestin group reported having cyclical mood changes prior to menopause. With hormone replacement therapy, there was a return of cyclic symptoms that was not seen in the estrogen only group. One cannot say from the results of this study whether a past history of PMS makes a woman more susceptible to the side effects of hormone replacement therapy,

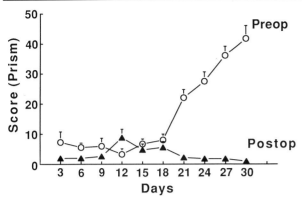

Fig. 2 Score on Prospective Record of the Impact and Severity of Menstrual Symptomatology (PRISM) calendars for the 14 women with severe PMS before (pre-op; 0) and (post-op; ▲) hysterectomy and oophorectomy with continuous estrogen replacement. (Reprinted from Casper RF, et al[18], with permission.)

since women with histories of PMS were not analyzed separately.

Magos et al[21] studied postmenopausal women taking subcutaneous estradiol and testosterone implants, who were given cyclic norethisterone or placebo. At a norethisterone dose of 5 mg, symptoms relating to concentration, behavioral changes, water retention, and mood were all worsened. Almost all symptoms worsened with placebo as well, although less than with norethisterone. No information about possible reactivation of PMS with hormone replacement therapy is given since we do not know how many of these women had PMS in the past.

Historically, PMS was thought to be caused by a deficiency of progesterone.[22] However, it is recognized that the incidence of PMS is markedly decreased in anovulatory cycles in which luteal phase levels of progesterone are completely absent. More recently, the studies of Magos et al[21] and Hammarback et al[20] suggest that PMS is associated with the addition of progestin in an estrogenic milieu. Further information is obtained from the studies using estrogen replacement therapy in PMS patients after hysterectomy.[17,18] Estrogen replacement given daily continuously either as conjugated equine estrogen or micronized 17-β estradiol did not result in the return of PMS symptoms in any of the patients.

PRESENT MANAGEMENT
OF SEVERE PMS

At the present time, in our clinic, women with severe PMS documented by 2 months of prospective daily charting, and who have failed conservative therapy as outlined elsewhere in this book, are started on GnRH-agonist therapy to induce a "medical oophorectomy." This treatment is continued for at least 3 months, during which time prospective charting is again recorded. Each woman is then reviewed, ideally with her husband present, to assess the degree of improvement in PMS symptoms that occurred with interruption of cyclic ovarian function. Those women who do not improve are referred to a psychiatrist associated with our program for assessment and treatment of possible underlying psychopathology. The majority of women, however, have complete resolution of PMS symptoms with GnRH-agonist therapy, and long-term management of their condition is discussed.

In a few cases, the knowledge that their PMS symptoms can be cured relatively easily is comforting enough for the patient to find new coping strategies and to obviate the immediate necessity for further treatment. Most patients desire treatment however, and if childbearing is complete, one option they are offered is hysterectomy with bilateral salpingo-oophorectomy and estrogen replacement as described. If future pregnancy is still a consideration or if the patient does not wish to undergo surgical therapy, we offer participation in one of our research protocols involving long-term GnRH-agonist treatment with low-dose hormonal replacement therapy. Hormone replacement in these women involves the use of strategies for progestin administration that avoid reintroduction of cyclic menstrual bleeding, and hopefully prevent recurrence of PMS. More work is needed to determine whether such long-term medical therapy for severe PMS is practical.

SUMMARY

The etiology of PMS is complicated and likely heterogeneous. Until the precise pathophysiology of PMS is understood and a selective, conservative therapy aimed at the etiologic mechanism is available, only suppression of cyclical ovarian activity is consistently effective in relieving PMS symptoms. At present, the options available to us to create a medical menopause are limited and none are satisfactory for long-term use. There exists a small percentage of patients with PMS who are psychologically and socially crippled by their problem, and to whom maintenance of fertility is no longer a concern. In these patients whose PMS does not respond to conservative measures, surgical therapy involving hysterectomy and bilateral salpingoophorectomy is indicated. The addition of hysterectomy, although an absolute barrier to future pregnancy, allows continuous estrogen replacement without progestin to avoid long-term sequelae of hypoestrogenism and to prevent recurrence of PMS symptoms. However, the risk:benefit ratio for any therapy must be assessed for the individual patient. Surgical therapy for severe PMS is warranted in a very small group of women in whom premenstrual symptoms are debilitating and other forms of therapy have failed.

REFERENCES

1. Frank RT. The hormonal causes of premenstrual tension. *Arch Neur Psych*. 1931;26:1053.
2. Magos A. Advances in the treatment of the premenstrual syndrome. *Br J Ob Gyn*. 1990;97:7.
3. Johnson TM. Premenstrual syndrome as a western culture-specific disorder. *Cult Med Psych*. 1987;11(3):337.
4. Backstrom CT, Boyle H, Baird DT. Persistence of symptoms of premenstrual tension in hysterectomized women. *Br J Ob Gyn*. 1981;88:530.
5. Silber M, Carlstrom K, Larsson B. Premenstrual syndrome in a group of hysterectomized women of reproductive age with intact ovaries. *Adv Contra*. 1989;5:163.
6. Siddle N, Sarrel P, Whitehead N. The effect of hysterectomy on the age at ovarian failure: identification of a subgroup of women with premature loss of ovarian function and literature review. *Fertil Steril*. 1987;47(1):94.
7. Lefler HT. Premenstrual syndrome improvement after laser ablation of the endometrium for menorrhagia. *J Reprod Med*. 1989;34(11):905.
8. Toth A, Lesser ML, Naus G, et al. Effect of doxycycline on premenstrual syndrome: a double-blind randomized clinical trial. *J Int Med Res*. 1988;16:270.
9. Muse KN, Cetel NS, Futtermean LA, et al. The premenstrual syndrome: effects of medical ooporectomy. *N Engl J Med*. 1984;311:1345.
10. Bancroft J, Boyle H, Warner P, et al. The use of an LHRH agonist buserelin, in the long-term management of premenstrual syndromes. *Clin Endocrinol*. 1987;27:171.
11. Hammarback S, Backstrom T. Induced anovulation as treatment of premenstrual tension syndrome. *Acta Obstet Gynecol Scand*. 1988;67:159.
12. Casper RF, Graves GR, Reid RL. Objective measurement of hot flushes associated with the premenstrual syndrome. *Fertil Steril*. 1987;47(2):341.
13. Watts JF, Butt WR, Logan Edwards R. A clinical trial using danazol for the treatment of premenstrual tension. *Br J Obstet Gynaecol*. 1987;94:30.
14. Sarno AP, Miller EJ, Lundblad EG. Premenstrual syndrome: beneficial effects of periodic, low-dose danazol. *Obstet Gynecol*. 1987;70:33.
15. Derzko CM. Role of danazol in relieving the premenstrual syndrome. *J Reprod Med*. 1990;35:97.
16. American College of Obstetrics and Gynecology. Prophylactic oophorectomy. *Tech Bull*. 1987;111.
17. Casson P, Hahn PM, VanVugt DA, et al. Lasting response to ovariectomy in severe intractable premenstrual syndrome. *Am J Obstet Gynecol*. 1990;162:99.
18. Casper RF, Hearn MT. The effect of hysterectomy and bilateral oophorectomy in women with severe premenstrual syndrome. *Am J Obstet Gynecol*. 1990;162:105.
19. Smith S, Schiff I. The premenstrual syndrome—diagnosis and management. *Fertil Steril*. 1989;52:527.
20. Hammarback S, Backstrom T, Holst J, et al. Cyclical mood changes as in the premenstrual tension syndrome during sequential estrogen-progestagen postmenopausal replacement therapy. *Acta Obstet Gynecol Scand*. 1985;64:393.
21. Magos AL, Brewster E, Singh R, et al. The effects of norethisterone in postmenopausal women on oestrogen replacement therapy: a model for the premenstrual syndrome. *Br J Obstet Gynecol*. 1986;93:1290.
22. Dalton K. *The Premenstrual Syndrome and Progesterone Therapy*. Chicago: Yearbook Medical Publishers; 1984.

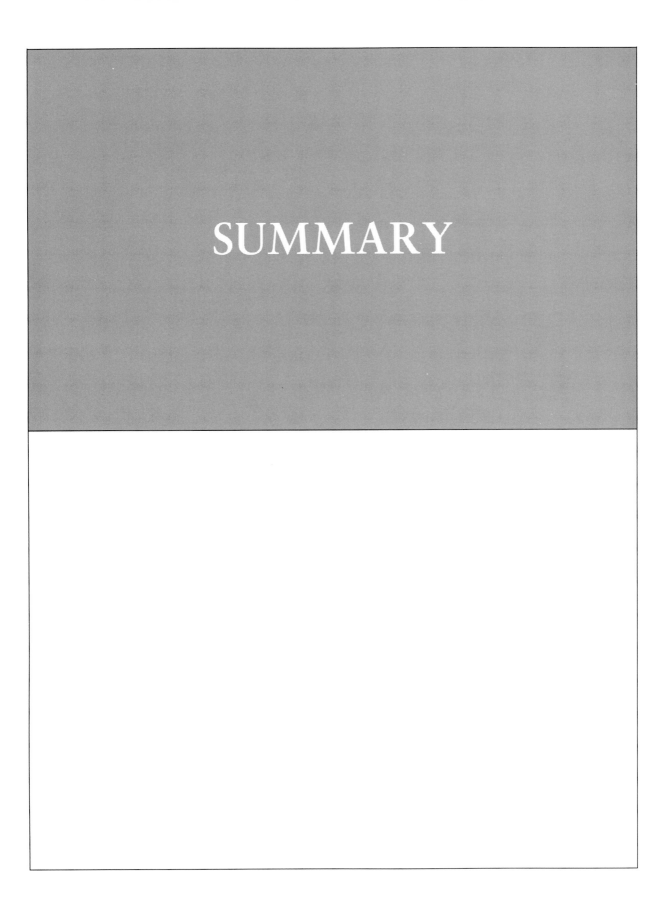

SUMMARY

CHAPTER 17

Practical Approach to Evaluation and Management of Premenstrual Syndrome

Samuel Smith and Isaac Schiff

Millions of American women are affected by premenstrual syndrome (PMS), and understandably, there is tremendous public awareness of this disease. In the past, there was great uncertainty regarding the cause(s) and cure(s) for PMS. Consequently, some fad cures appeared and disappeared, and many women were inappropriately treated. Furthermore, many women with PMS were never evaluated by a physician. These circumstances exist, in part, because of lack of information about PMS. As physicians become more knowledgeable, they will be better able to educate their patients about PMS, and more able to offer rational treatment approaches.

This chapter reviews the evaluation and treatment of patients presenting with premenstrual complaints. Guidelines are presented for conducting the patient interview, diagnosing PMS, and managing the disorder in a systematic and clinically sound manner.

INITIAL INTERVIEW

Most patients have experienced disturbing symptoms for many years before seeking medical evaluation. Consequently, their complaints are long-standing. It is important to collect as much information as possible during the initial interview. A detailed history of the present illness (HPI), a review of past medical, surgical, obstetrical, gynecologic, and psychiatric history, family history, social/lifestyle history, and review of systems is necessary.

History of Present Illness

The HPI should focus on the most disturbing emotional and physical symptoms, their relationship to the menstrual cycle, the level of interference with activity, and the change in symptoms over the years. Previous diagnostic methods should be assessed, since many women have been labeled with a diagnosis of PMS without prospectively documenting their symptoms. Past treatments for the condition should be reviewed in terms of their efficacy, side effects, and the duration of therapy.

It is essential to find out why the patient is seeking help now, as opposed to some other time. Patients usually seek help when they experience symptoms that frighten them, such as suicidal thoughts, violent behavior, or loss of a relationship or a job.

The HPI should include details about the woman's level of functioning, what aspects of her lifestyle are being compromised, and how many days per month she experiences impaired function. Information regarding social maladjustment is sought as is information about sexual dysfunction. PMS patients demonstrate significantly greater levels of social maladjustment in work roles, social roles, and parenting roles.[1] Child abuse may be more common in these women. There is also a significantly higher prevalence of psychosexual dysfunction, usually inhibited sexual desire.[1] It is controversial whether marital distress is more common in PMS patients; some researchers[2] have found this, but others have not.[3] Women who have a high degree of social maladjustment, or sexual dysfunction, should be appropriately referred for counseling and therapy. Suicidal thoughts also warrant psychiatric referral.

Past Medical History

Women who seek evaluation and treatment for PMS frequently have significant medical histories. In one survey, 12 of 68 respondents had previously undetected medical or gynecologic disorders, despite being under medical supervision.[2] This suggests that some physicians simply dismiss these patients as complainers.

Since PMS patients have a higher than expected prevalence of postpartum depression, obstetrical history should be detailed and inquiry made about postpartum depression-like symptoms.

Psychiatric history is important, and detailed information regarding past or current psychiatric problems is necessary. Data indicate that PMS patients demonstrate oversensitivity to criticism, a tendency to externalize blame,[2] and in general, more psychopathology than is reported in control subjects.[1] Many of these women develop a major psychiatric illness sometime during their life span.[4,5] Thirty to 50% of women presenting for PMS evaluation are found to have a major psychiatric illness rather than PMS at the time of their presentation.[6] These findings suggest that women presenting with severe psychiatric premenstrual symptoms should have a comprehensive mental health evaluation by a psychiatrist, since many will be diagnosed with a major affective disorder at the time of evaluation for PMS, or in the future.

It is clear that careful and direct questioning of patients is needed to identify those with significant social maladjustment, and those who may be a danger to themselves or others. In addition, these women should be questioned about past or current history of sexual, physical, or emotional abuse, which are important factors contributing to the vulnerability to PMS.

Family History

Very little has been written regarding family history of PMS. However, Freeman et al[7] reported that the severity of PMS correlated significantly with the presence of PMS in the patient's mother. This suggests a familial tendency toward PMS. The correlation may be due to undetermined biologic variables or shared psychologic factors, such as expectations about menstruation.[8]

Social History/Life Style History

It is important to obtain a complete social history in all patients. Recent changes in a woman's job, health, and/or relationships, and knowledge of her life style, coping strategies, mechanisms for emotional support, exercise level, and sleep and dietary habits are important. Low level of exercise correlates with high levels of symptom severity.[7] Sleep is frequently disturbed in PMS patients, in part because of disturbed circadian rhythms.[9] PMS patients tend to have more tossing and turning, frequent awakenings, difficulty falling back to sleep, and oversleeping. Disturbed sleep can lead to fatigue and increased irritability, thus contributing to PMS symptom severity. Patients frequently report that they have a poorly entrained biologic clock, and that they do not have a fixed time to go to sleep or awake.

Nutrition influences the prevalance and severity of PMS symptoms.[10,11] The consumption of caffeine-containing beverages, chocolate, and other sweets, and alcoholic beverages is associated with PMS, and the amounts of these substances consumed correlate with symptom severity.[10,11] However, no etiologic relationship is proven or presumed. Nevertheless, it is important to acertain information about dietary habits, including vitamin and mineral intake.

Mental Status Assessment

It is important to assess the patient's appearance, mood, effect, thought process and content, insight, and judgment. Cognitive functioning, concentration, and distractability should also be evaluated. The mental status assessment is influenced by the phase of menstrual cycle. Patients who are first interviewed during the follicular phase should be seen in follow-up consultation during the luteal phase, and vice versa.

Physical Examination

A complete physical examination should be performed with height, weight, posture, and body language recorded. Women complaining of abdominal bloating should have abdominal circumference checked in the resting, maximum expanded, and maximum contracted position. An assessment of abdominal muscle tone is made, and the presence of absence of diastasis recti is recorded. Pelvic examination should also include cervical cultures in light of a recent report suggesting an association between pelvic infection and PMS.[12] Pelvic examination should also seek evidence of additional pelvic pathology. In fact, 12% to 50% of PMS patients have associated gynecologic pathology.[2,6]

Labwork

Complete blood count (CBC), blood chemistry, serum prolactin, and serum thyroid-stimulating hormone (TSH) are usually assessed. The CBC may uncover anemia which may contribute to fatigue. Serum chemistry may reveal occult renal or liver disease, or calcium, phosphorus, and lipoprotein abnormalities. In addition, the blood urea nitrogen (BUN) and electrolytes can be used to screen for diuretic abuse. Prolactin excess may be seen in PMS patients and can contribute to physical symptoms, such as irritability. Lastly, serum TSH determined by immunoradiometric assay is sensitive enough to screen for both hyperthyroidism and hypothyroidism. Thyroid dysfunction affects approximately 5% of women and can cause symptoms indistinguishable from PMS. If any of these parameters are abnormal, medication should be prescribed to correct the anemia, thyroid dysfunction, or hyperprolactinemia.

PROSPECTIVE DIAGNOSIS

PMS may be suspected from the patient's history but can be confirmed only by prospectively documenting the temporal relationship of symptoms to menstruation. Patients are thus advised to maintain a daily symptom calendar (DSC) as described in Chapter 2. They are asked to return in 4 to 8 weeks for follow-up. They are simultaneously given PMS literature to review, which explains the nature of the illness, its pathophysiologic features, and management. Patients are encouraged to write down questions to streamline telephone calls and future visits.

At the follow-up appointment, 4 to 8 weeks of prospectively documented symptoms are assessed. PMS is diagnosed if the symptoms demonstrate the proper relationship to menstruation and are sufficiently severe. A presumptive diagnosis of PMS is made after reviewing 4 weeks of symptoms, and a concrete diagnosis can be made when 2 months of symptoms are reviewed.

Approximately 50% of patients demonstrate symptom calendars that are inconsistent with PMS. Most commonly, these patients demonstrate emotional symptoms throughout the month, perhaps with some worsening in the premenstrual week. These patients often have a chronic affective disorder and should be referred for comprehensive psychiatric evaluation. Some patients show evidence of PMS superimposed on a chronic affective disorder. These women also need a complete psychiatric evaluation, even if they insist that their follicular phase symptoms are a consequence of their PMS. These women may be very reluctant to undergo a formal psychiatric evaluation; nevertheless, they should be repeatedly encouraged to do so, since the usual medical management for PMS is unlikely to benefit them.

Another problematic group of women are those who present for PMS evaluation and are taking oral contraceptives. These women may demonstrate symptom calendars that are indistinguishable from those of PMS patients. They should be encouraged to discontinue their oral contraceptives so that they may be evaluated in their natural hormonal state. On occasion, these women refuse to discontinue taking hormonal contraception. This makes diagnosing PMS impossible, since all current PMS research protocols exclude patients who are on oral contraceptives, and there is little in the medical literature to guide management of these patients. On occasion, changing to a lower dosage monophasic preparation helps. Usually, however, these patients require moderate to large dosages of psychotropic medications to control their emotional symptoms. Referral for comprehensive psychiatric evaluation is recommended.

MANAGEMENT OF PMS

The key to managing PMS is early and correct diagnosis using prospective methods of documentation.

Education, Support, Stress Reduction, and Exercise

Initial management consists of education, support, and stress reduction. PMS patients and their families need to understand that PMS is a reproductive endocrine disorder of undetermined etiology. PMS is not caused by "raging hormones" and it is not "something in the woman's head." These common notions should be discarded. PMS patients need to understand that the blood levels of their reproductive hormones are not different than those of other women; however, their hormones are interacting with brain neurochemicals, prostaglandins, and other body systems differently. Patients generally understand the concept of vulnerability factors that make them susceptible to PMS, and they should be given examples; for instance, disturbed circadian rhythms (biologic clock), history of emotional/physical/sexual abuse, physiologic abnormalities (serotonin deficiency), and poor nutrition.

Support measures involve listening, reassurance, and open discussion of the emotional impact of PMS, including responses of family members to the patient. Physician support, empathy, and patience are very helpful.[13,14] Setting realistic goals is also important. A reasonable goal is to educate the patient about her illness, and to reduce symptom severity so that she can function without interference. An unrealistic goal is the complete eradication of symptoms; patients with unrealistic expectations are very likely to be disappointed.

Quite often, simply educating the patient about PMS and having her prospectively record her symptoms is satisfactory treatment. Up to 30% of patients may have sufficient improvement in their symptoms and not require additional treatment.[6]

Stress appears to exacerbate premenstrual complaints. Many women need advice on how to manage stress. Stress reduction techniques can be taught by a wide range of health care personnel, including physicians, social workers, psychologists, and occupational therapists. Topics include ways to avoid and/or cope with stress, and relaxation therapy.[15,16] Many women find relaxation techniques very effective in reducing symptom severity. Reading, listening to music, meditation, yoga, hypnosis, and exercise have all been used successfully, and should be encouraged. PMS patients may also need to learn strategies to control their feelings of anger, irritability, and overemotionality. Behavior modification is effective, and new coping strategies can be learned from psychologists and other professionals.

Women with PMS frequently complain about a lack of control over their emotions and their lives. A menstrual symptom calendar can afford an opportunity to schedule work, social, and family activities on days of the cycle that she expects to be relatively symptom-free. External life stress can be modified by using the symptom calendar intelligently, and this gives the patient a greater sense of control over her life.

Regular exercise should be encouraged because women who exercise have fewer symptoms and an improved sense of well-being. Although regular exercise does not usually improve the emotional symptoms associated with PMS, it does reduce some of the physical symptoms.[17] Regular exercise affords a woman some time to herself and improves her general health. An exercise program should be sensible and gradual, so that the patient can master the program and develop a sense of accomplishment and control. Aerobics, jogging, bicycling, weight-training, treadmilling, dancing, swimming, ice skating, and horseback riding are all acceptable, and each woman should be encouraged to exercise. Strenuous exercise that leads to secondary amenorrhea is not advised because of the adverse effects of a chronic hypoestrogenic environment. However, those women who do develop hypoestrogenic amenorrhea secondary to their exercise schedule uniformly find that their PMS symptoms disappear.

Some women also benefit from group therapy and PMS support groups. These methods reinforce the principles of education, support, and stress reduction, and are invaluable to many women (Chapter 15).

Many women respond to these self-help measures with satisfactory reduction in symptoms and do not require further therapy. Others, however, require additional intervention, usually dietary modification followed by medication if nutritional changes are also inadequate.

PMS Management: Dietary Modification

Dietary modification has never been evaluated in a controlled scientific manner. Nevertheless, it is widely recommended.

Women are encouraged to eat regular, well-balanced meals; adequate protein, fiber, and complex carbohydate intake, and low fat intake are recommended. Carbohydrate-rich meals and snacks can temporarily improve depression, anger, tension, alertness, and fatigue, perhaps by increasing central nervous system (CNS) serotonin biosynthesis.[18] Low-fat diets are reported to significantly improve symptoms of water retention.[19] Consequently, PMS patients are no longer instructed to avoid high carbohydrate foods premenstrually as long as they maintain a low-fat diet of less than 50 to 60 g per day. In past years, women were instructed to avoid carbohydrates and sweets premenstrually because of their proposed association with abnormal changes in blood glucose concentration and mood.[20] PMS patients, however, do not demonstrate abnormalities in glucose and insulin metabolism.[21,22]

Foods that are high in salt and simple sugar should be avoided because they can promote water retention, weight gain, and physical discomfort.[23] Methylxanthine-containing beverages (coffee, tea, cola) should be eliminated from the diet because caffeine is a stimulant that may worsen irritability, tension, and insomnia. After PMS symptoms are under control, small amounts of caffeine may be added back to the diet, to see if symptoms recur.

Calcium and magnesium supplementation has been incorporated into the diet with modest success.[24,25] Calcium supplementation at a dosage of 1000 mg per day significantly reduces both physical and emotional symptoms of PMS; depression, irritability, headache, mood swings, abdominal bloating, and back pain were reduced by 50% in one controlled trial.[24] The mechanism for calcium's benefit is unknown. Magnesium, 360 mg per day, significantly reduces the water retention and negative affect associated with PMS; however, 2 to 4 months are required in order to see the benefit.[25] It is currently unknown whether supplementing calcium and magnesium simultaneously has a greater benefit than either mineral alone.

Alcoholic beverages and illicit drugs should be avoided in PMS patients because these agents may actually worsen emotional symptoms. PMS patients may drink in order to relieve symptoms, only to find themselves more emotionally labile, tense, and angry than expected.

Lastly, pyridoxine, vitamin B₆, is commonly prescribed to PMS sufferers. Since pyridoxine is an important cofactor for enzymes involved in the synthesis of various neurotransmitters, it has been theorized that pyrodixine may correct central imbalances in neurotransmitters associated with PMS. Dosages of 500 mg per day have been shown to improve PMS.[26] Dosages of 100 to 200 mg per day, however, are generally ineffective in reducing PMS symptoms.[27–29] Most recently, 50 mg per day was shown to significantly improve depression, irritability, and tiredness.[30] The existing evidence for a beneficial effect of pyridoxine, however, is weak.[31] Moreover, pyridoxine neurotoxicity was observed at dosages as low as 50 mg for 6 to 12 months duration; it manifests itself as paraesthesia, hyperaesthesia, muscle weakness, numbness, and bone pain.[32] Consequently, pyridoxine should be used at low dosage (50 mg) and discontinued if there is no evidence of improvement in PMS symptoms over several months. In addition, anyone who is using pyridoxine should be questioned about neurologic side effects.

Education, stress reduction, maintaining a DSC, exercise, and nutritional modification have been the first-line of therapy for many years. Regulation and improvement of sleep habits is also important and may occur as other life style changes are taking place. Women are encouraged to sleep and awake at a similar time each day to help entrain a biologic clock, and perhaps correct abnormalities in circadian rhythms.

More than 30% of PMS patients have their symptoms reduced sufficiently by these measures that no additional therapy is needed. They should continue monitoring their symptoms daily, and have their progress monitored every several months. These patients tend to do well over the long term, although occasional months may demonstrate disturbing symptoms.

PMS Management: Medical

When symptoms persist despite the self-help measures, medical therapy can be initiated and tailored to the individual. The physician needs to very carefully assess the symptom calendars, looking at the evolution of symptoms during the cycle. It is important to observe which symptoms emerge first, when symptoms reach their maximum, which symptoms are most severe, and note the pattern of resolution. If the symptom calendars are skillfully interpreted, logical therapeutic decisions follow. Too often, however, physicians fail to use symptom calendars to guide management. Consequently, many physicians use one of several medications for all of their patients, without much individualization of care.

Progesterone and Progestins

In the past, progesterone was the most commonly prescribed therapy for PMS. Progesterone deficiency was once considered a leading etiologic factor for PMS, but this has now been refuted. Progesterone therapy is ineffective. To date, no placebo-controlled clinical trial has shown any clinical superiority of progesterone vaginal suppositories over placebo.[33,34] Consequently, a newly diagnosed patient with PMS is statistically unlikely to improve with progesterone suppositories. A minority, however, may respond well to progesterone. Data suggest that progesterone suppositories should not be considered an initial therapy for PMS, but can be offered as a trial prior to using medications that carry a moderate to high risk of disturbing side effects. The usual dosage is 200 to 400 mg daily, administered in divided dosages. There is no documented difference between these dosages in peak serum progesterone concentrations or area under the progesterone curve.[35]

Oral progestins are evaluated in a variety of controlled clinical trials.[36–41] Dennerstein et al[36] evaluated 300 mg per day oral micronized progesterone administered during the luteal phase and found that swelling of the hands, legs, and abdomen, and vasomotor flushes were improved compared to placebo. However, restlessness, headache, breast discomfort, depression, aggression, irritability, interest in sex, and general sense of well-being were not improved. Dydrogesterone is a synthetic, orally active progestin chemically similar to progesterone. It was not found to have any clinically relevant benefit for PMS.[37–39] Medroxyprogesterone acetate, 5 mg b.i.d. from cycle day 19 to 26, improves premenstrual depression, but not tension, sadness, lethargy, aggression, bloatedness, headache, or breast tenderness.[40] A higher dose of medroxyprogesterone acetate, 15 mg daily for 21 days each menstrual cycle, suppresses ovulation in many women, and improves tension, irritability, and breast pain. However, almost 75% of cycles demonstrate breakthrough bleeding, which can be very disturbing to patients.[41]

Data regarding progesterone and progestins for PMS suggest that little or no benefit can be expected with their use. However, a minority of women may show improvement, and these agents are considered prior to initiating medication regimens that are likely to cause disturbing side effects.

PMS Management: Targeting Medication to Symptoms

There are two predominant methods of medically managing PMS. One method involves the use of medication to eliminate ovarian cyclicity, that is, ovulation. The second method involves selecting medication(s) that reduce particular symptoms, a symptom-targeted approach.

Physical Symptoms

Medication is indicated if disturbing symptoms are still present after several months. As a general rule, physical symptoms are treated first, since improvement in emotional symptoms frequently accompanies improvement in physical symptoms. This may be due to a shared pathophysiologic mechanism, a "domino" effect, or be a consequence of long-term self-help measures.

As described in Chapter 10, water retention symptoms can be well managed with diuretic therapy. Diuretics are administered in the luteal phase, beginning just before the onset of water retention and weight gain, and continued until menstruation. Diuretics should generally be reserved for women who document a premenstrual gain in weight. Physical symptoms and weight are monitored during therapy, and electrolytes,

BUN, and creatinine are checked intermittently. Virtually any diuretic may be used to treat PMS. No diuretic has been shown to be more effective than another.

Prostaglandins mediate many of the pain-related symptoms of PMS, and prostaglandin inhibitors effectively treat the pain associated with PMS. Nonsteroidal antiinflammatory drug (NSAID) therapy is initiated 1 to 2 days prior to the onset of pain-related symptoms, and are continued until, and perhaps throughout, menstruation. Improvement in emotional and behavioral symptoms, as well as pain symptoms may occur. Almost any NSAID may be used, but caution must be used in patients with a history of peptic ulcer disease, and in those who are taking diuretics concurrently (see Chapter 10).

Bloating without weight gain is a very difficult symptom to treat, but limited success is achieved with bromocriptine, 2.5 mg daily. Diuretics may be successful also. However, care must be taken to identify those women whose bloatedness is related to poor abdominal muscle tone, cyclic dieting, and diuretic or laxative abuse (see Chapter 10).

Mastalgia may be treated with diuretic therapy if water retention and weight gain are also seen. Bromocriptine, 2.5 mg daily, and danazol, 100 to 200 mg daily are also effective, but have more side effects (Chapter 10).

Emotional Symptoms

Several psychotropic agents, such as alprazolam, fluoxetine, and buspirone, have documented superiority over placebo for treating the emotional symptoms of PMS.

ALPRAZOLAM

Alprazolam (Xanax) is a triazolobenzodiazepine with anxiolytic, antidepressant, and smooth muscle relaxant properties. Low dosages significantly reduce nervous tension, mood swings, irritability, anxiety, depression, and fatigue.[42] The half-life of alprazolam is 12 to 15 hours, and dosing is usually daily to t.i.d. The most common side effect of alprazolam is drowsiness. Other side effects include dry mouth, headache, tachycardia, constipation, dizziness, and nasal congestion, but these are uncommon at low dosages.

The onset of affective symptoms can be predicted by examining past daily symptom calendars. Alprazolam is administered daily, from 2 days prior to the onset of symptoms until menstruation occurs. The first dose is usually 0.25 mg in the evening. If undue sedation occurs, subsequent dosages are 0.125 mg. If sedation is not a problem, alprazolam is next administered the following morning and each morning thereafter. Patients can titrate this daily dosage up to 0.25 mg t.i.d.; most patients respond very satisfactorily to this or a lower dosage.[42] Sedation or other side effects occasionally limit the effectiveness. Alprazolam dosage is tapered during menstruation to minimize withdrawal side effects; however, withdrawal side effects are very rare unless larger dosages are used on a continuous basis. Alprazolam is generally administered for 5 to 18 days per month; cyclic, low-dosage therapy is only rarely associated with tolerance.

Alprazolam can also be used at higher dosages. Harrison et al[43] titrated dosages for each patient and used a maximum of 4 mg daily. Since the safety of alprazolam in pregnancy is not determined, effective nonhormonal contraception is advised. Lastly, alprazolam is one of the most abused drugs in the United States. Therefore, it is imperative that patients be dispensed small prescriptions, seen at frequent intervals, and be monitored for compliance and the amount of medication used with DSC. The authors tend to see patients monthly for 6 to 12 menstrual cycles before lengthening the follow-up interval to 2 to 4 months. By following these guidelines, patients can be safely maintained on cyclic, low-dosage alprazolam therapy for many years. Daily dosage requirements tend to remain stable over time and many patients may require lower dosages as they develop additional coping strategies for their stresses. Patients who begin to require alprazolam in the follicular phase should be evaluated for a chronic affective disorder; women with PMS are at increased lifetime risk to experience an Axis I psychiatric disorder.

Fluoxetine

Fluoxetine (Prozac) is an effective and well-tolerated treatment of severe PMS. Several controlled clinical trials demonstrate that it improves a variety of symptoms (labile mood, irritability, anxiety, depression, fatigue, and appetite increases) at a 20-mg daily dosage.[44–46] Side effects are few, and include decreased appetite nausea, insomnia, fatigue, drowsiness, dizziness, anxiety, and nervousness.

Fluoxetine selectively inhibits the reuptake of serotonin at presynaptic neuronal membranes, which causes increased synaptic concentrations of serotonin in the CNS, and enhanced serotonergic neurotransmission.[46] In addition, fluoxetine's principal metabolite, norfluoxetine, has a similar effect on serotonin-reuptake inhibition. There is little or no effect of fluoxetine on other neurotransmitters.

There are currently no studies of fluoxetine in pregnant women. Fluoxetine has a prolonged elimination half-life and can cross the placenta in animals. Consequently, the drug must be used with caution in patients contemplating pregnancy, and effective nonhormonal contraception is generally advised.

Fluoxetine 20 mg daily is usually satisfactory to control PMS symptoms. Improvement may be seen within 1 to 2 weeks or may require 4 to 8 weeks. Some patients may require higher dosages, but because optimum clinical improvement may not be observed for at least 4 weeks, dosage increases should not occur at less than 4-week intervals.

Prescriptions of fluoxetine should be written for the smallest quantity of capsules that is consistent with good patient management, and patients should be seen at monthly intervals for 6 to 12 months prior to lengthening the follow-up interval.

Lastly, in recent months the lay media have suggested that there is a relationship between fluoxetine and suicidal ideation. Scientific data, however, do not support a causal relationship between fluoxetine and suicidality (ideation or acts). Clinicians must nevertheless be sensitive to patients communicating suicidality, since the possibility of suicide is inherent in depression and PMS.

Buspirone

Buspirone (Buspar) is a nonsedating, nonbenzodiazepine antianxiety medication that is effective in PMS.[47] Buspirone is generally administered at a dosage of 10 mg b.i.d to t.i.d. It is unique among anxiolytic agents because it does not promote abuse or physical dependence. Buspirone exerts a differential influence on monoaminergic neuronal activity, suppressing serotonergic activity while enhancing dopaminergic and noradrenergic activity. In contrast to benzodiazepines, which potentiate γ-aminobutyric acid (GABA) neurotransmission, buspirone demonstrates an antagonist effect on GABAergic transmission.[48]

Buspirone has a slow onset of action. It may be administered cyclically in the luteal phase or continuously throughout the menstrual cycle. The most common side effects are nausea, lightheadedness, headache, dry mouth, drowsiness, insomnia, and nervousness.[49]

d-Fenfluramine

In addition to alprazolam, fluoxetine, and buspirone, d-fenfluramine was shown to improve the emotional symptoms of women with PMS. Subjects receiving 15 mg twice daily during the luteal phase demonstrated a

60% reduction in depression scores as well as suppression of luteal phase carbohydrate, fat, and calorie intake.[50] Serotonin mediated neurotransmission is enhanced by d-fenfluramine's ability to selectively release CNS serotonin and block its neuronal reuptake.

d-Fenfluramine is not commercially available in the United States. However, dl-fenfluramine (Pondimin) is available and is used as an anorectic agent. Therefore, dl-fenfluramine may be administered at a dosage of 15 to 30 mg b.i.d. in the luteal phase to patients with PMS. Unfortunately side effects seem to be more common with dl-fenfluramine because the levoisomer has a direct antidopaminergic action that is not associated with the dextroisomer. The usual side effects with fenfluramine are nausea, anorexia, dry mouth, and headache.[50]

PMS Management: Ovulation Suppression

Patients who do not respond to symptom-directed medical management usually respond to medications that suppress ovulation.

Although oral contraceptives eliminate ovulation, they do not treat PMS effectively. In fact, many women report that their affective and physical symptoms worsen while on oral contraceptives. Anecdotal experience suggests that only a minority of women with PMS improve with low-dose oral contraceptives. Clinicians should encourage nonhormonal forms of contraception for women whose PMS symptoms are exacerbated by oral contraceptives.

Transdermal Estradiol

Transdermal estradiol (Estraderm), 0.2 mg daily, inhibits ovulation and is combined with cyclic progestin administration to induce menstruation. It effectively reduces PMS symptoms despite high circulating hormone levels.[51] Although effective, danazol and GnRH agonists are currently preferred by most physicians in the United States.

Danazol

Danazol (Danocrine) is not frequently used to treat PMS, but it demonstrates good therapeutic efficacy. Danazol suppresses ovulation in a dosage- and duration-dependent manner. Approximately 50% of women report ovulation suppression at 200 mg/day dosage, and 80% to 99% report anovulation at 400 mg daily.[52,53] However, ovulation suppression may not be observed during the first month of treatment.

Women who become anovulatory on danazol have excellent symptomatic improvement. Emotional, physical, and behavioral symptoms may all improve, and some patients become completely asymptomatic.[52,53]

Danazol is generally used at 200 to 400 mg daily.[52,53] The potential for androgenic side effects, such as weight gain, oiliness of the skin, and unwanted hair growth, makes many PMS patients reluctant to use danazol. The lowest effective dosage should be used to minimize the androgenic and hypoestrogenic side effects of danazol. Side effects are usually tolerable at 200 mg daily. Women should use effective barrier contraception while taking danazol, to prevent unintended pregnancy and the potential for virilization of a female fetus. Danazol 200 mg can also be administered only in the luteal phase, with good results.[54] In this case, effective contraception is essential.

GnRH Agonists

GnRH agonists (GnRH-a) are used by a variety of investigators to eliminate ovulation, create a hypoestrogenic environment, and treat PMS.[55,56] GnRH agonists are currently the most effective treatment for PMS, and they are not associated with disturbing androgenic side effects. In the United States, leuprolide acetate for depot injection (Lupron Depot) and nafarelin acetate (Synarel) for intranasal spray administration are most popular. However, there are other commercially available preparations and still more are undergoing research and development.

GnRH-a therapy dramatically improves symptoms in PMS patients who fail to respond to other therapies. An acyclic hypoestrogenic environment is achieved 2 to 4 weeks after the initiation of therapy. The first dose is usually administered in the late luteal phase after a negative serum pregnancy test, or during the first few days of menstruation. Patients are advised that they may experience a worsening of emotional and/or physical symptoms during the first 2 weeks of therapy because of the initial "flare" phases of GnRH-a therapy. Ovarian steroid hormone secretion increases during the flare and may be associated with symptom exacerbation. However, once down-regulation and desensitization of pituitary gland GnRH receptors occur, an anovulatory hypoestrogenic environment ensues, and PMS symptoms disappear.

The usual dosages of GnRH-a therapy are 3.75 to 7.5 mg leuprolide acetate depot as a monthly intramuscular injection, and nafarelin acetate, 200 μg intranasal spray b.i.d. to t.i.d. Serum estradiol concentration should be checked to document complete hypothalamic-pituitary-ovarian suppression. Most patients report vasomotor flushes and other hypoestrogenic side effects.

Patients utilizing GnRH-a therapy must understand that osteoporosis and premature coronary artery disease are important risks associated with their therapy.[57] Consequently, patients should have their bone density and lipoprotein-cholesterol panel checked prior to therapy and at appropriate intervals, usually 6 to 12 months. Currently, quantitated digital radiography (QDR) examinations provide the most precise measurement of bone mineral content. Women whose pretreatment bone density is 10% to 20%, or greater, below the mean for young white women are at significant risk for osteoporosis; GnRH-a therapy must be used with caution in these women.

GnRH Agonist with Estrogen-Progestin Add-Back

The long-term use of GnRH-a therapy is limited by the risks associated with a chronic hypoestrogenic environment. Consequently, estrogen-progestin add-back is recommended after the second or third month of unopposed GnRH-a treatment. Oral estrogens such as conjugated equine estrogen (Premarin), micronized estradiol (Estrace), estropipate (Ogen), and transdermal estradiol (Estraderm) may be used to treat vasomotor flushes and prevent genitourinary atrophy and loss of bone mineral content. Progestins, usually medroxyprogesterone acetate (Provera, Cycrin) are administered at dosages of 5 to 10 mg daily for 7 to 14 days each month, to induce cyclic withdrawal bleeding, and to prevent the development of endometrial hyperplasia. Some women are sensitive to the hormone replacement therapy and develop PMS-like symptoms, usually during the progestin phase. This is usually a dosage-dependent phenomenon, and is most often observed with 19-nor progestins such as norethindrone.[58,59] Hormone dosages may be titrated on an individual basis to minimize the recurrence of PMS-like symptoms. Bone mineral content should be assessed by a sensitive method to identify those women who lose bone even with calcium supplementation and estrogen-progestin replacement. Whenever possible, exercise should be recommended since strenuous exercise can reverse postmenopausal bone loss.[60,61]

At present, the use of GnRH-a in combination with standard regimens of postmenopausal hormone replacement provides a safe, long-term therapy for patients with severe PMS. As with other regimens, these women should be seen monthly for at least 6 months prior to lengthening the follow-up interval. Although

GnRH-a are extremely effective in eliminating the physical and emotional symptoms of PMS, symptoms tend to recur when the GnRH-a therapy is discontinued and ovulatory menstrual cycles resume. At this point, surgical management may be considered as an alternative to continuation of medical therapy.

PMS Management: Surgical

Severe intractable PMS responds well to hysterectomy with bilateral ovariectomy.[62,63] In general, a trial of GnRH-a therapy or danazol is recommended prior to surgical management of PMS patient. Surgical castration is unlikely to be effective if medical ovariectomy with GnRH-a is ineffective.

Surgical castration may appear to be a radical treatment for PMS, but the literature supports its use in a subset of women with severe PMS unresponsive to other measures.[62,63] Estrogen replacement therapy is recommended postoperatively to reduce the risk of osteoporosis, heart disease, and genitourinary atrophy.

Hysterectomy without bilateral ovariectomy may improve PMS in some women, but not all.[64] It is well documented that PMS can persist after hysterectomy; symptoms are cyclical in nature and appear in the luteal phase of the cycle. Consequently, hysterectomy with preservation of the ovaries is not considered the surgical treatment of choice for PMS. Neither is hysteroscopic endometrial ablation.[65]

PMS Management: Approach

The initial treatment for PMS consists of some combination of education, support, stress reduction, exercise, and dietary modification. Many women have satisfactory improvement in symptoms with these measures alone (Fig. 1).

Medical management is indicated when the aforementioned self-help measures are unsuccessful. There are two general approaches to medical management (Table 1). The first is symptom-directed medical management in which therapy is tailored to an individual patient's symptom complex. For example, emotional symptoms are treated with psychotropic agents and water retention symptoms may be treated with diuretics (Fig. 2). Combinations of medications are frequently used.

Another approach to medical management is ovulation suppression. Danazol, GnRH-a and high dosage transdermal estradiol may all be used to eliminate ovulation and treat PMS. GnRH-a therapy seems ideal for the perimenopausal patient with severe PMS. Ovulation

A

Name:																														
Day of cycle:	1	2	3	4	5	6	7	8	9	10	11	12	13	14	15	16	17	18	19	20	21	22	23	24	25	26	27	28	29	30
Date *Feb/Mar*	7	8	9	10	11	12	13	14	15	16	17	18	19	20	21	22	23	24	25	26	27	28	1	2	3	4	5	6		
Menses 2-7-91	MM	MM	MM	MM	S	S	S	S																						
Irritability	1	1	1	1																				1	2	2	3	3		
Anxiety	2	2	2	2											1	2								1	2	2	3	3		
Nervous tension	1	1	1	1																					1	1	2	2		
Mood swings	2	1	1	1																					1			2		
Depression	1	2	2	2																				1	1	1	2	3		
Crying easily	1	2	1	1																				1	1	1	2	2		
Abdominal bloating	2	1	1	1									1	1										1	2	2	2	2		
Headaches	2	2	1	1																		1	1	1	1	1	1	2		

B

Name:																														
Day of cycle:	1	2	3	4	5	6	7	8	9	10	11	12	13	14	15	16	17	18	19	20	21	22	23	24	25	26	27	28	29	30
Date *Oct/Nov*	23	24	25	26	27	28	29	30	31	1	2	3	4	5	6	7	8	9	10	11	12	13	14	15	16	17	18	19	20	
Menses 10-23-91	MM	MM	MM	S	S	S	S																							
Irritability																														
Anxiety																														
Nervous tension																														
Mood swings																														
Depression																														
Crying easily																														
Abdominal bloating																														
Headaches	2																									1				
Therapy:																														
Nutrition																														
B-6 50 mg																														
Calcium 1000 mg																														
Motrin 800 mg	3																									1				
Exercise	✓	✓	✓		✓	✓	✓	✓			✓	✓	✓		✓	✓	✓	✓		✓	✓	✓		✓	✓	✓	✓	✓		

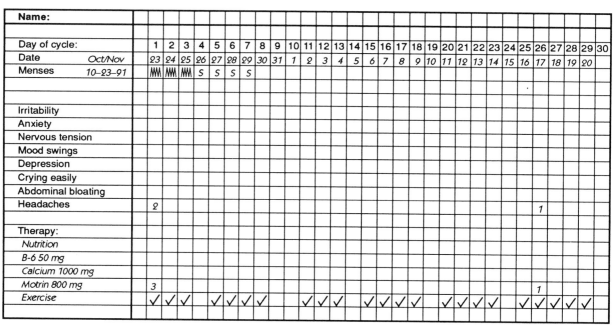

Fig. 1 **A,** Excerpts from a symptom calendar of a woman with premenstrual syndrome; **B,** Excerpts from a symptom calendar of the same woman treated with conservative measures, including education, stress reduction, and nutritional modification.

suppression treats both physical and emotional symptoms simultaneously (Fig. 3). In addition, medical disorders that are menstrually entrained, such as severe irritable bowel syndrome, respond to GnRH-a therapy.[66] Thus, there are many advantages to ovulation suppression as a treatment for PMS, and many advocate its routine use for patients with severe PMS.

The treatment of PMS is still largely empiric. Although tremendous progress has been made in our understanding of PMS, the pathophysiologic mechanism for an individual patient is seldom known. Detailed patient interviewing helps to identify vulnerability factors such as diet, history of abuse, current levels of stress, learned attitudes and expectations about menstruation, and past history of a major affective illness. If these factors are considered very important to a patient's disease expression, initial management should focus on life style modification, psychological support, and counseling.

That some women with PMS respond to endometrial ablation procedures[65] suggests that physiologic and psychologic factors related to menstruation contribute to

Table 1

Medical Management of Premenstrual Syndrome

Symptom-Directed Approach	Ovulation Suppression
Diuretics	Danazol
Nonsteroidal antiinflammatory drugs	GnRH agonists
Danazol	Transdermal estradiol
Bromocriptine	Progestins
Psychotropic agents	

PMS in some women. For these women, therapy aimed at controlling menstrual bleeding and perhaps counseling regarding menstruation are logical. Hysterectomy may be helpful in these women but there is no way to predict which women will respond to hysterectomy without concomitant bilateral ovariectomy.

Selecting medication for a patient can be guided by history and prospective symptom calendars. Craving

Fig. 2 **A,** Excerpts from a symptom calendar of a woman with premenstrual syndrome; **B,** Excerpts from a symptom calendar of the same woman treated with alprazolam, 0.25 mg daily, from cycle day 20 until menstruation.

Name:																														
Day of cycle:	1	2	3	4	5	6	7	8	9	10	11	12	13	14	15	16	17	18	19	20	21	22	23	24	25	26	27	28	29	30
Date Jan/Feb	18	19	20	21	22	23	24	25	26	27	28	29	30	31	1	2	3	4	5	6	7	8	9	10	11	12	13	14	15	
Menses 1-18-88	ΜΜ	ΜΜ	ΜΜ	ΜΜ	ΜΜ	S																								
Irritability																											2	3	3	
Anxiety	2		2																		2	2	2	2	2	2	2	2	2	
Nervous tension																											2	3	3	
Mood swings																					2	1	1	1	2	2	2	2	3	
Depression																					2	2	2	2	2	2	2	2	3	
Headaches	1				2																				1	1	1	1	1	
Food cravings																					2	2	2	2	2	2	2	2		

A

Name:																														
Day of cycle:	1	2	3	4	5	6	7	8	9	10	11	12	13	14	15	16	17	18	19	20	21	22	23	24	25	26	27	28	29	30
Date Dec/Jan	30	31	1	2	3	4	5	6	7	8	9	10	11	12	13	14	15	16	17	18	19	20	21	22	23	24	25	26	27	
Menses 12-30-88	ΜΜ	ΜΜ	ΜΜ	ΜΜ	ΜΜ	S	S																							
Irritability																														
Anxiety																					2									
Nervous tension																														
Mood swings																														
Depression																														
Headaches																														
Food cravings																					2	2								
Therapy:																														
Nutrition																														
Xanax 0.25 mg	1/2	1/2	1/2	1/2																	1	1	1	1	1	1	1	1	1	1

B

for sweets is generally regarded as a marker for central serotonin deficiency. When observed as part of the PMS complex, a physician may select serotonin agonists, such as fluoxetine and fenfluramine, as initial medications. When anxiety and irritability symptoms predominate, or when carbohydrate cravings are absent, alprazolam, or perhaps buspirone, may be the initial psychotropic therapy. Unfortunately, although these guidelines seem sensible, there are no scientific data to guide clinicians in their choice of psychotropic agents. Therapy remains largely empiric and intuitive.

Fig. 3 **A,** Excerpts from a symptom calendar of a woman with premenstrual syndrome; **B,** Excerpts from a symptom calendar of the same woman treated with the GnRH-agonist leuprolide acetate for depot injection. Anovulation was achieved during the first cycle of therapy. PMS symptoms remitted. Vasomotor flushes became more pronounced as the month progressed.

Name:

Day of cycle:	1	2	3	4	5	6	7	8	9	10	11	12	13	14	15	16	17	18	19	20	21	22	23	24	25	26	27	28	29	30	31
Date *May*	4	5	6	7	8	9	10	11	12	13	14	15	16	17	18	19	20	21	22	23	24	25	26	27	28	29	30	31			
Menses *5-4-89*	MM	MM	MM	MM	S																										
Irritability	2																							2	2	2	2	2			
Anxiety	2																							2	2	2	2	2			
Nervous tension	2																								2	2	2	2			
Mood swings	3																						2	2	3	3	3	3			
Anger/Rage	3																							2	2	3	3	3			
Depression	2																							2	2	2	2				
Swelling (legs, hands)																										2	2				
Breast tenderness																								2	2	3	3				
Abdominal bloating	2																							2	2	3	3				
General aches/pains	2																					3	3	2	2	2	2	3			
Hot flushes																															
Food cravings	3																					3	3	3	3	2	2	3			

A

Name:

Day of cycle:	1	2	3	4	5	6	7	8	9	10	11	12	13	14	15	16	17	18	19	20	21	22	23	24	25	26	27	28	29	30	31
Date *May/June*	31	1	2	3	4	5	6	7	8	9	10	11	12	13	14	15	16	17	18·	19	20	21	22	23	24	25	26	27	28	29	30
Menses *5-31-89*	MM	MM	MM																												
Irritability	2	2																													
Anxiety	2	2																													
Nervous tension	2	2																													
Mood swings	3	3																													
Anger/Rage	3	3																													
Depression	2	2																													
Swelling (legs, hands)	2	2																													
Breast tenderness	3	3																													
Abdominal bloating	3	3																													
General aches/pains	3	3																													2	2
Hot flushes						1	1	1	1	1	1	1	1	1	1	1	1	1	1	1	1	1	1	1	1	1	1	1	1	2	2
Food cravings	3	3																													
Therapy:																															
Lupron depot		7.5																													

B

SUMMARY

PMS research continues to focus on pathophysiologic mechanisms, and is now beginning to look at clinical predictors for response to medication. Meanwhile, physicians are being reeducated with regard to the diagnostic methods, pathophysiologic mechanisms, and the nutritional, psychologic, and medical aspects of PMS management. Communication between psychiatrists, reproductive endocrinologists, and gynecologists is better than ever, which promotes collaboration in research and clinical practice. PMS care is truly multidisciplinary, and can involve physicians, psychologists, counselors, support groups, dietitians, and physical education specialists. We seem to have broken away from the fad cures for PMS, and now view PMS as a complex reproductive disorder that can be managed intelligently and effectively.

REFERENCES

1. Chandraiah S, Levenson JL, Collins JB. Sexual dysfunction, social maladjustment, and psychiatric disorders in women seeking treatment in a premenstrual syndrome clinic. *Int J Psychiatry Med.* 1991;21:189.
2. Keye WR, Hammond DC, Strong T. Medical and psychological characteristics of women presenting with premenstrual symptoms. *Obstet Gynecol.* 1986;68:634.
3. Stout AL, Steege JF. Psychological assessment of women seeking treatment for premenstrual syndrome. *J Psychosom Res.* 1985;29:621.
4. Graze KK, Nee J, Endicott J. Premenstrual depression predicts future major depressive disorder. *Acta Psychiatr Scand.* 1990;81:201.
5. Halbreich U, Endicott J. Relationship of dysphoric premenstrual changes to depressive disorders. *Acta Psychiatr Scand.* 1985;71:331.
6. Gise LH, Lebovits AH, Paddison PL, et al. Issues in the identification of premenstrual syndromes. *J Nerv Ment Dis.* 1990;178:228.
7. Freeman EW, Sondheimer SJ, Rickels K. Effects of medical history factors on symptom severity in women meeting criteria for premenstrual syndrome. *Obstet Gynecol.* 1988;72:236.
8. Brooks-Gunn J, Ruble DN. The development of menstrual-related beliefs and behaviors during early adolescence. *Child Dev.* 1982;53:1567.
9. Mauri M, Reid RL, MacLean AW. Sleep in the premenstrual phase: a self-report study of PMS patients and normal controls. *Acta Psychiatr Scand.* 1988;78:82.
10. Rossignol AM. Caffeine-containing beverages and premenstrual syndrome in young women. *Am J Pub Health.* 1985;75:1335.
11. Rossignol AM, Bonnlander H. Prevalence and severity of the premenstrual syndrome. Effects of foods and beverages that are sweet or high in sugar content. *J Reprod Med.* 1991;36:131.
12. Toth A, Lesser ML, Naus G, et al. Effect of doxycycline on premenstrual syndrome: a double-blind randomized clinical trial. *J Int Med Res.* 1988;16:270.
13. Lurie S, Borenstein R. The premenstrual syndrome. *Obstet Gynecol Surv.* 1990;45:220.
14. Pariser SF, Stern SI, Shank ML, et al. Premenstrual syndrome: concerns, controversies, and treatment. *Am J Obstet Gynecol.* 1985;153:599.
15. Morse CA, Dennerstein L, Farrell E, et al. A comparison of hormone therapy, coping skills, training, and relaxation for the relief of premenstrual syndrome. *J Behav Med.* 1991;14:469.
16. Goodale IL, Domar AD, Benson H. Alleviation of premenstrual syndrome symptoms with the relaxation response. *Obstet Gynecol.* 1990;75:649.
17. Prior JC, Vigna Y, Sciarretta D, et al. Conditioning exercise decreases premenstrual symptoms: a prospective, controlled 6-month trial. *Fertil Steril.* 1987;47:402.
18. Wurtman JJ, Brzezinski A, Wurtman RJ, et al. Effect of nutrient intake on premenstrual depression. *Am J Obstet Gynecol.* 1989;161:1228.
19. Jones DY. Influence of dietary fat on self-reported menstrual symptoms. *Physiol Behav.* 1987;40:483.
20. Abraham GE. Premenstrual tension. *Curr Prob Obstet Gynecol.* 1981;3:1.
21. Reid RL, Greenaway-Coates A, Hahn PM. Oral glucose tolerance during the menstrual cycle in normal women and women with alleged prmenstrual "hypoglycemic" attacks: effect of naloxone. *J Clin Endocrinol Metab.* 1986;62:1167.
22. Spellacy WN, Ellingson AB, Keith G, et al. Plasma glucose and insulin levels during the menstrual cycles of normal women and premenstrual syndrome patients. *J Reprod Med.* 1990;35:508.
23. Reid RL. Premenstrual syndrome. *Curr Prob Obstet Gynecol Fertil.* 1985;8:1.
24. Thys-Jacobs S, Ceccarelli S, Bierman A, et al. Calcium supplementation in premenstrual syndrome: a randomized crossover trial. *J Gen Intern Med.* 1989;4:183.
25. Facchinetti F, Borella P, Sances G, et al. Oral magnesium successfully relieves premenstrual mood changes. *Obstet Gyncol.* 1991;78:177.
26. Abraham GE, Hargrove JT. Effect of vitamin B6 on premenstrual symptomatology in women with premenstrual tension syndromes: a double-blind crossover study. *Infertility.* 1980;3:155.
27. Hagen I, Nesheim BI, Tuntland T. No effect of vitamin B6 against premenstrual tension—a controlled clinical study. *Acta Obstet Gynecol Scand.* 1985;64:667.
28. Williams MJ, Harris RI, Dean BC. Controlled trial of pyridoxine in the premenstrual syndrome. *J Int Med Res.* 1985;13:174.
29. Kendall KE, Schnurr PP. The effects of vitamin B6 supplementation on premenstrual symptoms. *Obstet Gynecol.* 1987;70:145.
30. Doll H, Brown S, Thurston A, et al. Pyridoxine (vitamin B6) and the premenstrual syndrome: a randomized crossover trial. *J Royal Coll Gen Pract.* 1989;9:364.
31. Kleijnen J. Riet GT, Knipschild P. Vitamin B6 in the treatment of the premenstrual syndrome—a review. *Br J Obstet Gynaecol.* 1990;97:847.
32. Dalton K, Dalton MJT. Characteristics of pyridoxine overdose neuropathy syndrome. *Acta Neurol Scand.* 1987;76:8.
33. Smith S, Schiff I. The premenstrual syndrome—diagnosis and management. *Fertil Steril.* 1989;52:527.
34. Freeman E, Rickels K, Sondheimer S, et al. Ineffectiveness of progesterone suppository treatment for premenstrual sydrome. *JAMA.* 1990;264:349.
35. Vargyas JM, Nakamura RM. Plasma progesterone levels after the administration of vaginal suppositories [Abstract No. 50]. In: Program of the 42nd annual meeting of the American Fertility Society, Toronto, Ontario, Canada, September 29–October 2, 1987.
36. Dennerstein L, Spencer-Gardner C, Gotts G, et al. Progesterone and the premenstrual syndrome: a double-blind crossover trial. *Br Med J.* 1985;290:1617.

37. Dennerstein L, Morse C, Gotts G, et al. Treatment of premenstrual syndrome: a double-blind trial of dydrogesterone. *J Affect Dis.* 1986;11:199.

38. Sampson GA, Heathcote PRM, Wordsworth J, et al. Premenstrual syndrome: a double-blind crossover study of treatment with dydrogesterone and placebo. *Br J Psychiatry.* 1988;153:232.

39. Hoffmann V, Pedersen PA, Philip J, et al. The effect of dydrogesterone on premenstrual symptoms. A double-blind, randomized, placebo-controlled study in general practice. *Scand J Prim Health Care.* 1988;6:179.

40. Helberg D, Claesson B, Nilsson S. Premenstrual tension: a placebo-controlled efficacy study with spironolactone and medroxyprogesterone acetate. *Int J Gynecol Obstet.* 1991;34:243.

41. West CP. Inhibition of ovulation with oral progestins—effectiveness in premenstrual syndrome. *Eur J Obstet Gynecol Reprod Biol.* 1990;34:119.

42. Smith S, Rinehart JS, Ruddock VE, et al. Treatment of premenstrual syndrome with alprazolam: results of a double-blind, placebo-controlled, randomized crossover clinical trial. *Obstet Gynecol.* 1987;70:37.

43. Harrison WM, Endicott J, Nee J. Treatment of premenstrual dysphoria with alprazolam: a controlled study. *Arch Gen Psychiatry.* 1990;47:270.

44. Stone AB, Pearlstein TB, Brown WA. Fluoxetine in the treatment of premenstrual syndrome. *Psychopharmacol Bull.* 1990;26:331.

45. Rickels K, Freeman E, Sondheimer S, et al. Fluoxetine in the treatment of premenstrual syndrome. *Curr Ther Res.* 1990;48:161.

46. Stone AB, Pearlstein TB, Brown WA. Fluoxetine in the treatment of late luteal phase dysphoric disorder. *J Clin Psychiatry.* 1991;52:290.

47. Rickels K, Freeman E, Sondheimer S. Buspirone in treatment of premenstrual syndrome. *Lancet.* 1989;i:777.

48. Eison As, Temple DL. Buspirone: review of its pharmacology and current perspective on its mechanisms of action. *Am J Med.* 1986;80(suppl 3B):1.

49. Newton RE, Marunycz JD, Alderdice MT, et al. Review of the side effect profile of buspirone. *Am J Med.* 1986;80(suppl 3B):17.

50. Brzezinski AA, Wurtman JJ, Wurtman RJ, et al. d-fenfluramine suppresses the increased calorie and carbohydrate intakes and improves the mood of women with premenstrual depression. *Obstet Gynecol.* 1990;76:296.

51. Watson NR, Savvas M, Studd JWW, et al. Treatment of severe premenstrual syndrome with oestradiol patches and cyclical oral norethisterone. *Lancet.* 1989;ii:730.

52. Halbreich U, Rojansky N, Palter S. Elimination of ovulation and menstrual cyclicity (with danazol) improves dysphoric premenstrual syndromes. *Fertil Steril.* 1991;56:1066.

53. Watts JF, Butt WR, Edwards RL. A clinical trial using danazol for the treatment of premenstrual tension. *Br J Obstet Gynaecol.* 1987;94:30.

54. Sarno AP, Miller EJ, Lundblad EG. Premenstrual syndrome: beneficial effects of periodic, low-dose danazol. *Obstet Gynecol.* 1987;70:33.

55. Muse KN, Cetel NS, Futterman LA, et al. The premenstrual syndrome: effects of "medical ovariectomy." *N Engl J Med.* 1984;311:1345.

56. Mortola JF, Girotn L, Fischer V. Successful treatment of severe premenstrual syndrome by combined use of gonadotropin-releasing hormone agonist and estrogen/progestin. *J Clin Endocrinol Metab.* 1991;71:252A.

57. Johansen JS, Riis BJ, Hassager C, et al. The effect of a gonadotropin-releasing hormone agonist (Nafarelin) on bone metabolism. *J Clin Endocrinol Metab.* 1988;67:701.

58. Watson NR, Studd JWW. Use of oestrogen in treatment of the premenstrual syndrome: a comparison of the routes of administration. *Contemp Rev Obstet Gynaecol.* 1990;2:117.

59. Kirkham C, Hahn PM, VanVugt DA, et al. A randomized, double-blind, placebo-controlled, cross-over trial to assess side effects of medroxyprogesterone acetate in hormone replacement therapy. *Obstet Gynecol.* 1991;78:93.

60. Dalsky GP, Stocke KS, Ehsani AA, et al. Weight-bearing exercise training and lumbar bone mineral content in postmenopausal women. *Annal Int Med.* 1988;108:824.

61. Notelovitz M, Martin D, Tesar R, et al. Estrogen therapy and variable-resistance weight training increase bone mineral in surgically menopausal women. *J Bone Min Res.* 1991;6:583.

62. Casson P, Hahn PM, van Vugt DA, et al. Lasting response to ovariectomy in severe intractable premenstrual syndrome. *Am J Obstet Gynecol.* 1990;162:99.

63. Casper RF, Hearn MT. The effect of hysterectomy and bilateral oophorectomy in women with severe premenstrual syndrome. *Am J Obstet Gynecol.* 1990;162:105.

64. Silber M, Carlstrom K, Larsson B. Premenstrual syndrome in a group of hysterectomized women of reproductive age with intact ovaries. *Adv Contraception.* 1989;5:163.

65. Lefler HT, Lefler CF. Ablation of the endometrium: three-year follow-up for perimenstrual symptoms. *J Reprod Med.* 1992;37:147.

66. Mathias JR, Ferguson KL, Clench MH. Debilitating "functional" bowel disease controlled by leuprolide acetate, gonadotropin-releasing hormone (GnRH) analog. *Dig Dis Sci.* 1989;34:761.

INDEX

Numerals in *italics* indicate figures; "t" following a page number indicates tabular matter.